D0267378

500

OF THE MOST IMPORTANT
HEALTH TIPS YOU'LL EVER NEED

Natricentre nutritionist 0207 436 5122

First published in Great Britain by
Cico Books
32 Great Sutton Street
London EC1V 0NB
(020) 7253 7960

Copyright © Cico Books 2001

Text copyright © Hazel Courteney 2001

Reprinted with corrections 2001

The right of Hazel Courteney to be identified as
the author of this work has been asserted by
her in accordance with the
Copyright, Designs and Patents Act 1988.

All rights reserved. No part of this publication may be
reproduced, stored in or introduced into a retrieval
system, or transmitted in any form or by any means,
electronic, mechanical, photocopying, recording or
otherwise, without the prior written permission of the
copyright holder and publisher.

10 9 8 7

A CIP catalogue record for this book is available from
the British Library

ISBN 1 903116 34 1

Jacket design by Alison Lee

Designed by Paul Wood

Printed and bound in Great Britain by CPD, Ebbw Vale

PUBLISHERS' NOTE:
Always consult a doctor before undertaking any of the
advice, exercise plans, or supplements suggested in
this book. While every attempt has been made to
ensure the medical information in this book is entirely
safe and correct and up to date at the time of
publication, the Publishers accept no responsibility for
consequences of the advice given herein. If in any
doubt as to the nature of your condition, consult a
qualified medical practitioner.

While every attempt has been made to ensure the
information in this book is entirely correct and up to
date at the time of publication, the publishers accept
no responsibility for changes in prices, stockist
arrangements and locations.

500

OF THE MOST IMPORTANT HEALTH TIPS YOU'LL EVER NEED

An A–Z of Alternative Health Hints to Help over 200 Conditions

Hazel Courteney

With Gareth Zeal

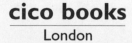

cico books

London

AUTHOR'S NOTE

Throughout the book, Gareth and I have in many instances suggested specific amounts of nutrients. This is to ensure that sufficient amounts of the nutrient are taken to benefit a specific condition. In places where no specific amounts are suggested, take the supplements daily, according to the instructions on the label or your health professional.

I have only mentioned books that I have found particularly useful, but whatever you are suffering from, believe me, there is a specialist book on it. Remember, you will only fail if you give up.

This book is not intended as a substitute for conventional medical counselling. Never stop taking prescribed medicine without first consulting your doctor. Always inform your doctor of any supplements or herbs you are taking in case these are contraindicated with your drugs.

During the last 20 years I have read hundreds of books and many phrases and facts have remained in my mind. Wherever possible, I have acknowledged the source of these phrases and facts and to those whose names I have forgotten, my apologies for any unintentional oversights.

Hazel Courteney is an award-winning, respected health writer and speaker based in the UK. In 1997, she was voted Health Journalist of The Year and continues to write regular features for numerous national newspapers and magazines. During her eight years as a weekly health columnist, Hazel answered more than 50,000 readers' health queries. This is her fourth health book, which is a sequel to her best selling *What's The Alternative?*

For more information on Hazel's work, log onto www.hazelcourteney.com

Other Books by Hazel Courteney:

What's The Alternative?

Mind and Mood Foods

Body and Beauty Foods

Divine Intervention

Gareth Zeal Bsc. is a nutritionist with 20 years' experience. As well as running a busy health practice, Gareth is a contributor to *Live Well* magazine. He regularly lectures at The College of Naturopathic and Complementary Medicine in Regent's Park, London and around the UK.

For Vicki
I Love You

Mum

Acknowledgements

A huge and heartfelt thank-you to my husband Stuart for his endless patience and support whilst I have spent up to 12 hours a day, seven days a week for over six months writing and researching this book.

To nutritionist Gareth Zeal for suggesting the most appropriate supplements for each condition, for hints, advice and help especially at the editing stage: a huge thank-you.

Thanks to nutritionist Patrick Holford for his anti-cancer diet and advice on the subject of depression.

Enormous thanks also to naturopath and homeopath Bob Jacobs and his wife Peta, for all your help in finalising the second half of the book, checking the manuscript and keeping me up to date with the latest research from America.

To naturopath Kerrin Booth, a million thanks for reading the finished manuscript and for adding your unique advice.

To my friend Dr John Briffa, for your expert knowledge regarding certain technical descriptions of some conditions.

To homeopath Fiona J. McKenzie, thanks for advising me on the most helpful homeopathic remedies. Grateful thanks to naturopath Harald Gaier for his advice on macular degeneration, also to *What Doctors Don't Tell You* and *Positive Health* for their wonderful websites and help.

To Dr Melvyn Werbach and your amazing research volume *Nutritional Influences on Illness* which has proven so useful.

To Said and Pat for all your wonderful, healthy food – and patience that has kept me going. Last but not least to my dear friend, Reiki healer and aromatherapist Debbie Flavell for keeping me sane. You are all true friends.

INTRODUCTION

WHY THERE IS AN URGENT NEED FOR THIS BOOK...

Four out of every ten people develop cancer at some point in their lives, which currently accounts for a quarter of all deaths in the UK: 155,000 people every year. Heart disease kills more than 140,000 people annually. Our rates of heart disease are 10 to 40 times above those in rural China. Half of all the adults in the UK are overweight and 80% of diabetes sufferers have the non-insulin dependent form, which is usually triggered by weight gain. Cases of arthritis, diabetes, asthma and eczema, to name but a few, are escalating at a rapid rate. Hence, in 1999, the number of prescriptions issued reached a staggering 656 million. That's almost 11 prescriptions for every person in England, Wales, Northern Ireland and Scotland every year. The toll of our escalating sickness cost the NHS £53 billion in 1999.

And yet, up to 85% of all chronic, degenerative conditions could be prevented. It continually amazes me that with such huge amounts of health advice now so freely available, the majority of people still do not realise just how much they can do to help themselves. With health services around the world at breaking point, the time has come to for us to begin taking far more responsibility for our own health.

For instance, do you know that if you have a consistently raised cholesterol level but eat a healthy diet you may have an underactive thyroid? As you read on, you will discover hundreds of such helpful tips.

Meanwhile, do you know where your pancreas is situated or what its function is? No? Well, join 90% of the population who have no idea either. But if your pancreas or any other part of your body were to malfunction in a life-threatening way, you would want to know everything and anything about your illness in order to become well. How much better it would be if we could learn more about our bodies to prevent them becoming sick in the first place. Unfortunately, too many people still hand total responsibility for their health to their overworked doctor. Most GPs are caring, hard-working people, but during their six years at medical school they are lucky to receive four hours' training in how diet and lifestyle can greatly improve and prevent many illnesses. Most of their courses are sponsored by drug companies – hence why prescribing a pill for our ills is usually their only answer. But this practice rarely addresses the root cause of the condition.

And we are not helping ourselves – in the UK in one year alone, we consume 8 billion litres of alcohol, smoke 76 billion cigarettes; also 43 million prescriptions are handed out for painkillers. In 1999, £277 million was spent on over-the-counter painkillers and 39 million prescriptions were issued for antibiotics – the residues of which are now found in all Western water supplies. Over 30 tonnes of fifty of the mostly extensively used pesticides were sprayed over our fruits, vegetables and grains last year.

31 million people now use mobile phones in the UK alone; add the effects of this to the microwaves, computers, and all electrical equipment which pulse us with harmful electromagnetic radiation. And you realise that without doubt it's the cumulative effects of these factors that is triggering the tidal wave of illnesses we are experiencing today. Our bodies were never designed to eat so much rubbish and ingest so many chemicals and they are telling us that they have simply had enough. We have caused most of the problems we face today – but the good news is that we can change or reverse many of them.

A small minority have woken up to the realisation that we are made of what we eat, but for the great majority, junk food is either more convenient or perceived to taste better and so still makes up part of the diet. The majority still do not treat the right food as being their best medicine. And it's not your last meal that makes you sick, but your last 1000.

Many conditions for which we consult our doctor can often be improved or alleviated when we change our thoughts, words and actions on an everyday level. We can also choose what we put in our mouths. Many of us now accept the idiom that we are what we eat; in reality we are what we can absorb – and fail to eliminate. If we do not absorb sufficient nutrients from our diet we can become malnourished and, in addition, failure to eliminate toxins can trigger a host of problems from diabetes to cancer.

Almost everyone is looking for a single magic bullet to help alleviate health problems. Most of us are in a hurry and yet happy to react to misleading health information which appears in the media with alarming regularity. But help is at hand.

In this book we have given numerous, simple but little-known solutions to many problems plus a host of rational, proven remedies, nutrients and ideas to improve your health on a day-to-day basis. We also offer alternative answers to many common symptoms that even your doctor may not recognise – to help you become your own health detective.

Modern illnesses require modern remedies, many of which are still being discovered from nature. In this book we share with you the most up-to-date, tried and tested remedies now known. The body is perfectly capable of healing itself – when given the right tools for the job.

May our work give you good health – today and all days.

Hazel Courteney

WHY YOU NEED NUTRITIONAL SUPPLEMENTS

How many times have you heard people say 'Surely if I eat a healthy balanced diet, I will not need to take vitamins and minerals'. 'Expensive pee' others say!

The truth is that as little as 5% of the Western population eats a truly healthy balanced diet. The majority talk about healthy eating, but in reality continue to eat far too much pre-packaged, refined junk foods that are often packed with salt, sugar, additives and saturated fats. A few people still do not comprehend that the human body is literally made of food molecules, so your body is largely made up from what you have eaten during the last year. To survive, the human body needs 50 factors, these are 13 vitamins, 21 minerals, 9 amino acids, 2 essential fatty acids, plus carbohydrate, fibre, air, water and light. As our bodies cannot manufacture these substances, we must take them in from external sources – through our diet and by taking the right supplements. If the body becomes deficient in nutrients, negative symptoms will eventually result.

We can all have treats and really enjoy them – but we must stop living on them. Many times I have watched people fill their supermarket trolleys with white bread, pre-packaged meals, cakes, chocolate bars and fizzy drinks. Almost all this refined, pre-packaged and processed food contains virtually no vitamins, minerals or fibre. We are bombarded with food advertisements claiming that products are 'packed with added vitamins'. Have you ever asked yourself why the manufacturers need to add vitamins, if the food is supposed to be nutritious in the first place?

Dr Richard Passwater, who has worked as a research scientist in Maryland, USA, for forty years, states that refined sugars have had 99.9% of all their natural nutrients removed, and the only reason that there is 0.1% nutritional value left is because these companies cannot figure out how to remove the last 0.1%. White flour and mass-produced oils are the same. Tinned foods are sterilised at high temperatures to kill any bacteria. How many nutrients do you think are left after these processes?

While many people can be negligent, preferring to spend their hard-earned wages on cigarettes rather than wholesome fruit, conversely I also have friends who are paranoid about their diet and worry constantly if their food contains pesticide and antibiotic residues. They are so fanatical about their diets, I have seen them become ill from worry, which is ridiculous. Balance – we keep forgetting about balance.

I definitely advocate organic farming and the more farmers who switch to organic methods, the fewer pesticides and herbicides will be in our food, water and air. Fewer chemicals means less acid rain, less pollution and less sickness. GM foods to my mind are another BSE/CJD scenario waiting to happen – I would never knowingly eat GM foods.

Intensive farming methods using pesticides, herbicides, additives, preservatives and overuse of antibiotics are definitely causing us health problems. Natural mineral levels in soil in many countries including the UK are dropping, and if vital nutrients such as selenium, known to reduce the incidence of cancer and heart disease, are not in our soil they are never going to make it into our fruits and vegetables. This is why, in countries like Finland, selenium has been added to all fertilisers since 1984. As a result sperm counts have risen and incidence of heart disease is falling.

Unfortunately some people compare vitamins, minerals and essential fats etc to prescription drugs once they are in capsule form – but remember that essential nutrients are essential to life.

As all these nutrients work synergistically, or together, inside the body, in a perfect world it is always preferable to ingest all the nutrients we need from a varied diet.

Unfortunately, our eating habits have changed drastically during recent years. As little as 50 years ago, it was routine for the family to sit and eat home-cooked meals with freshly picked vegetables and fruits from a local farm or allotment. Today, this tradition seems to have all but disappeared. Many fruits and vegetables that were once grown locally are often transported thousands of miles to reach our tables.

The longer fresh food is stored and cooked, the more nutrients are lost. If you leave an orange in a fridge for more than three days, up to 50% of the vitamin C content disappears. And, because the modern diet is less than perfect, we need to come to a compromise – hence why Gareth and I both take nutritional supplements and recommend specific nutrients in this book.

Many governments suggest minimum amounts of nutrients, called recommended daily allowances (RDAs); in America they are now called RDIs – Recommended Daily Intake. In Europe there are RDAs for 13 nutrients and yet there are 45 essential nutrients required for health. Confusion is rife as RDAs and RDIs vary from country to country, so who do we believe? Initially, the idea of RDAs was to prevent obvious signs of deficiency such as scurvy (vitamin C deficiency). However, they do not represent the quantities of nutrients we require for optimum health. Nor do they represent the levels of vitamins and minerals we need to protect our bodies from the pollutants and toxins in our modern environment. What is more, RDAs take no account of individual requirements such as age, gender or health status of the person. For example the current RDA for vitamin C is 60mg – but to ingest this amount from your diet you would need to eat 10 apples, 3 kiwi fruits or two large oranges. In the US, the RDI for the mineral chromium, which has been proven to halve the incidence of late-onset diabetes, is 120mcg – yet in the UK no RDA exists. Confused? Well, join the club.

But there is hope. A couple of years ago, I met a man aged 73 who had been refused heart surgery as his arteries were so blocked. He was deemed a lost case. He was so breathless, he could not even walk across the room. A nutritional physician friend took him on. Firstly, she completely changed his diet, then gave him supplements proven to thin blood naturally, lower cholesterol levels and to help clear some of the plaque that had built up in his arteries. Under medical supervision he was taught yoga and after several months, he slowly but surely regained his health. Today he climbs alpine slopes as a hobby. It's never too late to change. And as Western doctors are now seeing plaque in the arteries of children as young as ten, change is imperative.

We all need to start eating food that is as unprocessed and unrefined as possible. Natural organic food, without pesticides and additives, is the way forward. But we also need extra help. There are now more than half a million clinical research papers showing that taken in the right amounts nutritional supplements can and do work.

IMPORTANT HINTS TO NOTE BEFORE TAKING SUPPLEMENTS

If you are taking any prescription drugs you must advise your doctor of any supplements or herbs you wish to take in case of complications. For instance, the drug Warfarin thins the blood, but so does vitamin E and the herb *Ginkgo biloba*. If you decide to begin taking supplements you must check with your GP so that you can have regular blood tests. Then, in time and with your doctor's permission your drug intake can hopefully be reduced.

- It is important to note that vitamins, minerals and essential fatty acids are nutrients essential to life – but herbs are powerful medicines. Many prescription drugs are based on herbs. Herbs themselves are not essential to life but, when taken in the appropriate amounts and for the appropriate time, have proven to be of great benefit for many conditions. Generally, take herbs for no more than three months at a time, have a month or so without them and then, if you feel the need, begin taking them again

- Supplements taken regularly in the long term almost always produce beneficial effects, but don't expect miracles in a week. Supplements are not magic bullets, but stimulate the body's natural healing processes, giving long-term health benefits.

- Generally speaking, supplementation with nutrients produces improvements in health more slowly than prescription medication, which normally just suppresses symptoms. If you start a course of vitamins, minerals or any supplements, take them regularly for at least two months in order to see the benefits. Any changes in your health may be very subtle.

- Many supplements currently on the market have less than optimum quantities of beneficial ingredients. In general, you get what you pay for. Some low-priced supplements contain relatively small amounts of nutrients or forms of nutrients. The better quality and usually more expensive supplements generally provide better value for money in the long term.

- Most vitamins have a good shelf life but cease to be effective if you keep them for too long. Be aware of sell-by dates and always keep your vitamins in a cool, dry place – never expose them to direct sunlight.

- Supplements should be taken with food unless otherwise stated on the label, which ensures better absorption.

- Avoid taking any supplements with tea, coffee or alcohol as these can block absorption of certain nutrients, especially iron.

- Some people have reactions to certain supplements but this is quite uncommon. This is usually caused not by the nutrients themselves but by a reaction to one or more of the other ingredients contained in the supplement. In general, better quality supplements containing hypoallergenic ingredients are less likely to give rise to adverse reactions. If you suffer a negative reaction to any supplement or herb, stop taking it immediately. For example most Glucosamine supplements are derived from crushed crab shells – so, if you are highly sensitive to shellfish, avoid this supplement.

■ Vitamin C is more effective when taken in repeated small doses throughout the day. It should always be taken with food. Ask for a non-acidic ascorbate form, which is less likely to upset the stomach in cases of sensitivity.

■ The supplements suggested in this book can be taken by anyone over the age of 16. For children's dosages, seek professional guidance.

■ Probiotics (or friendly bacteria), more commonly known as acidophilus, should also contain bifidus strain bacteria. All probiotic preparations keep better in glass bottles and must be kept either in a fridge or freezer. Take these after meals. A few companies suggest these should be taken on an empty stomach – but research shows that the majority of the healthy bacteria would be destroyed by stomach acid.

■ Natural source vitamin E is better absorbed and retained by the body than synthetic forms.

■ If you are pregnant, or planning a pregnancy, do not take any supplement containing more than 5000iu of vitamin A. Most manufacturers state whether supplements are unsuitable to be taken during pregnancy.

■ Do not take separate iron supplements if you are over 50 unless you have been diagnosed with a medical condition that requires extra supplementation. Never leave iron tablets near children.

■ Keep all supplements away from young children. Any substance taken in excess can cause harm. Follow the manufacturer's instructions unless we have stated otherwise.

■ If you have any problem taking pills and cannot find liquid formulas at your health shop use an inexpensive tablet crusher. To order call **Health Plus** on 01323 737374. Website: www.healthplus.co.uk

■ The supplements we suggest should be taken in most instances until the condition is alleviated. For maintenance nutrients see under *General Supplements for Better Health*.

■ If you are in any doubt about the amount of supplements you or your children should be taking, always consult a qualified health practitioner.

THE CODES – HOW TO USE THIS BOOK

Throughout this book we have used codes to identify specific brands. The codes are included for each condition at the end of the Useful Remedies section. When a code is mentioned, the full details will feature here. If no code or other details are mentioned, then the listed supplements should be readily available from good health food stores worldwide.

No one is more aware than myself of the thousands of alternative supplements now available. In this book, Gareth and I have suggested many specific brands, which he and I have used regularly for some years. If I tried to mention every brand by name, this book would not be an easy-to-read book of hints, but a lengthy encyclopaedia. Our choices of specific brands in no way infers that they are better or more beneficial than others on the market. If you have specific brands you know and trust, check with your own suppliers or health shop who, I am sure, will stock similar supplements to those recommended. It is well worth noting that virtually every reputable supplement company has its own in-house qualified nutritionists who are happy to help you. Don't be afraid to call them. Most of these suppliers are happy to post orders anywhere worldwide.

BC
BioCare Ltd, Lakeside, 180 Lifford Lane, Kings Norton, Birmingham, B30 3NU
Tel: 0121 433 3727
Fax: 0121 433 3879
Sales fax: 0121 433 8705
Email: biocare@biocare.co.uk
Website: www.biocare.co.uk

BLK
Blackmores UK, Willow Tree Marina, West Quay Drive, Yeading, Middlesex, UB4 9TA
Tel: 020 8842 3956
Fax: 020 8841 7557
Email: sales@nhb-company.co.uk

Australia: Blackmores, 23 Roseberry Street, Balgowlah, NSW 2093, Australia
Tel: +61 (0)2 9951 0111
Website: www.blackmores.co.au

FSC
The Health and Diet Company, Europa Park, Stone Clough Road, Radcliffe, Manchester, M26 1GG
Tel: 01204 707420
Fax: 01204 792238
Website: www.gnc.co.uk

HN
Higher Nature Ltd, The Nutrition Centre, Burwash Common, East Sussex, TN19 7LX
Tel: 01435 882880
Fax: 01435 883720
Nutrition department Tel: 01435 882964
Email: sales@higher-nature.co.uk
Supply internationally/worldwide

NL
Nutrica Limited, Newmarket Limited, Newmarket Avenue, White Horse Business Park,
Trowbridge, Wiltshire, BA14 0XQ
Tel: 01225 711677
Fax: 01225 768847

NC
The NutriCentre, The Hale Clinic, 7 Park Crescent, London, W1N 3HE
Tel: 020 7436 0422
Fax: 020 7436 5171
Bookshop Tel: 020 7323 2382
Email: enq@nutricentre.com
Website: www.nutricentre.com

PN
Pharma Nord (UK) Ltd, Telford Court, Morpeth, NE61 2DB
Tel: 01670 519989
Fax: 01670 513222
Email: bhenriksen@pharmanord.com
Website: www.pharmanord.com

PW
Pharm West Inc. 520, Washington Blvd, Suite 401, Marina Del Rey, California,
USA 90292
Tel in UK: 00 800 8923 8923
Fax from UK: 001 310 577 0296
Website www.pharmwest.com and www.immunalive.com

S
Solgar Vitamin and Herb, Aldbury, Tring, Herts, HP23 5PT
Tel: 01442 890355
Fax: 01442 890366
Email: solgarinfo@solgar.com – for general/sales enquiries, not orders
Website: www.solgar.com

Solgar Vitamin and Herb Company, 500 Frank W Burr Boulevard, Teaneck, Jersey,
NJ 07666, USA
Tel: +1 201 944 2311, +1 201 944 7351.

For all other addresses and details, see the Index of Useful Information and Addresses on page 311

ACID STOMACH

(see also *Indigestion* and *Low Stomach Acid*)

Many people complain about having an acid stomach, often mistakenly presuming that they produce too much stomach acid – hydrochloric acid also known as HCl. In fact, sufferers from acid stomach regularly produce too much stomach acid at the wrong times – usually in response to stress, or overindulgence in caffeine, alcohol or sugar – which all leave the stomach with too little stomach acid for digesting foods. And as the average person eats 100 tons of food in their lifetime, which requires 300 litres of digestive juices to break it down, it's no wonder we are suffering more and more digestive disorders. Typical symptoms are feelings of heartburn, acid reflux, indigestion, bloating and general discomfort. When you are under prolonged stress or exhausted, your digestive system is further greatly weakened. Never underestimate how stress and chronic exhaustion can affect the body.

Foods to Avoid

- Reduce your intake of coffee, black tea, alcohol and sugar.
- Full-fat cheeses and rich creamy foods.
- Fried and very fatty foods.
- Oily, spicy foods (such as an Indian take away with lots of sauce) which are usually packed with cheap, refined vegetable oils.
- Concentrated fruit juices can exacerbate this problem especially oranges, lemon, grapefruit and raw tomato juice. Buy non-concentrates and dilute with water.
- Reduce your intake of wheat-based foods, which can be a problem for people with acid stomach (especially croissants, white bread and pre-packaged, mass-produced pies and cakes).

Friendly Foods

- Eat more whole grains such as brown rice, quinoa, kamut or amaranth, and try lentil, corn or spelt-based pastas, breads and cereals. Rice cakes, amaranth and spelt crackers are often easier to digest than wheat. If you adore bread, try wholemeal varieties.
- Include plenty of lightly cooked vegetables and fruits in your diet, which are easier on the digestive system.
- Try making more fruit compotes or lightly grilled fruit kebabs without sugar.
- Choose low-fat meats such as venison, and turkey, duck and chicken without the skin and include plenty of fresh fish in your regimen.
- Replace full-fat cow's milk with organic rice or soya milk, or use skimmed milk.

- Experiment with caffeine-free herbal teas such as fennel and liquorice which reduce acidity. Camomile and meadowsweet teas soothe the gut.
- Fresh root ginger is very calming to the gut as is lightly cooked cabbage or cabbage juice made from raw cabbage.
- Eat more live, low-fat yoghurts.

Useful Remedies

- De-glycyrrhized liquorice helps to protect and heal the lining of the oesophagus and stomach. Chew 1 to 2 tablets twenty minutes before a meal. It can also be used as an alternative to antacids after meals. Available from good health shops.
- **Herbcraft** make a *Peppermint Formula* containing peppermint, gentian, fennel and camomile – take either on the tongue or in water after meals. **FSC**
- *Gastroplex* is a supplement containing slippery elm, marshmallow and gamma oryzanol which all help to soothe the stomach lining. **BC**
- The mineral sodium phosphate helps to balance excess acidity. Take 200mg three times daily. **BLK**

Helpful Hints

- Chew all foods thoroughly and avoid drinking too much with meals, as this dilutes the stomach acid which you need to digest your meal.
- Eat little and often, avoiding large, heavy meals. The larger the meal, the greater the burden on your digestive system. Small meals are especially important if you are stressed, as stress increases stomach acid at inappropriate times.
- Take time out to eat your meals calmly – do not eat on the run. Never eat large meals when you are feeling upset.
- If you are prone to nervous conditions, join a yoga or t'ai chi class and learn to relax. Get plenty of exercise, but do not take strenuous exercise immediately after eating. Walking for 10–15 minutes after a meal will greatly aid digestion.
- Drink peppermint, fennel or camomile herbal teas after a meal.
- Food combining helps an acid stomach: this means separating proteins and starches to aid digestion. Basically if you are eating a protein such as meat or fish, eat this with salad or vegetables but not potatoes, pasta or bread; conversely, when you eat bread, pasta or potatoes, eat them with vegetables or salad, not protein. Read *The Complete Book of Food Combining* by Kathryn Marsden, Piatkus. Many people become reliant on antacids to control their symptoms, when making a few simple changes to the diet and eating pattern can produce very significant relief in most cases. Antacids can harm the body if used excessively and many contain aluminium, which has been implicated in Alzheimer's disease.

Remember digestion begins in the mouth – chew food thoroughly.

ACNE

(see also *Rosacea*)

Many adolescents experience acne due to the massive increase in hormone production, which often leads to overproduction of sebum, or naturally produced oils in the skin that cause blockages in the skin's sebaceous glands. For adults, acne often results from internal toxicity, which can be caused by many factors. Constipation, candida (a yeast fungal overgrowth) (see *Candida*) or food intolerances can all trigger this problem. Pre-menstrual women can also experience acne. The key factor in controlling and preventing acne is to look after your liver and ensure that toxins can be eliminated. Once the system becomes overloaded it begins dumping toxins into the skin, hence why constipation and poor skin often go hand in hand.

Foods to Avoid

■ Sugar and alcohol in any form. Most mass-produced pre-packed meals, cakes, biscuits and pies are high in sugar, salt and saturated fats, which place a great strain on the liver.

■ Full-fat cheeses and dairy produce, fried foods and greasy burger-type foods.

Friendly Food

■ Eat more beetroot, artichoke and dandelion (picked from a field well away from traffic fumes and thoroughly washed) which help to cleanse the liver.

■ Chickpeas, soya, black-eyed, haricot and cannellini beans as well as pulses help the body to excrete excess hormones.

■ Japanese and Thai foods which are rich in tofu and tempeh, that regulate hormone levels.

■ Include more fresh vegetables and fruits such as figs in your diet – this is especially true of teenagers who tend to eat a very poor diet. We can all do this for a certain time but symptoms will arise once the body becomes very toxic.

■ Drink at least 8 glasses of water daily.

■ Add a tablespoonful of linseeds and sunflower seeds to high-fibre, low-sugar breakfast cereals.

■ Snack on unsulphured dried apricots and dates as well as raw, unsalted nuts and seeds.

■ Raw wheatgerm and avocados are rich in the vitamin E, which feeds the skin.

■ See also *General Health Hints*.

Useful Remedies

■ Zinc has been shown to be as successful as taking certain antibiotics for this condition – take 30mg of zinc up to 3 times daily until the condition improves. For every 15mg of zinc, you should also take 1mg of copper to maintain a healthy balance within the body.

■ Take a good quality B-complex vitamin plus a multi-vitamin and mineral daily.

■ Tinctures containing dandelion and burdock cleanse the liver: 10 drops up to 8 times daily.

- Vitamin A is essential for healthy skin, if you are not pregnant or planning a pregnancy take up to 30,000iu taken daily for up to two months.
- Natural source vitamin E 200–400iu daily reduces the tendency to scarring and helps maintain healthy skin.

Helpful Hints

- *The Sher System* is a skin regime especially formulated for problem skin. Contact **The Sher System**, 30 New Bond Street, London, W1Y 9HD Tel: 020 7499 4022. Fax: 020 7629 7021 Website: www.sher.co.uk/skincare Email: skincare@sher.co.uk
- *Rosa Mosqueta*, a Latin American plant-based oil, can be used topically to heal scars. **NC**
- Tea tree oil is highly antiseptic. Add a few drops to bath water or use cream, soap or lotion on the affected areas.
- *Purifying Body Bath* by **Blackmores** contains tea tree oil and St John's wort which are both anti-bacterial and are especially useful if you have the acne on your back or chest. **BLK**
- *Kali Brom 6x* is a homeopathic remedy that helps if the acne is only on the face.
- Exercise encourages free flow of sebum and detoxification of the body through sweating.
- Many readers have benefited from taking aloe vera juice internally and using the gel externally.

Ageing is a state of mind –
Joan Collins

AGEING

Ageing is the normal wear and tear on the body that occurs as we grow older. We can reduce the affects of this wear and tear dramatically by watching our diet, taking more exercise and reducing stress levels in our everyday lives.

The actual mechanism of the damage from ageing is caused by free radicals, which are formed as the natural results of our bodies' metabolism and waste production. They can also enter the body from foods, air, water and exposure to environmental chemicals and factors including excessive sunlight, cigarette smoke, car exhaust fumes, electromagnetic fields and pollution. When you peel an apple it oxidises – it turns brown – this same process happens to our cells and genes as we age.

Our genes control the structure and function of our body – if our genes stay healthy, then our bodies stay healthy. If you live a healthy lifestyle, you can change which genes dominate. In other words, if your parents and grandparents died of heart attacks, you may well have a pre-disposition for heart problems at some point. But if you live a different lifestyle and eat healthier foods, you can change the chemistry within the body – you don't have to suffer just because they did. Genes are repairable and alterable – they adjust to our environment and state of mind.

Generally, people who live to a great age are positive, adaptable and hard working; they eat a good breakfast and consume plenty of freshly, locally grown fruits and vegetables. Jeanne Calment, a French lady, lived to 122; she gave up smoking at the age of 120 in 1995 saying 'it had become a habit' and died two years later. She was one in six billion, but there are always exceptions to every rule.

Never underestimate just how much your thoughts and stress levels can affect not only your health, but also the speed at which you age. If you keep saying over and over 'it's to be expected at my age', do not be surprised if you become sicker and age faster.

Some years ago, a group of 70-year-old men was installed in a university, which had been transformed to a replica of a 1950s building. The men were dressed in clothes that they wore in their fifties and were asked to behave as they had when they attended college. After 3 weeks, researchers found that their biological age had decreased an average of 3 years in just 3 weeks!

In my twenties and thirties I was obsessed with ageing and spent too much time rushing around having the latest anti-ageing therapies, instead of simply enjoying being young. Now I wish I had enjoyed the moment more.

Foods to Avoid

- Sugar ages the skin as much as smoking and sunbathing to excess. So reduce your intake of refined sugars in any form. Sugar turns to a hard fat within the body if not used up during exercise – which can trigger hardening of the arteries and cataracts.

- Reduce your intake of animal fats and refined carbohydrates.

- Fried and barbecued foods, and highly preserved foods.

- Reduce your intake of alcohol. One glass of red wine daily is fine.

Friendly Foods

- Eat plenty of organic fruits, vegetables and whole grains such as brown rice, millet, quinoa, amaranth, buckwheat, spelt – the greater variety the more benefits.

- Grow your own sprouts such as alfalfa, aduki or mung bean sprouts, and eat tofu regularly.

- Include plenty of sunflower, pumpkin, sesame seeds and linseeds in your diet which are all rich in fibre, minerals and essential fats.

- Use cold, unrefined, organic sunflower, walnut and olive oils for your salad dressings.

- Drink at least 1 litre of water daily.

- Green tea is rich in antioxidants.

- Broccoli, strawberries, spinach, prunes, raisins, blueberries, raspberries, papaya, sweet potatoes, cherries, spring greens, kale and cabbage are some of the most anti-ageing foods you can eat.

- See *Fats You Need to Eat*, plus *General Health Hints*.

Useful Remedies
Daily anti-ageing regimen for pre-menopausal women.

- A high-strength multi-vitamin and mineral made for your age.

- Grapeseed extract and *Pycnogenol* (pine bark extract) contain powerful antioxidants, which help clean free radicals from the cells. 100 mg daily.

- Alpha lipoic acid is a natural antioxidant found in every cell, but, as we age, the body produces less, which is quickly used up in today's polluted environment. It also removes free radicals and helps detoxify the liver: 30–50mg daily.

- Essential fats feed your skin, hair and nails from the inside out and are essential for every cell in the body. **Bio Care** make a powdered formula *Omega Plex* containing a correct ratio of essential fats, which do not need to be processed by the liver – half a teaspoon daily in water. **BC**

- If you suffer heavy periods, take an iron supplement such as *Spatone* or *Floradix*.

- 100mg of magnesium and 200mg of calcium in a citrate form should be taken as well as the multi-vitamin or mineral to help protect your bones.

- One gram of vitamin C with bioflavonoids to encourage healthy skin, bones and immune system – take daily.

- For post-menopausal women, see *Menopause*.

Daily anti-ageing regimen for men

- A high-potency multi-vitamin and mineral for men that contains at least 15mg of zinc, which helps protect the prostate and increases sperm count, plus 200mcg of selenium to reduce the risk of cancer. **S**

- *Lycopene* helps protect the prostate. 15mg daily.

- Also take 400iu of vitamin E daily to protect the heart.

- Carnosine and SAMe (s-adenosyl methionine) are two naturally occurring substances within the body – as we age levels decline. They protect the liver, improve joint flexibility and fight depression. Carnosine lengthens the life of cells and is highly anti-ageing. **NC**

Helpful Hints
- As we age the protective ability of cells to maintain healthy skin is severely compromised. In healthy tissues, cells called islets of Langerhans constantly clear the skin of debris, maintaining clear, more resilient skin. But, in a clinical study of *Beta-1 3- D Glucan*, with 150 women using a topical application, results showed a 27% improvement in hydration of skin, 56% improvement in facial wrinkles, a 29% improvement in skin dryness and a 74% improvement in skin elasticity/firmness within 8 weeks. A/V in tablets and creams. **NC**

- Get plenty of exercise, but not to excess. Stop smoking. Have fun – laugh a lot.

- Intravenous anti-oxidant therapy (also known as chelation) has anti-ageing properties, to help prevent cancer, and heart disease. For details, call **The Integrated Medical Centre** on 0207 224 5111 and ask for details of Dr Trossell or Dr Denning.

- Stop worrying – as Dale Carnegie once said '85% of things you worry about never happen'. Stop worrying about the things you can't change and concentrate on what you can change.

- Don't overeat. Generally in the West, we tend to eat 40% more food than the body needs. Having said that, there are some people who are living on 1,200 calories a day to try and delay the ageing process, but most of them look awful! And food is meant to be a pleasure. We can all enjoy treats and not feel guilty but we must stop living on treats.

- Meditation reduces stress, which can age us faster than any other condition (see *Meditation*).

- Too much sun is ageing but we do need some sunshine to produce vitamin D, which helps to keep bones healthy. Sunshine makes you feel good – everything in moderation – and wear a PABA-free sunscreen whenever you are outside to protect the skin.

- As moisture is so vital to ageing skin, invest in a humidifier and use it in the bedroom.

- An ioniser helps clean the air in the room, negative ions have a relaxing effect on the body and nervous system.

- Always use a body lotion after bathing – the **Body Shop** make some fantastic body creams based on nut oils. My favourite is *Body Butter* made from Brazil nuts. There are many fabulous organic vitamin creams now widely available from health stores.

- Vitamin and mineral injections help to regenerate sun-damaged skin. I have mine done at **The French Cosmetic Medical Co** at 25 Wimpole Street London, tel: 020 7637 0548.

- Laser therapy can help remove the visible signs of ageing, such as liver spots. Contact **Laser Care Clinics**, 1 Park View, Harrogate, North Yorkshire, HG1 5LY. Tel: 01423 563827. Fax: 01423 563158. Email: lasercare@btinternet.com Website: www.lasercare-clinics.co.uk

Constant tiredness can be due to a dependency on caffeine and sugar.

ALCOHOL

Moderate consumption – meaning a single unit: one shot of spirits, one glass of wine or half a pint of beer – of alcohol has been shown to be slightly protective against heart disease. If your cholesterol level is above 4.5, you can justify having an occasional drink – the ideal being a glass of aged red wine. The nutrient content of alcohol is very low, but many people have a drink believing they are protecting their heart and choose to forget they are elevating their risk of hormonal cancers, particularly breast cancer. Alcohol places an enormous strain on the liver, which reduces its ability to detoxify the body. Over-consumption of alcohol can lead to fatigue, dehydration as well as disruptive sleep patterns and depleting many vital nutrients from the body. Pregnant women risk foetal abnormalities if they consume more than one unit of alcohol a day during pregnancy; alcohol should be avoided if you are trying to become pregnant. During pregnancy, give up.

Foods to Avoid

- Avoid eating fresh or tinned grapefruit juice, if you are drinking, as this will increase the toxicity of the alcohol.
- Saturated fats also place a great strain on the liver. Avoid as much as possible fatty meals – especially sausages, burgers, pre-packaged meat pies and so on.
- Never ply anyone who is drunk with coffee, which will further dehydrate the body which can increase the concentration of alcohol in the system. See *General Health Hints*.

Friendly Foods

- Plenty of fresh fruits and vegetables especially broccoli, artichokes, cauliflower, beetroot, celeriac, celery, fennel and radiccio to help to detoxify the liver.
- Eat plenty of soluble fibres such as linseeds (flax), oat bran, psyllium husks and low sugar cereals such as muesli or porridge.
- Drink at least 8 glasses of water daily.
- Use unrefined olive, walnut or sunflower oils for salad dressings.
- See also *General Health Hints*.

Useful Remedies

- The herb *Chinese Kudzu* extract contains diadzin, which has been known to be beneficial for treating alcoholism. Not only does kudzu extract help reduce the craving for alcohol, but it also acts as a muscle relaxant which helps to overcome some of the withdrawal symptoms. Take 10–20 drops of the tincture or 2 tablets before you take a drink. **FSC**
- The herb *Milk Thistle* (silymarin) has been proven to help detoxify and regenerate the liver. Take 500mg of standardised extract up 3 times daily with meals for one month. During this time you need to cut down your intake of alcohol to give the liver time to repair. **BLK**
- If you are an occasional drinker, take 3 capsules of *Milk Thistle* before and after drinking.
- Take a good quality multi-vitamin and mineral daily.
- To avoid hangovers, take 2 grams of evening primrose oil, 1 gram of vitamin C, a B complex plus 500mg of milk thistle with a full glass of water before going out. Repeat this dosage the next morning upon waking.
- To help alleviate hangovers try the formula *Intox Rx*, containing vitamin C, the amino acid cysteine, the liver-friendly herbs kudzu and silymarin, plus lipoic acid and pyroglutamic acid. *Intox Rx* has been specifically designed to provide protection from the toxic effects of alcohol. Take one capsule twice daily. **BC**

Helpful Hints

- For every alcoholic drink, make sure you have a non-alcoholic one in between. Generally drink more water as alcohol severely dehydrates the body. Avoid alcohol when flying because the pressurised cabins cause considerable dehydration.

a

- Do not give a person coffee to sober them up as coffee is a diuretic which depletes fluid from the body and makes the alcohol content in the body even more concentrated.

- If you have a hangover – you need to raise your blood sugar quite quickly upon waking. Eat a banana or blend various fresh fruits including a banana and low-fat, live yoghurt and drink immediately, or drink some fruit juice.

- Drink 3 glasses of water immediately.

- Homeopathic *Nux Vomica 30c*. Take one before bed and another upon waking to help reduce a hangover.

- Bingeing on alcohol is extremely dangerous – it creates too much shock in the liver. Vomiting is an indication that the body has reached a danger level and you must stop drinking.

- If you must drink, have a couple of drinks daily – but do not drink to excess. Better quality red wine seems to confer the most health benefits, due to antioxidant substances called polyphenols, present in the skin of red grapes. The skin of white grapes is discarded during the processing of white wine.

- Dandelion root tea is excellent for cleansing the liver.

- Remember it takes 20 minutes for alcohol to have an effect and over one hour for the body to process each unit (one unit = half a pint of beer, a small glass of wine or a single measure of spirits). If you are concerned about the amount that you (or a member of your family) are drinking, call **Drinkline** on 0800 917 8282 for advice and information. The line is open from 9.00am to 11.00pm (Monday to Friday) and 6.00pm to 11.00pm (weekends). All calls are treated in the strictest confidence and **Drinkline** provides a full support service for people with drink problems as well as their families.

You will never fail unless you give up.

ALLERGIC RHINITIS

(see also *Allergies* and *Hayfever*)

Typical symptoms include a runny nose, sneezing, sinus congestion plus itchy and watering eyes. Unlike hayfever this tends to affect people all year round, although symptoms can worsen at certain times of year when pollen counts are high. In some individuals it is triggered by a food intolerance. This will need to be addressed for the problem to be resolved, otherwise you can take all kinds of herbs and supplements in efforts to relieve the problem, or worse still antihistamines but this will not address the root cause of the condition – see also Allergies.

Foods to Avoid
- Sugar, dairy products, white flour and pasta, orange juice, tomatoes and any other foods to which you may have an intolerance. Wheat and dairy produce from cows are known to be triggers for this condition, but it could just as easily be bananas.

Friendly Foods

■ Include plenty of garlic, onions, horseradish, root ginger, freshly squeezed fruit and vegetable juices (but not carton juice) in your diet.

■ If you have an intolerance to wheat – try rye, rice or amaranth crackers and oat cakes. Ask at your health shop for wheat-free bread and pasta.

■ Dairy alternatives include organic rice, soya or oat milk.

Useful Remedies

■ When the symptoms are acute take up to 5 grams of vitamin C in an ascorbate form daily plus 500mg to 2 grams of pantothenic acid (vitamin B5).

■ Take a Bioflavonoid complex: 500mg to 2 grams.

■ Take between 1000mcu (milk clotting units) to 4000mcu of bromelain – an enzyme from pineapple which helps to release mucous and reduce the allergic response which reduces the discomfort.

■ Nettle tincture or tea three times a day helps to alleviate symptoms.

■ Plant Sterols and sterolins help to boost immune function which reduces allergic reactions. Take 3 capsules daily on an empty stomach. Usually sold under the name of *Moducare*. **NC**

■ *Oralmat* is an extract of the rye plant. It contains beneficial, naturally occurring compounds such as Beta 1,3 glucan, matairesinol, genistein, squalene and co-enzyme Q 10. This liquid extract supports healthy respiratory function by strengthening the body's natural defences against allergens. Dr Princetta, an allergy specialist in Atlanta, Georgia, reports impressive results with allergy and asthma patients saying: 'The South-eastern United States, and Atlanta, Georgia, in particular, is a well-known allergy area of the world. Even some of my worst allergy patients responded very well to the drops and suffered a minimum of 50 percent less this past spring. It's certainly worth a try and you can take 3 drops under the tongue (hold 30 seconds or longer) 3 times daily. Children should use one drop.' **NC**

Helpful Hints

■ Until you are able to identify any food intolerance or external allergies, take 400mg of the bioflavonoid quercetin three times a day which helps to reduce the allergic response.

■ During an acute attack, a homeopathic nasal spray called *Euphorbium Spray* is extremely effective. It helps to relieve a runny nose, congestion and headaches. **NC**

■ Dust and other airborne allergens can be reduced in your immediate environment with an ioniser.

■ Try **New Era** tissue salts for allergic rhinitis from any good pharmacy or health food store.

Many canned fizzy drinks contain up to 10 teaspoons of sugar and if not used up during exercise this will turn to a hard fat inside your body.

ALLERGIES
(see also *Leaky Gut*)

Approximately one in three people in the West now suffer some form of food intolerance. Allergies from external sources such as pesticides, food additives, paints, pollution, perfumes, animal hairs, grass, plant and tree pollens are also widespread. There are more than 3,500 food additives in use today and an average person ingests six kilos a year. Symptoms appear when the system becomes overloaded with toxins and/ or stress. Many people only partially digest food proteins, which can sometimes break through the gut wall. The body treats these particles as it would an infection and attacks them as an enemy, which if left untreated can cause a myriad of allergic-type symptoms.

Foods to Avoid
- Eggs, dairy produce from cows, wheat, corn and soya are all very common allergens.
- All food additives.
- Caffeine, peanuts, chocolate, beef, yeast and shellfish.
- It is important to have an allergy test to find your worst offenders.

Friendly Foods

- This is a possible minefield until you know which foods are your problem but generally eat more brown rice, pears, lamb, cabbage and sweet potatoes.
- Include more linseeds, sunflower seeds, organic sunflower and olive oil in your diet. These foods are a good starting point that very few people react to.
- It's worth noting that the foods you crave the most are usually the ones that are causing you the most problems.
- Papaya is rich in digestive enzymes. Live, goat's or sheep's yoghurt contain friendly bacteria.
- Raw cabbage juice is high in L-glutamine, known to help to heal a leaky gut. Try making fresh juices daily that include a little chopped raw cabbage, a tiny piece of root ginger, celery, carrots, apples and add half a cup of aloe vera juice. Drink immediately after blending while all the enzymes and nutrients are still active.
- Drink liquorice tea, which helps heal the gut. Nettle tea helps reduce the allergic response.

Useful Remedies
- *Histazyme*, a complex containing calcium, vitamin C, zinc, bromelain, silica, vitamin A and manganese acts as a natural anti-histamine. **BC**
- *HEP 194* contains the herb silymarin (milk thistle), the enzyme lipase, the amino acid methionine and B vitamins which all help to cleanse the liver. **BC**
- Two acidophilus/bifidus capsules daily after food to help replenish healthy bacteria in the gut and aid digestion. **BC**

- Betaine hydrochloride – stomach acid – is often lacking in people suffering allergies, *HCl* is available from most health stores – take one capsule just as you begin eating your main meal. Not to be taken if you have active stomach ulcers. **FSC**

- The amino acid L-glutamine can help heal a leaky gut, take 500mg 3 times daily until symptoms ease.

- A good quality multi-vitamin and mineral daily.

- Once you have identified your intolerance the above can be reduced to the multi-vitamin and mineral and the *HCl* daily.

Helpful Hints

- It is vital to chew food more thoroughly.

- Avoid large meals which overload the digestive system and can trigger an allergic response.

- Many toothpastes, shampoos, soaps, detergents and perfumes contain a myriad of chemicals. Buy products in their most natural and unadulterated state. For anyone who suffers dermatitis or skin allergies, **The Green People Company** make organic skin, hair, body lotions, sun screens and toothpaste. Advice line Tel: 01444 401444. Email: organic@greenpeople.co.uk Website:www.greenpeople.co.uk

- Many allergic and chemically sensitive people can benefit enormously by switching from tap water to mineral or filtered water. Tests in the US found that 98% of environmentally ill patients improved by eliminating tap water. Reverse osmosis water is extremely pure and helps cleanse pollutants and chemicals from the body. For details call *The Pure H2O Company* on 01784 221188 email. info@purewater.co.uk website: www.purewater.co.uk

- To test if you have a food allergy, first take your resting pulse rate. Then for at least 14 days completely avoid the food you want to test , for example wheat. Then try eating the food you have avoided on its own, for example Weetabix in water or plain brown toast. Take your pulse at 15, 30 and 60 minutes after eating the specific food. If your pulse has increased by more than ten beats a minute, it is likely that you have sensitivity to the test food.

- Nutritionist Stephanie Lashford has specialised in allergy medicine for 20 years. Initially she asks all patients for 7 days to eat only foods and drinks they have not ingested for the previous 6 weeks – except for water – and even that has to be bottled. And during the first 7 days no flour, dairy or sugar from any source is allowed. This triggers a real detox, and for the first few days you may feel worse, but the benefits are profound. After the 7 days when any food to which you have an intolerance is re-introduced, symptoms are immediate. For details of *The Lashford Technique* log onto www.sandford-clinic.co.uk Stephanie has clinics in London, Manchester and Cardiff. Tel: 02920 747507.

- *Medivac Vacuum Cleaner* is an excellent and effective high-powered vacuum, which does not give out dust in its exhaust. Contact **Medivac Healthcare** on 01625 539401. Fax: 01625 539507. Email: medivacuk@aol.com Website: www.medivac.co.uk

- A company specialising in indoor air quality equipment is the **Air Improvement Centre Ltd**. They can be contacted at 23 Denbigh Street, Victoria, London, SW1V 2HF. Tel: 020

a

7834 2834. Fax: 020 7630 8485. Website: www.air-improvement.co.uk

■ *The Allergy Handbook* published by *What Doctors Don't Tell You* magazine is a good investment for anyone suffering allergies. WDDTY, Freepost, ND 6041, Market Harborough. LE16 7BR. Tel: 0800 146054, 01858 438894. Email: wallacepress@subscription.co.uk

■ Consult a kinesiologist to help you identify food intolerances (see *Useful Information*).

Energise and help de-stress your body by taking a really deep breath every 20 minutes.

ALZHEIMER'S DISEASE
(see also *Memory*)

Alzheimer's is a progressive, degenerative disease that attacks the brain, causing symptoms such as memory loss – especially short-term memory – and a decrease in intellectual functioning. It is the loss of memory of how to do everyday tasks that tends to make an ordinary life unmanageable. As we get older, memory and brain function often decline – but this does not automatically mean that we have Alzheimer's or dementia and many people are misdiagnosed. Many scientists predict that within 30 years, 20% of people over 65 will have this disease.

Excessive exposure to aluminium from cooking utensils and pots and mercury poisoning from dental fillings have been linked to this condition. Many scientists believe that free radicals and an excessive intake of refined, processed foods low in antioxidant vitamins such as vitamins C and E are a contributing factor. Basically, the more pollutants and refined foods we are exposed to, the more vital minerals and vitamins are excreted from the body and our brain function deteriorates. Eating the right foods, taking supplements that nourish the brain and taking more exercise increases circulation to the brain and memory can often be improved. See also *Memory*. Alzheimer's patients are often lacking in the vital brain nutrient acetylcholine, which is manufactured by the body and is also found in our diet, but unless you eat large amounts of organic meats, oats, soya beans, cabbage and cauliflower your levels are likely to be low. And as many elderly people eat a poor diet, levels decrease with age, which not only affects the memory but can trigger symptoms such as lethargy, decreased dreaming and a dry mouth. The main object is to prevent the acetylcholine breaking down in the first place.

Foods to Avoid
■ Foods known to contain traces of aluminium such as commercial chocolate, ready-made desserts, baking powders, processed cheeses, chewing gum and pickles.

■ Any food containing the food additive monosodium glutamate (MSG).

■ Ready-made meat pies, cakes, and pre-packaged meals that are stored in aluminium containers which also tend to be high in saturated fat, sugar and salt.

■ Reduce intake of saturated fats in fatty meats and full-fat dairy and other fatty produce.

■ Reduce your intake of caffeine, sugar and alcohol, which can interfere with brain function.

■ Avoid adding sodium-based salt to your foods.

Friendly Foods

■ Sprinkle a tablespoon of lecithin granules over breakfast cereal, over yoghurt or fresh fruit. Lecithin is rich in choline, but make sure the brand you choose contains at least 30%.

■ Other foods containing this nutrient are egg yolks and fish, especially sardines. Include salmon, herrings, mackerel and tuna in your diet, as they are rich in omega 3 essential fats.

■ Essential fats are vital for proper brain functioning. Use extra virgin unrefined olive, or sunflower oil for your salad dressings.

■ Eat linseeds, sunflower and pumpkin seeds, rich in healthy fats. (See *Fats You Need to Eat*)

■ Be sure to include plenty of fresh fruits, vegetables and whole grains such as brown rice and wholemeal bread and pastas in your diet

■ See also *General Health Hints*.

Useful Remedies

■ The B group vitamins are needed for the formation of acetylcholine and for the manufacture of neuro-transmitters within the brain, so take a high-strength B complex daily.

■ NADH, a derivative of vitamin B3 has been shown to improve memory function and reduce lethargy. Sold as *Enada*, 5mg can be taken 30 minutes before food. **NC**

■ Phosphatidylserine (PS) is another vital brain nutrient. The body can manufacture PS but only if you tend to eat lots of organ meats. 100mg can be taken 3 times a day.

■ Hyperzine A is an extract from a Chinese herb, which has been shown to prevent the breakdown of acetylcholine. Take 200mcg twice a day. **NC**

■ The herb *Ginkgo biloba*, taken as 120–240mg of standardised extract daily, which helps to increase circulation. In rare cases ginkgo can cause a rash, in which case stop taking it. **FSC**

■ Vitamin E 1000iu plus vitamin C 1 gram 3 times a day with meals have been shown to slow the progress of Alzheimer's and to help prevent onset of dementia. If you are on blood-thinning drugs see your doctor before taking the vitamin E which thins the blood naturally.

Helpful Hints

■ Stop smoking. Recent research from Holland indicates that smokers are twice as likely to develop dementia in later life. Avoid drugs such as marijuana and Ecstasy which are associated with memory loss if used in the long term.

■ Vigorous exercise under professional supervision has helped many sufferers restore some bodily functions, especially memory.

■ Certain prescription drugs cause side effects which appear similar to symptoms of senile dementia. Anyone who feels they may have the onset of dementia should immediately consult a qualified doctor, who is also a nutritionist (see *Useful Information*).

- In certain cases, the removal of mercury (amalgam dental fillings) has assisted with the recovery of some faculties (see *Mercury Fillings*). Because of the link between aluminium and Alzheimer's, avoid aluminium cooking utensils and pans, and food stored in aluminium containers. Use stainless steel or glass cookware. Many anti-perspirants contain aluminium, so use a natural deodorant such as *PitRok*, available from all chemists and health stores.

- Simple antacids are often based on aluminium salts and should also be avoided. Aluminium is also found in toothpastes, some cosmetics, processed cheeses, baking powder, buffered aspirin. Table salts often contain aluminium, which is added as a pouring agent.

- If our mineral levels are low, then the body tends to absorb more aluminium, therefore include a good multi-mineral in your everyday health regimen.

- The brain needs to be kept working. There is truth in the phrase 'use it or lose it' as far as the brain is concerned. Do crosswords and force the brain to work by counting down from 1,000 each day in multiples of various numbers, such as 1,000 less 7 = 993, less 7 = 986.

- Try writing and using the opposite hand to the one you normally use. Extend your arms out at shoulder level, rotate one hand clockwise and the other anticlockwise and then change them over. Learn lines from famous poems and recite them by heart a line at a time.

- Many pesticides have been linked to neurological problems and these chemicals along with aluminium are finding their way into our drinking water. Fluoride is a by-product of the aluminium process (see *Fluoride*). Use a good water filter that removes these residues. I recommend reverse osmosis water which is 99 per cent pure and this method is far more efficient than over-the-counter carbon filters. For details call *The Pure H2O Company* on 01784 221188 email: info@PUREH2O.CO.UK website: www.PURE H2O.CO.UK

- Many people have found good results after taking a herbal remedy called *Biostrath*, available from good health stores.

Time is a precious gift – use it wisely.

ANAEMIA

Anaemia tends to come in two forms – pernicious anaemia and iron deficiency. If you have pernicious anaemia, it is due to a lack of intrinsic factor needed to absorb vitamin B12. In the past it was always thought necessary to have B12 injections, however, research has now found that taking 1mg (1000mcg) of B12 can rectify this deficiency if taken daily. A number of disorders can create B12 malabsorption including Crohn's and coeliac disease.

If you have been diagnosed as suffering anaemia the normal procedure is to take a large amount of iron, but it is very important to make sure that the cofactors, which are vitamin B12, folic acid and vitamin C, are taken at the same time to optimise absorption.

Iron deficiency can be brought about by a number of factors, such as losing more blood than the body can replace naturally, common among women who suffer very heavy periods and which should always be investigated by a GP or a gynaecologist. Over-consumption of tea and coffee inhibit iron absorption from your food. Many people take an iron supplement when they are feeling tired, but it is always worthwhile having blood levels of iron checked before you begin supplementing iron. Common symptoms of low iron levels are fatigue, headaches, faintness and pale skin.

Generally, vegetarians eat less iron than non-vegetarians. However, in Israel they found that blood iron levels were actually higher in vegetarians, which is probably due to their high consumption of fruit and vegetables. Vegetarians who do not eat sufficient fruit and vegetables can be low in iron.

Foods to Avoid
■ Black tea and coffee, which reduce absorption of iron from food.
■ Excessive intake of high-fibre foods will have the same effect, but they are needed for good health so if you need iron supplements take them with low-fibre foods such as fruit juice.

Friendly Foods
■ Liver and most meats are rich in iron – especially lean steak. Chicken, pheasant, partridge, grouse, pigeon, kidneys, venison, hare and cockles are also good sources.
■ Wheat bran and wholewheat flour contain good amounts and most breakfast cereals contain added iron.
■ Dried fruits such as apricots, raisins and prunes are also a good source. As dried fruits are high in sugar, soak them for a few minutes in warm water to reduce the sugar content. Drain before serving.
■ Almonds, cocoa and curry powder and raw parsley contain moderate amounts of iron.
■ Leafy green vegetables such as spinach, cabbage and organic tomatoes are also rich in iron.

Useful Remedies
■ Take 1 gram of vitamin C, plus 400mcg of folic acid and 1000mcg of B12 daily as these help to increase absorption of the iron.
■ As B vitamins work together within the body, take a B complex with the above.
■ Iron ascorbate 14–56mg is a more easily absorbed form of iron. Do not take iron sulphate which may damage mucous membranes in the digestive tract and can cause constipation.
■ Vitamin A and iron together are more effective than taking iron on its own. 5000iu of vitamin A can be taken daily while symptoms last.

Helpful Hints
■ When taking an iron supplement it is generally best to take it with a glass of pure fruit juice, which seems to aid absorption due to the vitamin C content in fruit juice.
■ Iron is so vital for health that we store it in our bodies, but if taken in excessive amounts, it can become toxic and is known to cause constipation in some cases. The exception to

this is women who suffer from heavy periods and are feeling exhausted. Pregnant women can benefit from liquid formulas such as *Floradix* or *Spatone* – available from health stores.

■ There is a form of iron combined with lactoferrin which is a dairy protein that helps iron to be absorbed and reduces excess iron that otherwise would be stored in the body. **NL**

■ Many scientists now state that no-one over 50 should take a separate iron supplement unless they have a medical condition that requires it, as high levels of iron are linked to an increased risk of heart disease for both men and women. If large amounts of iron are recommended because of anaemia, then it is best to see a qualified nutritionist who can re-balance your diet and supplements (see *Useful Information*).

■ As we age, our stomach-acid levels fall, which means that nutrients are often poorly absorbed from the foods we eat. Taking a digestive enzyme with meals improves absorption.

■ There is a genetic disorder called haemochromatosis, which affects one in every 200 women, in which iron and large amounts of vitamin C should not be taken. A simple blood test can detect this condition.

It's not your last meal that made you sick – it's your last 1000.

Dr Udo Erasmus

ANGINA

(see also *Cholesterol*)

Angina is often experienced as a pain in the chest frequently after running up a flight of stairs, but in extreme cases after getting out of a chair. It is brought on by an inadequate supply of oxygen via the blood to the heart muscle. Over many years arteries begin laying down sticky deposits, which harden and eventually cause a narrowing within the blood vessels. Typical symptoms include pain in the centre of the chest, which sometimes spreads to the neck/jaw area and down the left arm. The pain can be accompanied by breathlessness, feeling faint, sweating and or nausea. If you have these symptoms seek medical attention as a matter of urgency. See also *Cholesterol*.

Foods to Avoid

■ Drinking 5 or more cups of coffee daily can increase the risk. Try to avoid it completely.

■ Cut down on alcohol which in the long term depletes the body of B vitamins. When you ingest alcohol, levels of homocysteine, a toxic amino acid linked to heart disease, are raised. Beer contains folate and vitamin B6 – so try an occasional beer instead of spirits and wines.

■ Reduce your intake of animal fats, including full-fat dairy produce, pre-packaged cakes, meat pies, sausages and chocolates.

■ Avoid sodium-based salt – use magnesium, potassium-based salts such as *Solo Salt* available from health stores.

■ Reduce your intake of refined sugars found in cakes, biscuits, fizzy drinks and desserts, which convert to hard fats inside the body if not used up during exercise.

■ Avoid all foods that contain hydrogenated or trans fats and fried foods. Never used highly refined cooking oils. (see *Fats You Need To Eat*)

Friendly Foods

■ Oily fish such as salmon, tuna or mackerel are rich in omega 3 fats, which help to thin the blood naturally, as do onions and garlic.

■ Use a little extra virgin olive oil on salad dressings.

■ Include plenty of fresh root ginger in your diet, which improves circulation.

■ To help lower cholesterol, often a contributing factor of angina, eat plenty of soluble fibre either from fruit, vegetables, oats, psyllium husks or linseeds (also known as flax seeds).

■ Dried beans such as haricot, kidney, chick peas, soya beans and whole grains such as brown rice, buckwheat, millet and barley are all rich in fibre and help to control cholesterol.

■ Margarines such as *Biona* and *Vitaquell* are healthier alternatives for spreading.

■ Use non-dairy organic rice or soya milk or skimmed milk.

■ If you can follow a vegan diet with the addition of fish, (preferably oily), this would be the ideal solution (see *General Health Hints*).

■ Sprinkle lecithin granules over cereals and salads to help lower LDL cholesterol levels

Useful Remedies

a

■ The amino acid L-carnitine taken 1–3 grams daily helps improve functioning of the heart and reduces symptoms associated with angina.

■ Co-enzyme Q10 150mg a day has helped angina patients manage more exercise with less symptoms. **PN**

■ Natural source vitamin E 400–500iu a day taken for at least 1 or 2 years thins blood naturally. If you are taking blood-thinning drugs have your blood checked regularly by a doctor.

■ Fish oils supply EPA and DHA which are essential fats that thin the blood naturally. Take 3 grams daily to help reduce chest pain.

■ The herb remedy Hawthorne, 1–2mls tincture or 1–2 grams in tablets daily, helps protect blood vessels and improves heart function.

■ Take 2 grams of vitamin C daily with 1 gram of the amino acid lysine, which work together to help reverse atherosclerosis. **HN**

■ Magnesium helps regulate the heartbeat. Begin on 200mg daily and increase to 400mg.

■ Include a good quality multi-vitamin and mineral in this regimen.

■ Begin using grapefruit pectin fibre called *Profibe*, over your breakfast cereals or in low-fat yoghurts. In numerous clinical trials regular intake has been shown to lower LDL levels (the bad cholesterol) and to gently remove some of the sticky plaque from artery walls. Available from all good health stores worldwide or call **The NutriCentre** (see page 15). **NC**

Helpful Hints

■ Smoking tends to constrict arterial flow – so give it up.

■ Remember that negative stress in the long term thickens the blood and constricts arterial flow.

■ Homeopathic *Arnica 6x* helps strengthen the heart. Take 1 twice daily for up to 3 months.

■ If you are overweight, then it is wise to lose weight. Rather than going on a strict diet, this is best achieved by eating healthily. See *General Health Hints*.

■ With your doctor's permission, embark on a programme of gentle exercise. Start by walking or swimming for 15 minutes daily, gradually building to 30 minutes or more.

■ Intravenous anti-oxidant therapy (chelation) helps to clear blocked arteries and is well worth a try. Call **Dr Keith Scott-Mumby** on 0700 0781744.

■ Watch *Linus Pauling's Theory of Heart Disease* video, from **The Institute of Optimum Nutrition**. Tel: 020 8877 9993. It explains how people have been helped by mega doses of vitamin C and the amino acid lysine. Website: www.ion.ac.uk

Learn to live in the moment.

ANTIBIOTICS

(see also *Candida and Thrush*)

Many people resort to the use of antibiotics whether they really need them or not. Antibiotics kill the friendly bacteria, which have an essential role to play in gut and general health. Bacteria are now mutating and many are becoming resistant to increasing numbers of antibiotics. In the long term, antibiotics suppress our immune system, and along with the loss of healthy bacteria in the gut they often allow fungal infections such as candida to flourish. Whenever you have taken an antibiotic you will need a probiotic. Antibiotics mean anti-life and probiotics the opposite – pro-life. Probiotics are supplements containing friendly bacteria called acidophilus or bifidus.

Foods to Avoid

■ If you have taken antibiotics, avoid foods such as alcohol, sugar and too much fruit (especially immediately after large meals) which trigger fermentation within the gut. This tends to lead to an overgrowth of unfriendly bacteria, which can trigger conditions such as thrush and candida.

■ Avoid mouldy cheeses which also cause fermentation in the gut.

■ Avoid yeast-based breads and foods such as *Marmite* and *Bovril*.

Friendly Foods

■ Pineapple contains the enzyme bromelain which increases the effectiveness of many antibiotics. It acts as a digestive aid – so eat a couple of fresh pineapple chunks before meals.

■ Eat plenty of live, low-fat yoghurt containing acidophilus and bifidus.

■ Artichokes and beetroots contain inulin, a substance which encourages the growth of friendly bacteria.

■ Garlic encourages the growth of friendly bacteria and also kills bad bacteria as well as helping to fight infections.

Useful Remedies

■ Acidophilus and bifidus are healthy bacteria. Take 2 capsules daily after food for at least 6 weeks after completing the antibiotics. Keep these sensitive, live, healthy bacteria in the fridge. **Bio Care** make *Replete* powder which can be dissolved in water, which will help the gut to rebalance quickly. **BC**

■ Take a B complex vitamin that includes 0.5–5mg of biotin daily. Biotin is greatly depleted by antibiotics. Lack of biotin affects your skin, hair and nails.

■ *Goldenseal* tincture 1ml taken twice a day for up to 2 weeks, or grapefruit seed extract, act like natural antibiotics, and can also be taken to avoid infections in the first place.

■ *Olive Leaf Extract* is an antibacterial, anti-viral and anti-parasitic plant extract which helps to dissolve the coating of bacteria and prevent viral replication. Up to 4 tablets daily. **NC**

■ Take 500mg of *Milk Thistle* 1 to 3 times daily with food to help detoxify the liver. **BLK**

Helpful Hints

■ If you feel awful when you are taking antibiotics, rather than wait until you have finished the course, start taking the acidophilus as soon as you feel below par, and also take a strong B vitamin. This will not negate the effect of the antibiotics but can make you feel better.

■ Bee propolis is a natural antibiotic used by bees to sterilise their hives. Many therapists and doctors find that two *Propolis* capsules taken every day with at least one gram of vitamin C can lead to a general improvement in health and enhanced resistance to infections.

■ A naturopath or nutritionist can help you restore your immune system (see *Useful Information*).

Sugar substitutes such as aspartame found in low calorie foods and drinks place a great strain on the liver and have been shown to add to weight gain.

APHRODISIACS, MALE

There are many causes for a man to lose either his desire for sex, or his ability to get and maintain an erection. Both problems are often linked to long-term stress and, by dealing effectively with stress, sexual desire and function can, in many cases, be restored. The related problem of 'brewer's droop' is mainly due to excessive alcohol consumption which can interfere with the ability to maintain an erection quite severely.

Smoking has been linked with reduced ability to maintain an erection; smoking constricts blood flow that is essential for erectile function. Anyone with erectile problems would do well to consider a cholesterol lowering diet. Some men find that strenuous exercise reduces their libido, while others find the opposite. Many couples who have been together for many years find the passion often dissipates over time.

Foods to Avoid

■ Avoid saturated fats found in red meat, full-fat dairy produce, sausages, meat pies and related products which over time clog the arteries and slow circulation.

■ Excessive alcohol and coffee can lower libido and prevent maintaining an erection.

■ Avoid foods high in sodium-based salt, which is linked to poor erectile function.

Friendly Foods

■ Pumpkin and sunflower seeds, linseeds and oysters are rich in zinc – vital for a healthy sex life.

■ Plenty of garlic and onions in your diet improve circulation and help lower LDL, also known as the 'bad' cholesterol.

■ Sprinkle cayenne pepper and turmeric over your food to add spice to your life – you can also take them in tincture or capsule form.

■ Eat more fresh fruits and vegetables and replace red meat with fresh fish and chicken.

■ See *General Health Hints*.

Useful Remedies

■ The herb remedy *Ginkgo biloba* when taken regularly improves circulation. Take 60mg standardised extract 1–2 times a day for 3 months. Then break for a month and begin again, making a cycle of 3 months on, 1 month off.

■ Take 2 grams of the amino acid L-arginine daily.

■ *Korean Ginseng* taken 500–1000mg a day helps reduce the underlying stress that is often linked to this problem. This is shown to be more effective when taken for a month, then stopped for a month and so on.

■ Suma, the South American root can help restore libido. 500–1000mg daily for up to 3 months.

■ Damiana, a herb from Mexico and India, is a natural aphrodisiac; take 125–500mg a day until libido is restored.

■ Stress reduces B vitamins in the body – therefore also include a good quality multi-vitamin and mineral for men that includes a full range of B vitamins. **S**

■ *Muira Puama*, a South American herb, is considered nature's most potent Viagra. A daily dose of 1–1.5 grams of a standardised extract has been proven to be effective. In one study of 100 men with impotence problems, 66% had increased frequency of intercourse, while 70% reported intensification of libido. The stability of the erection was restored in 55% of the patients and 66% reported a reduction in fatigue. **NC**

■ *Natura-Viga* is a combination capsule containing damiana, Mexican yam, ginseng, lecithin (which lowers cholesterol), vitamin E, vitamins B1 and B3, grapeseed extract and zinc – it has worked well for many men. For details in the UK, call 0870 787 9253. Fax: 0870 787 9254. Website: www.natural-sex.co.uk

Helpful Hints

■ Measures to alleviate stress are often very effective. Take regular exercise and learn to laugh more. This releases natural endorphins, which lower stress levels and help you feel more positive. Learn to breathe more deeply.

■ People who use a large amount of marijuana or take steroids may also find their erectile function diminished.

■ By constantly worrying about your lack of sex drive, you often make the situation worse. Studies show that a lack of vitamins C, E, A, B and the minerals zinc and selenium can cause a low sperm count and lack of sex drive. Anyone taking regular antidepressants or sleeping pills may be lacking in these nutrients.

■ If the condition continues, or you are worried about infertility as well as impotency, see a doctor who is also a nutritionist (see *Useful Information*).

Rather than using sugar substitutes such as aspartame, try a little honey. To reduce sugar cravings, take 200mcg of the mineral chromium daily.

ARTHRITIS, OSTEO

Osteoarthritis is characterised by progressive degeneration of the body's cartilage which cushions and surrounds the joints. In most cases it affects the load-bearing joints: hips, knees, spine and hands. There is a popular misconception that exercise makes you more prone to developing osteoarthritis. In reality, the reverse appears to be true, so long as the exercise does not involve contact sports like rugby, football or hockey where the joints might get damaged. Regular exercise, of the sort which doesn't impact too much on the joints, such as walking or swimming, is one way of keeping the joints in good shape long term.

The majority of people who suffer osteoarthritis eat too many acid-forming foods, in common with many other health problems. Proteins such as meat and dairy produce from cows as well as refined carbohydrates such as white bread and pizzas are acid-forming – whereas fresh vegetables and most fruits and millet are alkalising. If we could all eat less acid-forming foods, many illnesses could be eradicated. Arthritis can be triggered following a joint injury and by overuse of laxatives. I broke my knee in 1991 and I have to keep up my exercises or my joints and spine become really stiff.

People who develop osteoarthritis are frequently told that they should avoid the nightshade family of vegetables, which includes tomatoes, potatoes, peppers and aubergines. Out of these, tomatoes seem to be the worst offender for sufferers. It has been shown that 60–70% of people who avoid these foods for at least 6 months or more see benefits. Being overweight places more stress on joints, which will add to the problem in later life.

Foods to Avoid

■ Reduce intake of black tea, coffee, alcohol, fizzy drinks, shop-bought cakes, pies, pastries, bread and pasta that are made with refined white flour, all of which are acid forming.

■ Avoid known triggers such as tomatoes, potatoes, aubergines, peppers, oranges, plums and rhubarb – and their juices.

■ Eggs are hard to digest for some people with arthritis, and can also trigger joint pain in sensitive individuals.

■ Greatly reduce any full-fat foods and cow's milk, red meats, fried foods, sausages, meat pies and chocolate.

Friendly Foods

■ Cherries are rich in bioflavonoids and reduce uric acid levels in the body.

■ Pineapple contains bromelain which is highly anti-inflammatory and also aids absorption of nutrients from the rest of the diet.

■ Eat oily fish such as mackerel, tuna, salmon, herrings or sardines 3 times a week.

■ Sweet potatoes are rich in vitamin A, fibre and make a good alternative to potatoes.

■ Grains such as millet, brown rice, amaranth, spelt, barley and quinoa are all preferable to refined wheat products. Choose wholemeal bread and try pastas made from corn, buckwheat, rice and lentil flours. Try 100% rye crisp bread, sugar-free oatcakes and sugar-free muesli or porridge.

■ Eat far more fresh green vegetables to re-alkalise your system. One of the quickest ways to do this is to blend raw cabbage, watercress, celery, a little root ginger plus any fresh fruits and vegetables you have to hand in a juicer. Add to this a teaspoon of any good quality green powder supplement found in all health shops and drink immediately after juicing. Add aloe vera juice for extra benefits.

■ Use organic, unrefined olive, sunflower, walnut or sesame oils in your salad dressings.

■ Eat at least 1 tablespoonful of linseeds, sunflower, pumpkin or sesame seeds daily, as they are rich in the essential fats that are vital for healthy joints. Hazelnuts, cashewnuts, almonds and walnuts are all rich in essential fats. Here's an easy way to eat more of them; add 2 tablespoons of each into a blender, whizz for 1 minute and store in an air-tight jar. Simply sprinkle over breakfast cereal, fruit salads or into low-fat yoghurts daily.

■ Try herbal teas such as *Devil's Claw* and nettle tea and also make the change and try dandelion coffee.

■ Add more turmeric and cayenne pepper to savoury foods as they help reduce inflammation

■ See also *General Health Hints*.

Useful Remedies

■ One of the best nutritional supplements known to help arthritic conditions is the amino sugar glucosamine sulphate. A number of studies have found that 500mg three times a day taken for three months or more can substantially reduce pain and improve mobility.

■ Initially, take 500mg of glucosamine 3 times daily until symptoms improve and then lower the dose to 500mg daily. Glucosamine is usually derived from crab shells, so if you have a severe intolerance to shellfish, avoid this supplement. **NC**

■ MSM (methylsulfonylmethane) is a form of organic sulphur which is involved with many key functions in the body. Extraordinary results are being reported in terms of pain relief from taking around 2–3 grams in tablets daily. It is also available in creams. **HN**

■ *Nutricol* powder, developed by Brian Welsby who designed the health programmes for most of the UK Olympic athletes, contains glucosamine, MSM and hydrolysed collagen. Call **Be-Well Products** on 01778 560868. Fax: 01778 560872.

■ Niacinamide (ask for **no-flush** vitamin B3) 500mg 3–4 times daily is a great alternative to glucosamine, which helps reduce joint pain. Some people reap the benefits in 4–5 weeks, but 3–12 months is a good time scale to see if it is going to benefit you. Incidentally, people who take niacinamide over a sustained period of time have an improved sense of humour! Ask for the **no-flush** variety as common niacin can cause a flushing effect that can be shocking if you are unprepared. The B group vitamins work together, so add a B complex to your daily regimen.

■ Take a couple of teaspoons of cod liver oil daily to help reduce arthritic pain. The vitamin D in cod liver oil or capsules also helps with pain relief. Or take 3 capsules daily.

■ Natural source vitamin E taken 400–600iu daily helps reduce pain.

■ Take 1–3 grams of vitamin C daily in an ascorbate form with meals, which will not irritate the gut and acts as an anti-inflammatory. Vitamin C is vital for the production of healthy synovial fluid, the substance that surrounds the joints.

■ Ginger, curcumin and boswelia are herbs with highly anti-inflammatory properties. Take 3–4 tablets a day. **FSC**

■ The formula *Ligazyme Plus* contains vital minerals such as calcium, boron, magnesium, rutin, silica as well as vitamins A and D and digestive enzymes, all of which support connective tissue and encourage healthier bones. **BC**

■ *Zinaxin* is a supplement made from Chinese ginger, very beneficial for bursitis, rheumatism and arthritis. Take two capsules per day for the first month, then 1–2 capsules daily. **NC**

■ Homeopathic *Rhus Tox 6x* helps relieve stiffness when you first move around.

■ See also *Helpful Hints*, page 41.

Enthusiasm is contagious – try it and see.
Dr Richard Bandler

a

ARTHRITIS, RHEUMATOID (RA)

Rheumatoid arthritis is primarily an inflammatory disease. It is an autoimmune disorder whereby the body's own immune system starts attacking joint tissue. A chronic disease, it tends to progress over time but many people find the pain and stiffness come and go for varying periods of time. RA affects three times as many women as men. It is now thought that over-acidity in the body and uric acid deposits in the joints are major contributing factors.

Researchers in England have found that at least one third of people can completely control their rheumatoid arthritis by eliminating foods to which they have a sensitivity (see *Allergies*). The most common culprits are any foods and drinks containing cow's milk as well as the nightshade group of fruits and vegetables (see *Arthritis, Osteo*).

Heavy exercise may cause the disease to progress faster, but gentle exercise such as swimming, t'ai chi, yoga, stretching and walking are more helpful. Researchers have found that all rheumatoid arthritis sufferers are deficient in the major antioxidant nutrients, vitamins A, C, E plus the mineral selenium – but particularly vitamin E. The majority of rheumatoid arthritis sufferers also appear to be low in stomach acid, and so supplementing with betaine hydrochloride capsules (stomach acid) can help. This makes sense as betaine helps to digest proteins and most people who suffer from allergies have a problem digesting certain proteins. If you have active stomach ulcers do not take betaine; use a digestive enzyme capsule instead.

Foods to Avoid

- Animal fats eaten to excess tend to aggravate rheumatoid arthritis. Avoiding dairy produce, as well as meat, sugar and eggs helps some people.

- Avoid known triggers such as tomatoes, potatoes, aubergines, peppers, oranges, plums and rhubarb – and their juices. Lectins, found in dried beans, can also exacerbate RA.

- Tea, coffee, chocolate, peanuts, spinach, rhubarb and beetroot are all high in oxalic acid, which seems to further aggravate rheumatoid arthritis.

Friendly Foods

- Eat more pineapple, which is a rich source of bromelain.

- People who are not prepared to eat oily fish are going to need to swallow a lot of fish oil capsules or take a good couple of teaspoons of fish oil daily. For those who don't or won't eat fish then a dessertspoon or two of linseed oil as well as using unrefined olive oil in salad dressings can help.

- A vegan diet has been shown to help some individuals.

- Root ginger and turmeric and the herb boswelia have anti-inflammatory properties. They will not alleviate the problem but can substantially reduce pain and this results in better mobility.

- Eat plenty of cherries and garlic and use rice, oat or organic soya milks as alternatives to dairy produce from cows.

- Avocado is rich in vitamin E and essential fats – eat twice weekly.
- Eat lots more green vegetables and add a green food powder such as Dr Gillian McKeith's *Living Food Energy* to cereals, juices and desserts. **NC**

Useful Remedies

- For those who don't like pineapple, bromelain is available as a supplement. Bromelain's activity is normally measured either as mcu (which are milk clotting units) or gdu (gelatin digesting units). You will need 2000–6000 mcu or 1000–4000 gdu daily. Take the bromelain on an empty stomach to increase its effectiveness.
- There is good research on the effectiveness of evening primrose oil but the amounts you need to take are high, somewhere in the area of 10 grams daily.
- EPO is taken for its GLA (gamma linolenic acid) content – GLA is highly anti-inflammatory and is available as a supplement. Take 1–2 grams daily. **BC**
- Take vitamin C 1–3 grams daily plus 400–800iu of natural source vitamin E.
- Take a multi-mineral containing 30mg of zinc, 70mcg of selenium plus traces of copper, known to help reduce pain. **NC**
- Take EPA–DHA fish oil 1–2 grams daily.
- Many sufferers of rheumatoid arthritis benefit from taking vitamin B5 (pantothenic acid). 500mg can be taken four times a day. As B vitamins work together, include a B complex in your regimen.
- The herbs curcumin and boswellia are also available in tablet and capsule formulas: 200–600mg. **HN**
- Take 300mg celery seed extract daily to reduce uric acid levels.
- Plant fats, sterols or sterolins (*Moducare*) extracted from fruits and vegetables, help balance the immune system. If the immune system is overactive, as it is in rheumatoid arthritis, the plant fats inhibit the damaging effects of antibodies that attack the body tissues. Take one capsule three times a day. **NC**

Helpful Hints for all types of arthritis

- Improving bowel function and gut flora using soluble fibres like linseeds and supplementing acidophilus can improve a number of symptoms associated with rheumatoid arthritis.
- Numerous people have experienced tremendous benefits after taking pure aloe vera juice daily for several months. For details call 020 8875 9915; Email: alasdairaloevera@aol.com
- Nettle tea taken regularly has helped reduce the pain and swelling for many people.
- To re-alkalise your system take a good quality green powder such as *Alkalife* daily. The same company also make *Alkabath* salts which help eliminate toxins from the joints. For your nearest stockists call **Best Care Products**, Tel: 01342 410 303. Fax: 01342 410909. Website: www.bestcare-uk.com

a

- *Boswelia Joint and Muscle Balm* or *Boswelia Complex* applied topically helps to relieve pain and inflammation, call **Higher Nature**, Tel: 01435 882880.

- Sufferers of rheumatoid arthritis should consider having a blood test to check for possible food intolerances. Removing of food allergens may reverse symptoms in many types of arthritis. For details contact **Dr Keith Scott-Mumby** Tel: 0700 078 1744.

- Wearing magnets has given pain relief to many people. Now a new super magnet is available that is 8,000 times more powerful than the earth's magnetic field. Magnets placed on the painful area will increase blood flow, which brings more oxygen to an injury or area of pain, thus helping to reduce swelling and inflammation. For details of *Super Magnets* call **Coghill Laboratories**, Tel: 01495 752 122. Website: www.cogreslab.demon.co.uk

- The Chinese exercise regimes of t'ai chi or qigong have helped many sufferers. They are easy to practise, even with severely impaired mobility. Rheumatoid arthritis seems to be affected by stress, so make sure you stay as calm as possible (see *Stress*).

- For help, ideas and counselling on arthritis call the **Arthritis Care Helpline** between 12.00 to 4.00pm, Monday to Friday, Tel: 0808 800 4050. Website: www.arthritis.care.org.uk

- Call the **Arthritic Association**. This charity provides very good dietary advice – yearly membership costs £6 in 2000. Tel: 020 7491 0233 or 01323 416550 between 10am–4pm weekdays. Website: www.arthriticassociation.org.uk

A smile costs nothing and makes a huge difference to your and others' well-being.

ASTHMA

(see also *Allergies* and *Leaky Gut*)

Asthma is a disease which affects the bronchial tubes leading to our lungs resulting in periods of wheezing and shortness of breath. One in every seven children in the UK now suffers asthma and the problem is escalating rapidly. Pollution from traffic fumes is without doubt a contributing factor, as during school holidays incidences of attacks are reduced as there is less traffic. Other atmospheric pollutants such as pollen, cigarette smoke and car exhaust fumes can all be triggers. Stressful situations and chronic exhaustion can also trigger an attack as can eating foods to which you have a sensitivity (such as sulphur dioxide, used as a preservative in many dried fruits). You can also suffer exercise-induced asthma. People who take paracetamol every day are twice as likely to suffer asthma, and if you take it twice weekly you are 80% more likely to be affected.

Foods to Avoid

- Salt is often a trigger for asthma.

- There is a strong association between asthma and dairy products, especially in children.

- Any foods to which you have an intolerance will make you more susceptible to attacks.

- Reduce intake of meat, eggs and full-fat dairy produce, which increase mucous production.

- Sodium-based salt in any foods (some people can have an attack after eating too many crisps).
- Some mass-produced, ready-prepared salads, dried fruits, wines and beers contain sulphur dioxide, which is known to trigger problems in sensitive individuals.
- Avoid sodium benzoate, which is frequently found in soft drinks.
- Generally avoid all mass-produced pre-packaged foods. See *General Health Hints*.

Friendly Foods
- Green leafy vegetables, fresh fruits and honey are rich in magnesium – a lack of which is linked to breathing problems.
- Include more beans and lentils plus garlic and onions in your diet.
- As asthma is often linked by nutritional physicians to a 'leaky gut' include plenty of fresh ginger in your diet which is very soothing. Cabbage also helps heal the gut (see *Leaky Gut*).
- Eat oily fish three times a week. This can reduce the severity and frequency of attacks.
- Use extra-virgin, unrefined olive and sunflower oils in salad dressings and include plenty of linseeds, pumpkin, sunflower and sesame seeds in your diet.
- Try rice or oat milks as non-dairy alternatives to cow's milk.
- Buy a juicer and make yourself a carrot, ginger, cabbage, radish, apple and celery mix – drink immediately. Try different mixes daily which is a great way to get health-giving nutrients into the body.

Useful Remedies
- Take a good quality multi-vitamin daily; plus a multi-mineral containing 200–400mg of magnesium; plus 200mcg of selenium as low levels leave you more at risk from an attack.
- Vitamin C in ascorbate form taken 1 gram 3 times a day with meals helps open the airways.
- Take vitamin B6, 150mg a day; B12, 1,000–2,000mcg a day; plus a B complex. Asthma medication depletes B vitamins, especially in people who are sensitive to sulphates.
- The enzyme bromelain taken 1,000–4,000 mcu a day helps to reduce mucous production and ease breathing.
- Take 60mg a day of natural-source beta-carotene if you suffer exercise-induced asthma.
- The herb *Ginkgo Biloba* 120–240mg standardised extract or 3-4ml of tincture taken daily has been shown to improve circulation and decrease asthma symptoms.
- *Oralmat* is an extract of rye grass in a liquid formula that has been shown to support healthy respiratory function by strengthening defences against toxins in the lungs. An Australian study in mild to moderate asthmatics showed considerable lessening of symptoms, for some after only a few days of use. Three drops should be placed under the tongue 3 times daily (hold 30 seconds or longer). Children should use one drop instead. **NC**
- Bronchial-dilating herbs such as euphorbia and grindelia help open the airways. Take 15 drops of each herb 3 times daily in juice. **NC**

Helpful Hints

- Use an ioniser in any room in which you are going to spend any length of time, as it can reduce the amount of pollen and dust in the air.

- Try to avoid antibiotics during the infant years, which have been linked to an increased risk of developing asthma in later life.

- Acupuncture has proved useful for many sufferers.

- To check for food and environmental allergens, consult a kinesiologist who can determine what foods and environmental agents you should avoid. Kinesiology is not 100% accurate but thousands have found it a good indicator of which foods and other factors are causing the most problems (see *Useful Information*).

- It's incredible how many people suffer breathing problems simply because they are not using their lungs properly. Most asthmatics benefit from tuition in proper breathing techniques. Every twenty minutes or so remember to take a deep breath down into your lower abdomen area.

- Shallow breathing is associated with being stressed. Learn relaxation techniques or consult a hypnotherapist who can teach you how to relax (see *Useful Information*). Try *Deep Relaxation,* a tape by hypnotherapist Paul McKenna. Tel: 01455 852233. Website: www.mckenna-breen.com

- Take gentle exercise such as yoga, t'ai chi, swimming or walking. Exercise reduces stress and helps you to breathe which should help to reduce the incidence of asthma attacks.

- The Buteyko method of breathing has helped many sufferers. Call the **Hale Clinic** in London. Tel: 020 7631 0156.

- Colonic irrigation or consulting a nutritionist have proved helpful for many sufferers. Homeopathy has proved especially helpful for children, but be sure to consult a qualified doctor who is also a homeopath (see *Useful Information*).

- Homeopathic *Pothos Foetidus 200c* can be used if an attack is triggered by animals. *Blatta Orientalis 30c* can be taken during an attack when catarrh is present. Deeper asthmatic treatment using homeopathy helps reduce the susceptibility for attacks (see *Useful Information*).

- Have a regular massage using essential oils of camomile and lavender.

- A company specialising in indoor air-quality equipment is the **Air Improvement Centre Ltd**. They can be contacted at 23 Denbigh Street, Victoria, London, SW1V 2HF. Tel: 020 7834 2834. Fax: 020 7630 8485. Website: www.air-improvement.co.uk

- Read *Asthma, The Complete Guide* by Prof. Jonathan Brostoff and Linda Gamlin, Bloomsbury.

- Consult the Asthma Helpline, Tel: 08457 010203, 9am–7pm, Monday–Friday.

- For a further range of asthma information contact the **National Asthma Campaign**, Tel: 020 7226 2260. Website: www.asthma.org.uk

Your body is only as strong as its weakest point.

ATHLETE'S FOOT

Athlete's foot is caused by a fungal infection of the skin and is characterised by itchy, flaking and cracked skin, especially between the toes and on the soles of the feet. This problem can be transmitted in public places such as swimming baths where people walk barefoot, and in moist atmospheres. Wear socks made from natural fibres such as cotton and silk that allow the skin to breathe and change footwear regularly. It is important that feet are dried properly after bathing or exercise. Persistent athlete's foot is often associated with an overgrowth of candida in the gut (see also *Candida*).

Foods to Avoid

- Avoid sugar in any form when symptoms are acute.Sugars ferment and feed yeast in the body.
- Avoid foods containing yeast such as cheese, wine, yeasty breads, beer, mushrooms, vinegar, soy sauce and yeast-based drinks such as *Bovril* and *Marmite*.
- Grapes are high in sugar and may have moulds on the skin.
- Peanuts should also be avoided.

Friendly Foods

- Eat plenty of garlic and onions, which are anti-bacterial and anti-fungal.
- Live, low-fat yoghurt containing acidophlius and bifidus – eat at least 250 grams a day.
- The herb *Pau D'Arco* is anti-fungal – take 6 capsules daily or drink several cups as tea.

Useful Remedies

- Apply tea tree oil externally or grapefruit seed and tea tree oil – *Citricidal*. **HN**
- *Black Walnut and Calendula Tincture,* applied topically and taken internally twice a day is effective. **FSC**
- *Kolorex* cream contains powerful anti-fungal agents, and is effective against resistant fungal infections, particularly when it fails to respond to standard treatments such as tea tree oils and grapefruit-seed extract. The cream can be applied twice daily for up to a month. **NC**

Helpful Hints

- *Pau D'Arco* is the bark from a South American tree which boosts immune function and helps fight fungal infections. It makes a very pleasant tasting tea and is easily available in capsules. It can also be added to a foot wash made with tea tree oil.
- Homeopathic *Sulphur 6x* will help if eruptions are getting worse, itching and becoming hot.
- Add 5–10 drops of citricidal liquid to a footbath and soak feet twice daily. **HN**

Have you called your mother lately?

AUTISM

This is a disorder which tends to develop in early childhood. Its numerous symptoms include an inability to communicate and concentrate, disturbed sleep patterns, hyperactivity, abnormal social relationships, rituals and compulsive behaviour. Some doctors say that autism is genetic and this is undoubtedly a factor in some cases, but reports are now accumulating which link the huge increase in autism to toxic overload either from vaccines (especially MMR – measles, mumps and rubella), pesticides or chemicals in food. Many autistic children have also been given large doses of antibiotics which in the long term can trigger gut problems – which in turn trigger sensitivities to many foods especially gluten and dairy produce from cows (see also *Candida* and *Leaky Gut*). I have heard of several cases where autistic children have been referred to psychiatrists and when given mind-altering drugs the children's symptoms worsened considerably.

Foods to Avoid

■ Removing all gluten found in most mass-produced breads, biscuits and cereals from the child's diet has been shown to be very helpful in many cases. Remember that rye, barley and oats also contain gluten. Some children suffered withdrawal-type symptoms and became worse before their parents noticed improvements. Many doctors are now happy to prescribe gluten-free products on the NHS.

■ Dairy produce from cows should also be avoided.

■ Wheat, soya, fish, eggs, peanuts, tree nuts and shellfish have been found to cause the most problems.

■ Avoid all pre-packaged junk-type foods and drinks that are packed with additives, salt, sugar and animal fats. Keep a food diary and note when symptoms become worse. To make sure that your child does not suffer nutritional deficiencies work with a qualified nutritionist or a nutritional physician (see *Useful Information*).

Friendly Foods

■ As far as possible, give your child only organic, whole foods that are free from pesticides and rich in magnesium, vitamin B6 and folic acid; especially green leafy vegetables, beans, fresh fruits and liver.

■ Gluten-free cereals, carrots, broccoli, baked beans, parsley, spinach, watercress and almonds – are all high in calcium, which helps reduce the incidence of self-injury.

■ Essential fats are vital for healthy brain functioning. Give your child oily fish, if this is not one of their problem foods – at least twice a week – and add cold organic sunflower and olive oil to cooked foods and use in salad dressings.

Useful Remedies

■ Take magnesium 15mg per kilo of body weight and vitamin B6 10mg per kilo of bodyweight. Many children with autism have also been found to be low in folic acid – part of the B group of vitamins, so try to include a B complex daily. As children do not tend to like tablets try adding liquid B vitamins to their food. **BC**

■ Some parents have found that adding an essential fatty acid like *Efamol's Efalex* or *Udo's Choice Oil* on a regular basis has helped their children. **NC**

■ Dissolve an additive-free vitamin C tablet into water daily to boost immune function.

■ As children can find pills hard to swallow use liquid multi-minerals and vitamins daily and make sure the supplement contains 5000iu of vitamin A. Or use a pill crusher and then sprinkle the powder over cooked foods. To order call **Health Plus**, Tel: 01323 737374. Website: www.healthplus.co.uk

Helpful Hints

■ Try to remove all chemicals from the child's environment such as perfumes, chemical cleaning products and toiletries.

■ Many parents have had some success in using homeopathy to minimise vaccine damage.

■ **What Doctors Don't Tell You** have an excellent book on this subject (see *Useful Information*).

■ Because each case of autism is so unique, I strongly suggest that before embarking on this programme you consult a nutritional physician. To find your nearest practitioner see *Useful Information* on page 317.

■ For further help call **Allergy Induced Autism** on 01733 331 771. Check their website at www.kessick.demon.co.uk/aia.htm

It's never too late to change – begin today.

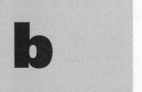

BACK PAIN

Twenty million working days in Britain alone are lost every year thanks to back pain, which affects 80% of people at some point in their lives. This is partly due to poor posture but more frequently to poor lifting habits. Most companies now train their staff how to lift properly; without doubt prevention is better than cure. Until recently most people thought that bed rest was the most sensible option, but 'right and light' exercise under the supervision of a professional is definitely preferable. The centre of the back can be thought of as a column made up of 33 pieces of bone called vertebrae. The spinal column is strengthened by ligaments, which run the length of the spine, and is supported by muscles, which attach to the vertebrae though tendons. It is important to have back pain diagnosed and, in an ideal world, you should see a chiropractor or an osteopath on a regular basis. I have seen people with ME and chronic fatigue receive huge benefits by having their back and necks manipulated back into place. I have also seen people who have ended up on crutches or even in a wheelchair when all they needed was a good chiropractor. One lady was given such strong painkillers after continually complaining of back pain that she ended up wandering the streets suffering memory loss. Doctors need to refer more patients with back pain as soon as possible to an osteopath or chiropractor. And if they won't, I suggest you find your nearest practitioner and pay privately. Chronic low level back or loin pain can also be due to a kidney infection.

Foods to Avoid

■ If you are in pain, it is worth avoiding foods and drinks containing caffeine, which reduces our ability to make endorphins that are the body's natural pain-killing chemicals.

■ Reduce your intake of meat which will exacerbate any inflammation.

Friendly Foods

■ Eat oily fish at least twice a week for its anti-inflammatory properties

■ Add fresh rosemary to meals to improve circulation and aid healing.

■ Ginger, turmeric and cayenne pepper can all improve circulation and have anti-inflammatory effects.

■ Cauliflower, berries, sweet potatoes, potatoes, fresh fruits (especially cherries) and green leafy vegetables are all rich in vitamin C which helps to produce collagen which makes up 90% of the bone matrix and also acts as a mild anti-inflammatory.

■ See *General Health Hints*.

Useful Remedies

■ While symptoms are acute take 1–3 grams of *Glucosamine* daily. This amino sugar helps to restore the thick gelatinous nature of the fluids and tissues around the joints and in between the vertebrae. Once the pain is eased, lower the dose to a maintainance intake of 500mg daily. If you suffer a severe sensitivity to shellfish do not take this supplement which is usually made from crushed crab shells. Many companies now blend the glucosamine with MSM, an organic form of sulphur which helps maintain healthy joints and aids pain relief. **HN**

■ Taking 3-4 tablets a day of a combination formula containing ginger, curcumin and boswelia should help to reduce the pain and inflammation. **FSC**

■ Calcium 500–1,000mg and Magnesium 200–600mg daily – many companies make them in one tablet. These minerals are known as nature's tranquillizers and reduce muscle spasm. **FSC**

■ Take 3 grams of vitamin C daily, in an ascorbate form – this vitamin helps to produce collagen.

■ Try *Ligazyme Plus*, a supplement devised by a chiropractor containing calcium, vitamin C, bromelain, magnesium and rutin, which all help support the skeletal system. **BC**

Helpful Hints

■ As soon as possible after any injury, consult a chiropractor or osteopath. To help reduce the immediate pain and muscle spasm, wrap some ice cubes or a bag of frozen peas in a towel and place on the painful area for 10 minutes every hour.

■ Back pain often has its root in poor posture. This is compounded by the fact that we now tend to lead very sedentary lives, which weakens the supporting structures of the spine and makes them much more prone to injury. Much severe back pain is caused by muscle spasm. Before agreeing to any surgery, always consult a chiropractor or osteopath for a second opinion (see *Useful Information*). Severe and persistent back pain should always be reported to your doctor. Also if you are extremely tired and under stress, not only does your immune system begin to fail but also your body in general. In other words when you stop supporting your body, it stops supporting you. If this is the case, then you need to take a long, hard look at your lifestyle and get more rest. Acupuncture is known to help in many cases.

■ For general back maintenance, yoga can be very beneficial as it improves flexibility and strengthens the spine and improves posture, protecting it from injury in the long term.

■ *Alexander Technique* and *Pilates* teaches individuals how to maintain their back and general health through better posture and exercises (see *Useful Information*).

■ Sports exercise is important too. It is generally accepted that swimming is the best form of exercise, because although the back muscles are worked, they are protected from jarring by the support given by the water.

■ Many people report good results from using a wooden 'backstretcher' for ten minutes each day. For a brochure, send a large SAE to **Enanef Ltd**, Beechwood House, King George's Hill, Abinger Bottom, Dorking, Surrey, RH5 6JW. Tel: 0700 222 5724 or 01306 731651. Website: www.thebackcoach.co.uk (for product information) or www.backbook.com (for book details).

■ **Obus Forme** based in Canada make extremely comfortable padded inserts for all chairs which really helped me after a recent back problem – they enabled me to sit at my desk without pain. For details in the UK call 01491 577129 or Email: clinic@activate.com To find your nearest stockists contact **Obus Forme Ltd**. Website: www.obusforme.com or write to them at 550, Hopwell Ave. Toronto. Ontario. M6E 2S6 Tel: (toll free) 1-888-225- 7378.

■ *Empulse* is a pulsed electromagnetic treatment – the setting is governed by an analysis of the brain's electrical activity. It is a non-invasive, non-drug based preventative treatment. Contact **Natural Health Works Ltd**, Felaw Maltings, 44 Felaw Street, Ipswich, IP2 8SJ, Tel: 01473 407333. Email: info@natural-health-works.co.uk Website: www.natural-health-works.co.uk

- A new device called the *Scenar* invented by Russian scientists has proved highly effective for reducing pain. The treatment takes an hour and costs £40–£70. Many people I interviewed found it so successful at controlling pain that they have bought their own baby *Scenar*. To find your nearest therapist in the UK call **Life Energies**, Tel: 01722 741111.

- Wearing magnets has given relief from the pain to many people. Magnets placed on the painful area will increase blood flow, which brings more oxygen to an injury or area of pain, which helps to reduce swelling and inflammation. A new super magnet is 8,000 times more powerful than the earth's magnetic field. For details of *Super Magnets*, contact **Coghill Laboratories** Tel: 01495 752 122 or log onto www.cogreslab.demon.co.uk

- Use good bath salts such as *Epsom* salts or *Alkabath* to help reduce muscle spasm. Alkabath salts are more powerful than *Epsom* salts and help eliminate toxins from the joints and re-alkalise the body. For your nearest stockists call **Best Care Products**. Tel: 01342 410 303. Fax: 01342 410909. Website: www.bestcare-uk.com

Have a weekly aromatherapy massage – the oils penetrate into the bloodstream and really help calm the muscle spasms. Roman camomile, lavender, and eucalyptus oils all help reduce pain.

For further help contact **BackCare**, 16 Elmtree Road, Teddington, Middlesex, TW11 8ST, or call 020 8977 5474 and ask for their helpline which is open 10.00am–2.00pm, Monday to Friday. Website: www.backpain.org Email: back_pain@compuserve.com

The spice turmeric aids digestion, helps purify your blood, acts as a natural antiseptic and antibiotic and reduces joint pain.

BAD BREATH

(see *Halitosis*)

BEREAVEMENT

During the past 10 years, I have written regularly about life after death and have received hundreds of letters from people of all ages who have lost a loved one. Their sense of loss and grief is often overwhelming. But how different we might all feel if we knew that our loved ones live on...

In April 1998 I went through a near death experience with a medical doctor present (this is well documented in my book *Divine Intervention*, Cima Books). I now write from a totally different perspective as I have an absolute personal 'knowing' that we all go on. Physicists have long known that matter cannot be created or destroyed, so everything that dies simply changes into a different material form. That material form itself is composed of energy. We are all electrical (energy) beings in a physical body.

Ask anyone who has had the privilege to be with a loved one at their moment of passing. Every single time they say that the 'essence' or spark that made that individual unique disappears once the physical shell is dead. Where it goes has been asked since the beginning of time.

If you choose to believe me – I will tell you where we go. We simply move to another frequency or dimension. When you turn on your radio or TV you can tune to hundreds of different channels or stations and receive or see huge amounts of information. The spirit realms are also on various frequencies. The human brain is both a transmitter and receiver. I have interviewed and met dozens of people who by learning to meditate, and stilling their minds into a receptive alpha state, have after time heard messages for themselves. Obviously, some people are better at this than others, but we all have the capability to hear other realms. When some people suddenly begin hearing voices they are labelled as mentally ill – some are – but others have simply begun hearing the spirit world and it is vital that the medical world begins to recognise this possibility.

Immediately after a loved one's passing, it is vital for you to express your feelings and let your emotions out. Grief, anger and guilt have a tremendous impact on the physical body. Tears shed in trauma contain high levels of stress chemicals – let them out and don't be afraid to break down. When my mother died in my arms in 1991 I was inconsolable and like millions of others I turned to good mediums who were able to give me specific messages that only the two of us knew. These days I can hear my mother for myself and this has brought me huge comfort. Some people say that talking to the 'dead' is wicked, but Jesus died over 2,000 years ago and we still talk to him.

Foods to Avoid
- As much as possible avoid junk, sugary, pre-packaged meals, which place a strain on your immune system, which is already under great stress.
- Especially avoid stimulants such as caffeine, alcohol and sugar which put a great strain on your adrenal glands, which further increase the feelings of total exhaustion.

Friendly Foods
- At times of extreme emotional stress it is easy to forget our own health. It is important to eat as healthily as possible, which will not only help your nervous system to cope but also boost your immune system. You help no one by allowing yourself to become ill. Try to eat one meal daily containing quality protein such as fish or chicken with fresh vegetables and fruit.
- See also *General Health Hints*.

Useful Remedies
- Take homeopathic *Ignatia 30c* and the **Bach Flower Remedy** *Star of Bethlehem* which help to reduce the feelings of shock and grief.
- Take a B complex daily to support the nerves.
- Take a good quality multi-vitamin and mineral. **S**
- The *Australian Bush Essence* – red suva frangipani – is excellent for relieving grief. **NC**
- *Stabilium (Garum armoricum)* has been used in relieving depression, anxiety and fatigue in bereavement. *Garum's* primary effect is to increase the amount of calming endorphins

made within the body. Four capsules can be taken on an empty stomach in the morning for 15 consecutive days. After two weeks, the dose should be reduced to two capsules every morning. **NC**

Helpful Hints

■ If you have a friend, colleague or relative who is dealing with the death of a loved one, take time out to shop and prepare the odd meal for them. Not only will this help to support their physical needs but also by having someone to talk to, it also supports their emotional needs.

■ **Cruse Bereavement Care**, a charity founded in 1959, has 180 branches in the UK. Write to **Cruse Bereavement Care**, 126 Sheen Road, Richmond, Surrey, TW9 1UR. Tel: 020 8940 4818 (9.30am – 5.00pm weekdays). Website: www.crusebereavementcare.org.uk

■ I found the book *A Free Spirit* by Patrick Francis, a medium who began hearing voices at the age of 44, very comforting. Patrick 'channels' a nun, Margaret Anna Cusack, known around the world as the nun of Kenmare, who died in 1899. Whether you believe in life after death or not – this book gives real hope. To order Tel: Dublin (Ireland) 00 353 (0)1 452 3793. By post send £7.95 (inc P & P) payable to Auricle Enterprises, 30 Old Court Manor, Fir House, Dublin 24. Ireland.

■ **The Compassionate Friends** is a nationwide organisation of bereaved parents offering understanding, support and encouragement after the death of a child or children. Members of TCF receive regular issues of **TCF News** and a quarterly Newsletter. For further information, contact **The Compassionate Friends**, 53 North Street, Bristol, BS3 1EN or call their helpline. Tel: 0117 953 9639, 9.30am–10.30pm every day. Website: www.tcf.org.uk Email: info@tcf.org.uk

■ To find a medium in your area contact, the **Spiritualist National Union**, Redwoods, Stansted Hall, Stansted, Essex, CM24 8UD. Tel: 0845 458 0768. Website: www.snu.org.uk If they are unable to locate a medium, they are happy to give details of your nearest spiritualist church.

Have you done your good deed for today yet?

BLADDER PROBLEMS

(see *Cystitis, Incontinence and Prostate*)

BLEEDING GUMS

(see also *Fluoride*)

Bleeding gums can be triggered by over-enthusiastic brushing, but they are frequently an indication of a lack of vitamin C or bioflavonoids either in the diet or through supplementation. To make sure you are not suffering with anything more serious, you should see your dentist on a regular basis. Make sure you see an oral hygienist at least twice a year for a proper scale and polish. When plaque builds up gum disease such as gingivitis can take hold. If left unchecked you can lose your teeth. Believe me, after all the problems I have suffered with my teeth during the last decade, your own teeth are very precious and should be taken care of at all costs.

Foods to Avoid

■ The plaque-forming bacteria that cause chronic gum disease thrive on sugar. Young children especially should only be allowed small amounts of fizzy drinks, sweets and puddings that are high in sugar.

■ Keep refined carbohydrates including biscuits, cakes and sweets to a minimum.

■ Avoid all foods and water containing fluoride, which is a by-product of the plant fertiliser industry. Fluoride may have reduced the number of cavities, but it is a poison and in my opinion should not be allowed into our drinking water. This is mass medication without consent.

Friendly Foods

■ Foods containing plenty of fibre such as leafy green vegetables, brown rice, fresh fruits like apples, figs and cherries are all rich in vitamin C, which supports healthy teeth and gums.

■ Chew liquorice sticks regularly to keep teeth and gums clean and reduce bacteria in the mouth.

■ Drink at least 6 glasses of filtered water daily.

Useful Remedies

■ *Co-enzyme Q10* is well known to improve gum health. Take 60mg a day.

■ Vitamin C with bioflavonoids, 1 gram a day with food.

■ A good quality multi-vitamin and mineral. **HN**

Helpful Hints

■ Mercury from amalgam fillings is also known to cause swollen, bleeding gums (see *Mercury*).

■ Eat a piece of fruit after main meals. This increases saliva production, which is alkaline and neutralises the acid produced by the bacteria, which are responsible for dental decay. Apples are excellent.

■ Toothpaste containing sodium lauryl sulfate can thin the lining of the cheeks and may weaken gum tissue.

■ Try squeezing the *Co Q10* from a capsule onto your toothbrush and brushing it onto your gums.

■ vitamin C supplements containing sugar when chewed will attack tooth enamel and weaken the lining of the mouth.

■ Use a good electric toothbrush.

■ Practise good daily dental hygiene by using floss and a natural tea tree mouthwash. Clean your teeth and gums daily using a water jet and appliance, adding a few drops of tea tree oil and one drop of clove oil, which is an excellent antiseptic, to the warm water. Water Tooth Cleaners are available from large chemists. Use a good herbal toothpaste like *Aloe Dent* available from all health stores.

If you have a high cholesterol level – but eat a healthy diet –
you may have an underactive thyroid.

BLOATING

(see *Candida*, *Constipation* and *Flatulence*)

BODY HAIR, EXCESSIVE (HIRSUTISM)

Many women suffer this problem after going through the menopause; some can be affected when they are much younger. It is normally due to an excess of male hormones called androgens, which are produced by the ovaries or the adrenal glands. It is important to consult your doctor if you have an unexplained excess body hair. It often helps if you can balance your hormones naturally (see *Menopause*). The condition is often related to polycystic ovarian syndrome.

Foods to Avoid

- Alcohol
- Animal fats have an adverse affect on hormone levels within the body which can make symptoms worse.
- If you cook food in plastic containers, chemicals which have an oestrogen or building effect within the body can leach into your food. Avoid drinking from plastic bottles.

Friendly Foods

- Include more hormone-regulating foods such as organic tofu, soya, chick peas and fennel.
- Eat more beans, lentils and leafy greens including broccoli, cauliflower, cabbage, artichoke and beetroot, all of which help cleanse the liver of toxins and balance hormones.
- Eat more linseeds, rich in essential fats which also balance hormones.

Useful Remedies

- The herbs that have proved most useful for reducing excess body hair are *Dong quai* and *Agnus castus*, which help to regulate hormonal levels. Take 500mg of either or both daily. Also available as a tincture. Try the *Agnus castus* in the first instance. **FSC**
- Black cohosh taken 500mg twice a day has been used successfully to inhibit and reverse facial hair growth in women. Many companies now sell all these herbs in one formula – try 500mg twice daily or take 1ml of a tincture. **BLK**

■ Herbs used for the related condition polycystic ovarian syndrome are liquorice, saw palmetto, paeonia and *Agnus castus*. Take 5mls of each daily. **NC**

Helpful Hints

■ The amount of excess body hair you have may be related to the amount you are overweight. Losing weight therefore can often ease this problem.

■ Women who grow excessive body hair may be short of progesterone, which helps balance the male hormones that women also make in small quantities. Many women don't ovulate regularly (but still have periods) due to stress, excess pollution in the environment and foods containing herbicides, which have an oestrogen-like building effect. As progesterone is only produced after ovulation or during pregnancy, progesterone deficiency is becoming more common; hairy legs and chins are one sign. Natural progesterone, made from yams in a cream called *Pro-Juven*, can reduce hairiness when used for some time. It is available on prescription in the UK (but freely available in America). You can order this for your own use by calling **Pharmwest**. **PW**

■ For a list of doctors in the UK that work with natural progesterone send an SAE to: NPIS, PO Box 24, Buxton, SK17 9FB.

If your nose begins running within a few seconds of eating a certain food – you may have an intolerance to this food.

BODY ODOUR

We are all covered in bacteria and in certain parts of the body such as under the arms and between our legs bacteria can accumulate. Unpleasant body odour is usually associated with poor hygiene habits but it can also indicate internal toxicity. Also if you eat too much garlic, the smell begins to ooze through your pores. It's very healthy for the person who has eaten it, but not so pleasant for those around you!

Foods to Avoid

■ Reduce the amount of low-fibre foods you eat such as jelly, ice cream, white breads and pastas, cakes, biscuits etc.

■ Avoid full-fat dairy produce which triggers mucous production and can exacerbate constipation.

■ Any foods that ferment in the gut (see p.34) can eventually trigger body odour. Cut down on sugar and alcohol and eat fruit in between meals.

■ Red meat and heavy fatty meals are hard to digest and slow your digestion and elimination.

Friendly Foods

■ Drink at least 6 glasses of filtered water daily to help flush toxins from the body.

■ Add a tablespoon of soluble fibre to your breakfast cereals such as linseeds, hemp seeds, psyllium husks or oat or rice bran – all available from health stores.

■ Treat yourself to a blender and a juicer. To help cleanse your system whizz any selection of fruits you like with a tablespoon of added linseeds (flax), plus a dessertspoon of a good quality green food powder. My favourite is blueberries, strawberries, a banana, a chopped pear and a kiwi, to which I add some linseeds, sunflower seeds, Dr Gillian McKeith's *Living Food Energy Powder* and some organic rice milk. If you drink this cocktail instead of an evening meal, it really helps to clear you out! If you add half a teaspoon of powdered essential fats it helps even more. *Omega Plex EFA* formula is available from **Bio Care**. **BC**

■ On alternate days, juice any green foods, plus artichoke, celery, apple, raw beetroot, a little fresh root ginger and aloe vera juice, which will all help to detoxify your system.

■ Adding fresh coriander to these juices and meals helps keep the bacteria which can cause unpleasant body odour under control.

■ Eat more pineapple and papaya, which are rich in digestive enzymes.

Useful Remedies

■ Healthy bacteria acidophilus/bifidus help improve gut functioning – take two capsules daily after meals. **BC**

■ A deficiency of the mineral zinc is related to excess perspiration – take a multi-vitamin and mineral daily, which usually contains 15mg of zinc, and then take a further 15mg before bed.

■ Any organic green food supplement powders containing chlorella and/or wheat grass is a great way to increase elimination. **NC**

■ The mineral silica really helps to reduce body odour. Take 75 mg daily. **BLK**

Helpful Hints

■ When the bowels are moving frequently the body doesn't have to try and eliminate toxins through the skin.

■ Fresh live yoghurt with acidophilus and bifidus eaten on a regular basis keeps gut flora in good shape.

■ Take a shower every day and change underwear regularly.

■ Wear cotton or silk next to the skin which enable the skin to breathe.

■ If persistent, body odour may indicate liver dysfunction, digestive problems and/or yeast infections, which are probably best investigated by a qualified nutritionist or a doctor who is also a nutritionist (see *Useful Information*).

■ Try *PitRok* – the natural odourless mineral salt deodorant, which prevents bacterial growth without the use of harsh chemicals or aluminium. Just wet the crystal and glide it over the skin. Also available in a spray. For your nearest stockist call **PitRok Ltd**, Tel: 020 8563 1120 Website: www.pitrok.co.uk

If you have poor digestion avoid drinking too much liquid with meals, which dilutes the stomach acid you need for digestion.

BOILS

(Furuncle)

Boils are normally due to an acute bacterial infection of a hair follicle caused by the bacteria staphylococcus aureus. If you suffer from boils on a regular basis, it's the body's way of telling you that your immune system is run down, you're consuming a very poor diet and you are full of toxins. Boils are more common in diabetics and Aids patients and may be accompanied by a slight fever.

Foods to Avoid

■ Any foods and drinks high in sugar which will lower immune function.

■ Reduce your intake of red meats and full-fat dairy produce especially cheese, chocolates, double cream and so on.

■ Avoid all pre-packaged meals, and mass-produced cakes, biscuits and snacks that are packed with hydrogenated or trans fats.

■ Eliminate mass-produced burgers, fried foods and oily take-away meals.

Friendly Foods

■ Eat more soluble fibres like linseed, oat or rice bran and psyllium husks to encourage faster elimination of toxins from the bowel.

■ Include more garlic and onions as they have antiseptic properties that cleanse the gut.

■ Eat more fresh beetroot, fennel, celeriac and artichokes, which help to cleanse the liver.

■ Eat plenty of fibre in the form of lightly steamed vegetables and fruits.

■ Eat low-fat live yoghurt with acidophilus and bifidus.

■ Drink at least 6 glasses of water daily.

■ See *General Health Hints*

Useful Remedies

■ Zinc is a vital mineral for healing the skin and stimulating the immune system. Take 30mg a day.

■ Vitamin C, take 1 gram in an ascorbate form 3 times a day with meals for one month and then reduce to 500mg daily for several months.

■ Vitamin A is also great for healing the skin. If you are not pregnant or planning a pregnancy, take up to 30,000iu for 7 days. Then reduce to 5000iu, which is also an acceptable dose if you are pregnant.

■ *Goldenseal* tincture on a cotton swab and apply it directly to the boil. *Goldenseal* helps to kill off the bacteria staphylococcus aureus. **FSC**

■ Apply a little tea tree oil on a cotton swab to the boil.

Helpful Hints

■ *Goldenseal* can be used as a poultice. The boils don't normally rupture if you use this herb.

■ If you do want the boils to come to a head and possibly rupture, 2 dessertspoons of Epsom salts in half a pint of hot water can be applied directly to the boil to enhance draining.

■ *Silica* – 75 mg daily internally – will also help to bring the boil to a head. If the boil is very severe and hasn't improved in 2–3 days, it's very important that you consult your doctor.

■ Get plenty of exercise, which helps detoxify the skin, and wash as soon as possible after exercise. Saunas help to clear blocked pores and drain toxins from the body.

■ A wonderful book for people suffering from skin problems is *Super Skin* by Kathryn Marsden (Thorsons).

Never sleep in a bra, which prevents the lymph glands from draining properly.

BREAST CANCER
(see *Cancer of the Breast*)

BREAST PAIN and TENDERNESS
(see also *Cancer of the Breast*)

Tender breasts are a common symptom of pre-menstrual syndrome (PMS) when they can become increasingly swollen and tender prior to menstruation. Breast pain is often associated with other symptoms such as fluid retention, abdominal bloating, and an excess of the hormone oestrogen. Tender breasts during the first few months of pregnancy are quite common. But if breasts are tender the whole month or if the discomfort becomes severe, it is important to see a doctor. If you find any lumps of any size or shape in your breasts seek medical attention immediately. Exercise is one way of reducing the symptoms of pre-menstrual syndrome as this encourages lymphatic drainage. On the other hand, wearing a bra for more than 12 hours a day can reduce the body's ability to drain the lymph nodes.

Foods to Avoid

■ Caffeine – complete avoidance can reduce the symptoms of breast pain. Moderate reduction doesn't always work; it does need to be complete elimination. Remember that caffeine is not just in tea and coffee but in cola, chocolate and some over-the-counter cold remedies.

■ Alcohol should be kept to a minimum as it can increase breast pain.

■ Sodium-based salt tends to aggravate fluid retention, which can exacerbate breast tenderness. Ask at your health shop for a magnesium-based salt and use sparingly.

Friendly Foods

■ Eat plenty of sunflower, sesame and linseeds, which all contain essential fatty acids, which should help reduce breast tenderness.

■ Eating organic soya-based foods like tofu, soya yoghurt and milk on a regular basis can again reduce the tendency or can help to relieve the symptoms and balance hormones.

■ Drink herbal teas and dandelion coffee.

■ Add kombu seaweed to bean dishes. It contains iodine, which helps reduce mastitis-type pains.

■ Eat more broccoli, cauliflower, kale and cabbage, which help to balance hormones naturally.

Useful Remedies

■ Take 400mg of magnesium for its muscle relaxing qualities.

■ Vitamin E 200–600iu a day for 3–4 months

■ A good quality B complex contains 50mg of B6 – take another 50mg of B6 separately. The dose should total 100mg daily.

■ Evening Primrose oil is useful for this problem, but you would need around 2–3 grams daily. Therefore it would be easier to take 250mg of *Mega GLA*. **BC**

■ The herb *Agnus castus* 500–2000mg a day or 2mls of tincture should help regulate hormone levels more naturally.

■ Take a good quality multi-vitamin and mineral for women. **BC**

Helpful Hints

■ Regular exercise (running or walking 1–3 miles a day) can relieve tenderness. Many women find it uncomfortable to run when their breasts are tender, but if you exercise on a regular basis tenderness should not be so much of an issue for 7–10 days prior to a period. Wear a sports bra.

■ Exercise improves circulation and aids drainage of the lymph system. Mini-trampolines are wonderful, as is any vigorous exercise such as fast walking, swimming or dancing.

■ Lymphatic drainage massage is known to improve drainage, thereby reducing swelling and pain (see MLD [manual lymphatic drainage] in *Useful Information*).

■ Sometimes breast pain is due to an imbalance between oestrogen and progesterone, which causes tender breasts and breast cysts, known as fibrocystic breast disease. It is becoming increasingly common because of the high levels of oestrogen pollutants we are exposed to. Using a natural progesterone formula found in creams and capsules may reduce the cysts and tenderness in a few months. You need a prescription for natural progesterone in the UK (but not abroad). For details of natural progesterone and a list of doctors who work with it write to **NPIS**, PO Box 24, Buxton, SK17 9FB. To order for your own use call **Pharm West**, Tel: 00 800 8923 8923 or check their Website: www.pharmwest.com

■ If, after three months, there is no improvement on the above regimen, see a qualified nutritionist who is also a doctor (see *Useful Information*).

Remember what you give out is what you get back.

BRITTLE NAILS

(see *Nail Problems*)

BRONCHITIS

This common problem is triggered when the bronchial tubes become infected. This can have a viral or bacterial origin and symptoms normally occur when you have an upper respiratory tract infection. Bronchitis is more common during winter months. If you contract a cold or flu, immune function can become very low indeed and the infection can then spread down towards the lungs. For some sensitive individuals, tobacco smoke is enough to set them off, but with other people exposure to pollens and other toxins they inhale can lead to an attack of bronchitis.

Some cases can be managed without the use of antibiotics, but if you find it painful to take a deep breath, have a temperature for more than 48 hours and can hear a rattle in your chest when you breath or cough, you must see your doctor. If the infection reaches your lungs it can become pneumonia. Having suffered bronchitis twice in the last 2 years which resulted from colds caught on long plane journeys I can assure you this condition is no laughing matter and once you have the weakness you really need to look after yourself if you get a cold or become run down. If my immune system had been in better shape I would have been more able to handle these infections. See also *Immune Function*.

Foods To Avoid

■ Greatly reduce your intake of any foods containing sugar – this includes concentrated fruit juices – as sugar reduces your immune system's ability to fight infections.

■ While symptoms are acute, avoid all dairy products from any source plus refined carbohydrates such as cakes, pastries and biscuits all of which create more mucous.

Friendly Foods

■ Eat plenty of fresh fruits and vegetables. When you feel this poorly, your digestive system can labour under the strain. Therefore eat fresh vegetable soups which can be thickened with sweet potatoes rich in Vitamin A, which helps boost your immune system.

■ Garlic and onions are really cleansing and have antiseptic properties.

■ Lightly stew or grill fruits, which make them easier to digest.

■ Eating fish regularly helps to reduce the frequency and severity of bronchial attacks and if you are undergoing one, the oils in fish can provide a strong anti-inflammatory effect.

■ As you are likely to be running a temperature, drink at least 6 glasses of water daily.

■ Make teas with fresh lemon juice, a small piece of root ginger and a little honey. Drink lots of herbal teas such as liquorice and elderberry.

Useful Remedies

■ Bromelain is extremely effective for bronchial conditions as it improves lung functions and softens and helps loosen the mucous. If you are frequently exposed to environmental toxins or cigarette smoke, taking vitamin C and vitamin E can reduce the damage and protect your lungs.

■ While symptoms are acute take 1,000–4,000mcu of bromelain, plus 1–4 grams of vitamin C in an ascorbate form with meals.

■ N-acetyl cysteine (NAC) helps to break up mucous and reduces the bacterial count for people suffering with bronchitis. Take NAC 600mg twice a day. Studies have shown that people who take NAC on a regular basis suffer less incidence of bronchitis. **S**

■ For 7 days, you can also take 25,000iu of vitamin A (if you are pregnant only take 5000iu) and 600iu of vitamin E.

■ Useful herbs for boosting immune function and reducing bacteria are echinacea, goldenseal and elderberry. **FSC**

■ Liquorice is anti-inflammatory, anti-viral and can be very useful with bronchial conditions. **FSC**

■ *Zinc Gluconate* lozenges really help to reduce the coughing and sore throat.

■ *Olive Leaf Extract* has powerful anti-bacterial qualities which have been shown to help with respiratory conditions – take 3 capsules daily to help boost your immune system.

■ Include a good quality multi-vitamin and mineral in your regimen

Helpful Hints

■ Inhaling steam is really helpful for opening up the lungs. Add a few drops of *Olbas Oil* or any pure eucalyptus oil into a bowl of boiling water. Place a towel over your head and really inhale the steam through your nose. If you do this 4–5 times daily it helps to loosen your chest.

■ Echinacea taken regularly helps prevent viral bronchitis from progressing into a more dangerous bacterial infection.

■ The herbs mullein, wild cherry bark, liquorice and lomatium are useful expectorants and have anti viral properties. These herbs are available as tinctures and taken on a regular basis can help loosen mucous, reduce the coughing and help fight the infection. **FSC**

■ If the infection becomes serious and you are prescribed antibiotics, as soon as you finish the course begin taking the healthy bacteria acidophilus/bifidus for at least 6 weeks to replenish healthy bacteria in the gut which in turn helps immune function.

■ In general terms, whenever you are suffering from a bronchial infection, you should stay in bed and rest for at least 2 days. The more you try to struggle on, the slower your recovery.

■ Use an *Ultrabreathe* – a small inexpensive device that helps to exercise the lungs. Tel: 0870 608 9019. Website: www.ultrabreathe.com

The average person in the West eats 40% more food than they need.

BRUISING

The discolouration of the skin is caused by blood leaking from damaged blood vessels into the tissues of the skin. It is a normal process but some people bruise excessively. Excessive bruising is often due to a deficiency of vitamin C and/or bioflavonoids the water-soluble pigment in fruits. But if you suffer regular bruising not associated with a hard knock or injury – it can indicate rarer underlying problems such as leukaemia, so if in any doubt check with your GP.

Foods to Avoid
■ Avoid all highly processed foods such as mass-produced cakes, biscuits and pre-packaged meals, which are generally lacking in any nutrients.

■ Don't cook foods for too long as cooking greatly reduces nutrient levels.

Friendly Foods
■ Eat plenty of foods high in vitamin C such as kiwi, cherries, peppers, blueberries, pineapple and papaya.

■ Include more leafy green vegetables in your diet.

■ See also *General Health Hints*.

Useful Remedies
■ Take 1–3 grams of vitamin C in an ascorbate form daily plus 500–2,000mg of bioflavonoids, to help strengthen capillaries.

■ *Rutin Complex* includes bromelain, a flavanoid extracted from pineapple. It has an anti-inflammatory effect. Take 500mg of bromelain daily until bruising disappears. Order from **Country Life** Tel: 020 8614 1411 Website: www.country-life.com

■ The herb *Horse Chestnut* is excellent for bruises. Take 500–1000mg until symptoms disappear.

Helpful Hints
■ For bruising after a trauma such as surgery, homeopathic Arnica is a wonderful remedy. If you have had surgery of any kind, you can take *Arnica 30c* every 4 hours until the bruising fades. Arnica cream used topically is magical and really helps reduce the swelling. It can also be very helpful for the bruising undergone after surgery.

■ For deeper tissue damage use *Ledum 30c* three times daily for 4–5 days.

■ Comfrey ointment speeds up soft-tissue healing.

■ For sprains and injury-type swellings use an ice pack to help reduce the immediate swelling. In an emergency, I grab anything from the freezer such as a bag of frozen peas, wrap them in a towel and place directly over the swelling for ten minutes every hour.

You can choose your thoughts – change every negative thought to a positive one and your life and health will change for the better.

BURNS, MINOR

First-degree burns affect the very top layer of the skin. Second-degree burns leave blisters but usually heal without scarring. Third degree burns are far more serious and affect the full thickness of the skin, leaving it charred or white. These burns need urgent medical attention to reduce the risk of infection and scarring. If you come into contact with acid, solvents or chemicals that burn the skin, as quickly as possible dowse the area with running cool water to lessen the damage. If a child drinks any chemical such as bleach that burns the oesophagus, do not encourage vomiting as it will also burn on its way back up. If possible allow the patient to drink milk and seek immediate medical help.

Foods To Avoid
■ Avoid any foods and drinks containing sugar or alcohol, as they will slow the healing process.
■ Generally, avoid highly processed, refined foods which contain almost no nutrients.

Friendly Foods
■ High-quality protein is vital in the initial stages for tissue healing. Include plenty of organic free range chicken, fresh fish, beans and lentils or even a good quality whey protein shake which is a very digestible form of protein in your diet to speed healing.
■ Nuts and seeds are rich in essential fats and zinc which are vital for healing the skin. Wheat germ and wheat germ oil are rich in vitamin E, which aids skin healing and reduces scarring.
■ Eat plenty of fresh fruits high in natural carotenes to help heal the skin such as apricots, sweet potatoes, spinach. Cantaloupe melons, carrots and green leafy vegetables.

Useful Remedies
■ The herb *Gotu kola* has been used to aid healing of burns for centuries. You can either take 500mg daily or take 1–2ml of tincture. The tincture can also be applied externally.
■ Take natural source vitamin E 500iu twice a day.
■ Vitamin C is vital for the production of collagen, take up to 3 grams daily with food – buy a formula that also contains bioflavonoids.
■ Also take a good quality vitamin and mineral supplement that contains 30–60mg of zinc, which aids skin healing and boosts immune function.
■ MSM (organic sulphur) helps wound healing and is anti-inflammatory – take up to 400mg three times daily. **HN**

Helpful Hints
■ You can bathe the burn in cold water for up to 30 minutes, if necessary. Dry with a clean sterile dressing and smother with sterile aloe vera gel.

- Take *Bach Homeopathic Rescue Remedy* every few hours to reduce the feelings of shock.
- Cover the area with a thin layer of honey and cover this with a sterile gauze. Honey is a very effective antiseptic, is anti-bacterial and can also speed the healing process.
- In India, fresh potato peelings are placed on burns. The wounds heal more quickly and infection is reduced.
- Papaya pulp has been shown to be effective in sloughing off dead tissue, preventing wound infection. Papaya is rich in enzymes that aid healing.
- Calendula cream helps to soothe the pain and promote tissue repair.
- Lavender oil helps to aid burn healing.
- Homeopathic *Cantharis 6x*, taken two or three times daily, will help to reduce the blisters.
- Aloe vera gel or calendula cream can be applied topically.
- MSM Cream (organic sulphur cream) containing vitamin A and E, B5, aloe vera and comfrey extract, can be applied topically to aid healing of minor burns. **HN**
- Once healing is underway, pierce a vitamin E capsule and apply directly to the affected area to promote healing.

Eating an apple daily helps to keep your lungs healthy.

BURSITIS

This is also commonly known as tennis elbow or housemaid's knee and is an inflammation of the bursa, the sac-like membrane containing the fluids responsible for lubricating the joints. It is most common in the shoulder, elbow, hip and knees and can cause severe pain or tenderness, particularly when the person places any weight on that joint. Orthodox medicine offers anti-inflammatory drugs and sometimes cortisone injections. My husband has suffered tennis elbow, which was triggered by too much weight lifting, and after the injections he found great relief – but within 3–4 months, the pain and tenderness returned even worse than before. He has found some relief by resting his elbow completely and when he is under less stress or on holiday the pain recedes.

Foods to Avoid
- Reduce your intake of caffeine and alcohol which can increase inflammation within the body.
- Cut down on animal-based foods and junk-type meals, which are very acid-forming.
- Avoid plums, rhubarb, oranges and asparagus, which are acid-forming.

Friendly Foods
- Eat more foods that re-alkalise the body such as fresh vegetables – the greener the better.
- Include plenty of fresh fruits in the diet.

■ Millet is alkaline – sprinkle the fine grain over your low-sugar breakfast cereal. Eat more fresh ginger and oily fish, which have anti-inflammatory properties.

■ Use turmeric and cayenne pepper in meals as they have anti-inflammatory properties.

■ See also *General Health Hints*.

Useful Remedies

■ Take 1–3 grams daily vitamin C with bioflavonoids until symptoms ease. **S**

■ Fish oils have anti-inflammatory properties: take 1–3 grams a day that contain EPA and DHA which are key essential omega 3 fatty acids.

■ Take 1,000–4,000mcu of the flavonoid bromelain for its anti-inflammatory properties.

■ *Boswelia Complex* contains the herbs boswelia, curcumin and black pepper which all have anti-inflammatory properties. Take up to 600mg daily. **HN**

■ *Glucosamine Sulphate*, an amino sugar with MSM (an organic form of sulphur), helps to restore the gelatinous fluids around the joints. Take 500mg three times daily and once symptoms are alleviated reduce to 500mg daily. If you are allergic to shellfish avoid this supplement. **HN**

■ *Zinaxin* is a supplement made from Chinese ginger, particularly beneficial for bursitis, rheumatism and arthritis. Two capsules can be taken daily for the first month, then 1–2 capsules daily. **NC**

Helpful Hints

■ *MSM Joint and Muscle Balm* contains boswelia, vitamin E, aloe vera, niacin and capsicum which used regularly may help reduce the pain. **HN**

■ Apply a bag of frozen peas wrapped in a tea towel to ice the painful area for ten minutes every few hours. This really does help to reduce inflammation and pain. You can alternate the cold compress with a warm ginger compress – simply add a piece of root ginger to boiling water. Let it steep for 10 minutes, soak a cloth in this mixture and press on the painful area for 10 minutes. Make the compress as warm as possible without burning yourself!

■ Use an elastic bandage during the day to limit swelling. Elevate the affected area above the level of the heart to encourage drainage of fluids out of the injured area.

■ Avoid weight training when pain is acute, as this will further aggravate the problem.

■ Many acupuncturists believe that bursitis results from muscle spasms, which pull joints out of line. If acupuncture does not give any relief after six treatments you are more than likely wasting your money. Consult a chiropractor or a physiotherapist.

■ Gentle aromatherapy massage using oils such as Roman camomile, ginger, marjoram and geranium can also help to relieve the pain.

Know right from wrong.

C

CANCER

(see also *Cancer of the Breast*)

There are more than 200 types of cancer, but the biggest four killers are lung, breast, bowel and prostate cancer. Cancer is a disease of the genes, but this does not necessarily mean it is inherited – but it's a defect of a gene that controls cellular reproduction. Genes are damaged by free radicals, radiation, viral infections and chemicals. Free radicals are unstable molecules that are formed within the body. Major risk factors for cancer are diets high in saturated fat, sunbathing to excess, exposure to toxic chemicals found in burnt food, petrol fumes, pesticides, preservatives, excessive hormones and over exposure to certain electromagnetic fields. Antioxidants such as vitamin A,C and E plus zinc and selenium remove free radicals from the body. By taking antioxidants on a regular basis we are given more protection from the negative effects of the free radicals on our tissues, cells and genes. It is now well-known that changing your diet can greatly reduce the likelihood of contracting cancer.

Various cancers have been linked to over-consumption of specific foods; for instance, people who regularly consume hot dogs and mass-produced burgers are more likely to develop bowel cancer. Excessive intake of dietary fats results in higher levels of oestrogens, which are a great risk factor for cancers especially of the breast and ovaries.

My mother died of cancer and I believe that her anger and bitterness after my father died at only 50 triggered her cancer. Emotions affect your health – how many times have you heard of a friend who suffers a shock and a year later they have cancer? It's imperative to heal emotional scars as well as physical ones. There are always exceptions. Some people eat healthily, exercise and really take care of themselves – but still develop cancer. Others smoke until they are almost 100 and are fine. No one has all the answers but we should all do what we can, where and when we can to practise more prevention.

The Alternative Anti-Cancer Prevention Diet

■ Avoid fried food. This is a good way to cut down on your exposure to free radicals. Boil, steam or bake food, eating most of your food raw or lightly cooked. Try 'steam-frying' food using a watered down soya sauce, plus herbs or spices for taste. Barbecued and char-grilled foods, especially if fatty, are also best avoided because they contain relatively high concentrations of cancer-causing substances called carcinogens.

■ Minimise pollution. Anything that is combusted produces free radicals. So the less time you spend exposed to car exhaust and other people's smoke, the better. Only use mobile phones for 10–15 minutes at a time. Reduce your exposure to electrical pollutants – microwaves, TVs and electrical equipment. Don't sleep with an electric clock by your bed. Never use chemical pesticides and herbicides in your garden and home.

■ Eat more organic food: soya, carrots, broccoli, Brussels sprouts, cauliflower and garlic all help to fight cancer. Carrots are rich in beta-carotene, high levels of which mean a low risk of cancer. Put two carrots, two heads of broccoli, half a pack of tofu (soya bean curd), a teaspoon of vegetable stock and some water in the blender for a delicious immune-boosting soup. Add soya milk if you want it creamy, and spices if you like it hot. Soya should always be eaten in its traditional form – Tofu, Tempeh, organic soya beans or soya milk, and the soya is best cooked. Soya contains anti-cancer compounds. A perfectly healthy, safe amount is around 50–100 grams of soya in total a day. Soya is without doubt beneficial to adults but it should not be given to small infants and children. Infant soya milk formulas give the infant a daily dose of phytoestogens, which helps to protect adults against cancer, but for infants the levels are too high. The obvious first choice is to breast feed infants for the first year. Soya lecithin granules are also a great food for adults, as lecithin lowers LDL (the bad cholesterol), improves memory and helps protect against many cancers.

■ Carrots, lettuce and many other healthy foods are overloaded with pesticides and herbicides that are associated with an increased risk of cancer. Throw away the outer leaves when preparing non-organic vegetables like cabbage or lettuce.

■ Just one serving of crisp or raw cabbage each week can help reduce the risk of colon cancer by as much as 50%.

■ Eat at least three pieces of fruit a day. Vitamin C and natural beta-carotene and lycopene are potent anti-cancer nutrients. Lycopene, a carotenoid found in tomatoes, has been shown to reduce the risk of many cancers, especially prostate cancer, but also reduces the risk of cancers in the colon, rectum, pancreas, throat, mouth, breast and cervix. If you are not allergic to tomatoes eat 6–10 servings weekly. When the tomatoes are heated in a little olive oil, more lycopene is released. Alternatively take *Lycopene Plus* a formula made by **Bio Care**.

■ Many patients with cancer have low levels of carotenes. Apricots, sweet potatoes, asparagus, French beans, broccoli, carrots, mustard and cress, red peppers, spinach, spring greens, watercress, cantaloupe melon, mangoes, parsley and tomatoes are all rich in carotenes. Fresh fruit contains lots of vitamin C. Eat fresh fruit as a snack throughout the day. A great way to take in a lot of nutrients quickly is to place your favourite fruits into a blender with a tablespoon of a good green food supplement powder, a teaspoon of mixed seeds (sunflower, sesame, flax and pumpkin) and whizz with a cup of organic rice milk. I drink this every day either for breakfast or as a meal replacement at supper. My favourite blend is blueberries, strawberries, raspberries, a kiwi and a banana. To ring the changes I add an unpeeled pear or apple to make sure I get plenty of fibre. It's delicious.

■ Eat whole foods, nuts, beans and seeds. Anything in its whole form, such as oats, brown rice, lentils, almonds or sunflower seeds are high in the essential anti-cancer minerals zinc and selenium. These protect the body from free radicals. Buy a pack of each of the following, sunflower seeds, pumpkin seeds, sesame seeds, hazelnuts, Brazil nuts, almonds, walnuts and linseeds – whizz them all together in a blender and keep in an air tight jar in the fridge. Sprinkle a tablespoon daily over fruits, cereals, soups and desserts. Wholegrains contain substances called phytates, which definitely offer us protection against cancer. They are now available as an isolated substance called *Inositol Hexaphosphate* or IP6 which is extracted from brown rice. See *Useful Remedies*. If you eat bran to keep your bowels regular, avoid wheat bran which can irritate the gut and try oat or rice bran instead.

■ Minimise alcohol. Alcohol is associated with an increased risk of cancer. Red wine does however contain antioxidant nutrients called polyphenols, which are associated with a reduced risk of heart disease. One glass a day is the recommended maximum. Red grape juice contains the same antioxidants without the alcohol.

■ Know your fats and oils. Animal fats are one of the biggest contributing factors in cancers. Greatly reduce your intake of saturated fats – from meat, full-fat dairy produce, chocolates, cheeses, sausages, meat pies, cakes and so on. Avoid any foods containing hydrogenated or trans fats. Once you start reading labels you will be appalled at how much hard, saturated fat you are ingesting. Never fry with mass-produced, highly refined oils. Use only organic sunflower, sesame, walnut or olive oils for salad dressings. Eat more oily fish, which is rich in omega 3 fats (see *Fats You Need To Eat*).

■ Cut down on sugar, which greatly lowers your immune function. Reduce caffeine – try herbal teas and dandelion coffee instead.

Useful Remedies if you suffer from cancer

■ *IP6*, a substance extracted from brown rice has been shown to inhibit the growth of certain tumours. There is 20 years' medical research and trials behind *IP 6*, which have proven very exciting. Take 6 grams daily on an empty stomach, 30 minutes before food. **PW** or **NC**

■ Take vitamin C, 3 grams a day in an ascorbate form.

■ *MGN-3* is a blend of the outer shell of rice bran with extracts of shitake, kawaratake, and suehirotake mushrooms. These three mushroom extracts are the leading prescription treatments for cancer in Japan. They increase natural killer (NK) cell activity. It is the activity of NK cells that determines whether you get cancer or a virus infection, rather than their number. In studies NK activity increased by 1.3 to 1.5 times in 16 hours, by one week it increased by 8 times, and at the end of 2 months it increased by 27 times! In one study of 27 cancer patients the NK activity increased from 100% to 537%, depending upon the kind of cancer, in only two weeks. If you have cancer, take 4 capsules 3 times daily with meals for 2 weeks, then 2 capsules twice daily for maintenance. Two capsules twice daily may be taken for prevention. **NC**

■ Take selenium – 200mcg daily

■ Take a high potency food state multi-vitamin and mineral without iron – as iron has been linked to cancer cell growth.

■ Drink organic green tea – 6 cups daily.

■ Take 1200mcg of folic acid plus a B complex which helps to stabilise genes.

Useful Remedies to prevent cancer

■ Take *IP6* – 2 grams daily to be taken on an empty stomach.

■ Take 1 gram of vitamin C daily.

■ Take 200mcg selenium daily.

- Take 400iu of natural source vitamin E.

- Take a good quality multi vitamin and mineral. **NC**

- Take *Alpha Lipoic Acid* 50mg daily or 60–100mg of *Pycnogenol* (pine bark extract) or Grapeseed Extract which are all great immune boosters.

- Also see details of *MGN 3* above.

Helpful Hints

- Strict vegetarians seem to develop fewer cancers than non-vegetarians. People who live in Thailand and Japan have much lower incidence of most cancers, so adopting a Far Eastern diet may well be a good way of staying healthy.

- Drink more organic green tea.

- If you are already undergoing any type of cancer therapy, Dr Rosy Daniel (the ex Medical Director of the Bristol Cancer Help Centre) says that nutrition is vital to help bring back up the white blood cell count. She advises patients to eat plenty of organic fresh fruit and vegetables along with whole foods like brown rice and brown bread. All animal fats should be avoided. She also recommends that cancer patients take a good antioxidant formula, which contains vitamins A, C, and E plus natural beta-carotene complex, zinc and selenium. Dr Daniel stresses that fear drains energy levels and advocates any therapy that can reduce anxiety, such as spiritual healing, Reiki, relaxation exercises, visualisation, acupuncture or homeopathy.

- Flower essences especially *Rescue Remedy* are very useful

- Laugh a lot. Watch films and programmes that make you laugh; laughter boosts your immune system. Refuse to look at the downside. Stay as positive as possible – without doubt the patients with the more positive outlook tend to have a more positive outcome.

- Maitake mushrooms available in capsule form have been shown to stimulate the immune system and seem to reduce the effects of chemotherapy. **NC**

- Reduce your exposure to mobile phones and computers.

- Oxygen therapies are well worth looking into. Dr Otto Warburg won a Nobel prize for discovering that cancer cells cannot exist in a high oxygen environment. You can use an ozone cabinet or some doctors are working with hydrogen peroxide injections. Many therapists who offer these treatments have been harassed by the FDA in America and the Medicines Control Agency in the UK. I can only surmise that someone, somewhere would prefer people not to know that there is an inexpensive non-drug based treatment that really can help. In Mexico, Dr Kurt Donsbach has used intravenous hydrogen peroxide for years and claims that the majority of his patients make a full recovery. In the UK, these therapies are used by Dr Patrick Kingsley in Leicestershire, Tel: 01530 223 622; Dr Fritz Schellander in Tunbridge Wells, Tel: 01892 543 535. Mark Lester in London uses ozone therapies and a cabinet to treat patients. Tel: 020 8349 4730, or log onto: www.thefinchleyclinic.co.uk. Dr Julian Kenyon is in London on 020 7486 5588. I strongly suggest you read *Oxygen Healing Therapies* by Nathanial Altman, Healing Arts Press.

■ **The Cancer Alternative Information Bureau** (CAIB) has been founded by Tina Cooke to help people who want more help on the holistic approaches available to cancer patients: PO Box 285, 405 Kings Road, London SW10 0BB. Tel: 020 7266 1505. Website: www.caib.co.uk

■ Many associations offer help, counselling and advice including **Bristol Cancer Help Centre**, Grove House, Cornwallis Grove, Bristol, BS8 4PG. Helpline: 0117 980 9505, 9.30am–5.00pm weekdays. Website: www.bristolcancerhelp.org Email: info@bristolcancerhelp.org

■ Try reading *The Cancer Prevention Book* by Dr Rosy Daniel (Simon&Schuster, £10.99).This book is vital for anyone who wishes to help themselves and their families avoid cancer.

■ Read *Nutrition and Cancer – State of the Art* by Dr Sandra Goodman, Positive Health Publications.

■ A wonderful book *What To Do When They Say it's Cancer*, Allen and Unwin, is the story of Joel Nathan and how he survived cancer. This should be given to every cancer patient. Both these books can be ordered by calling Tel: 0117 983 8851.

Treat your body like a temple – not a rubbish bin

CANCER OF THE BREAST, PREVENTION OF

Breast cancer is the commonest cancer in Britain with around 35,000 cases a year. Around 1 in every 10 women will develop breast cancer at some point in their lives and it is the most common cause of death in women aged 35–54. It is not the death sentence that it used to be; today there is a lot we can do to help prevent and heal breast cancer.

A few women are so terrified of breast cancer, as their mother and sometimes their grandmother and other relatives died of this disease, they have their breasts removed as a precaution. My mother died from breast cancer – but I would never undergo such radical surgery unless I actually had cancer.

Our inherited genes control the structure and function of our body but if our genes stay healthy then our body stays healthy. If you live a healthy lifestyle, you can change which genes are expressed. In other words if your parents and grandparents died of heart attacks or cancers, you may well have a pre-disposition for heart problems and cancer, but if you live a different lifestyle and eat healthier foods, you can change the chemistry within the body – you don't have to suffer just because they did. Genes are repairable and alterable – they adjust to our environment and state of mind.

Meanwhile, risk factors for breast cancer are using HRT for too long, the contraceptive pill, excessive intake of saturated fats, dairy products, alcohol, pesticides, herbicides, and a low intake of fruit and vegetables.

Many young women overproduce oestrogen and this is one of the reasons they suffer with symptoms of the pre-menstrual syndrome. If you eat a healthy diet the body excretes these hormones via the liver. However, if the diet is high in saturated and

C

animal fats or alcohol, not only is it harder for the body to excrete these oestrogens, it tends to recycle them into an aggressive form, which begins attacking tissue.

Residues of pesticides and herbicides known to cause cancer are now in our food chain and drinking water and these toxins live in fatty tissue within the body – so the more you avoid contact with such substances the more you reduce your chance of contracting cancer.

Foods to Avoid

■ Reduce your intake of alcohol to no more than 1 unit a day.

■ Animal fats should be kept to a minimum; eat very lean organic meats. Dairy products especially from cows, sheep and goats should be very low-fat – fully skimmed milk or very low-fat yoghurt.

■ Pesticides and plastics act like strong oestrogens, hence why we advocate you eat organic food as much as possible. Never re-heat a pre-packaged meal in its plastic container as the chemicals can leak into the food. Transfer food to glass or stainless steel cookware before heating.

■ There has been a lot of misinformation in the media about soya, saying that it causes hormone activity, which is non-beneficial to health. This is not true. Soya acts like a weak oestrogen which blocks the stronger, negative oestrogens in our environment and within the body from binding to the breast cells, and is definitely beneficial in small amounts. Anything in excess can harm you.

Friendly Foods

■ Eat soya beans, chickpeas and soya products like tofu, soya milk and soya yoghurt. Japanese and Thai women have a much lower incidence of breast cancer and this appears to be due to their regular consumption of soya-based foods before puberty. One of the active ingredients in soya foods is genistein, an isoflavone. Genistein inhibits the growth of cancer cells.

■ Broccoli, cabbage, Brussels sprouts and alfalfa sprouts all contain chemicals which are protective against many cancers including breast cancer.

■ Raw linseeds sprinkled regularly onto meals contain a fibre called lignan, which helps to protect breast tissue.

■ My favourite way to ingest a lot of nutrients quickly is by juicing. Blend some organic raw carrots, cabbage, apple, fresh root ginger, raw beetroot, radish and celery, add to this a teaspoon of any organic greenfood supplement and some aloe vera juice and you will feel really energised. For breakfast I often mix a banana, an apple, a small box of blueberries, a tablespoon of soya lecithin granules, and some green food powder with a couple of fresh or dried figs. I throw in some sunflower seeds and linseeds and a cup of organic rice milk and whizz this for a minute – it makes the most deliciously healthy breakfast.

■ Replace full-fat margarines that contain hydrogenated or trans fats with healthier spreads such as *Biona* or *Vitaquell*.

■ Many patients with cancer have low carotene levels. Apricots, sweet potatoes, asparagus, French beans, broccoli, carrots, mustard and cress, red peppers, spinach, watercress, mangoes, parsley, tomatoes are all rich in carotenes.

Useful Remedies for prevention and healing of breast cancer.

■ *IP-6* 3–4 grams per day, available from **Twinlab**, Tel: 01159 897323 Website: www.twinlab.com

■ If you have cancer you can take up to 5–10 grams of vitamin C daily in an ascorbate form for a few weeks. In such doses you may experience loose bowels, in which case cut the dose a little. For maintenance take 1 gram daily.

■ Take a high-strength antioxidant formula that contains vitamins, A, C and E, zinc and selenium.

■ If you have cancer, take *Co-enzyme Q10* – 300mg twice a day. This important co-enzyme has been shown to inhibit cancer cell growth and protect breast tissue. To aid prevention take 100mg daily. **PN**

■ Reishi, shitake and maitake mushrooms are available either as tincture or as tablets and should be taken 3 times a day. They have been shown to have great immune enhancing properties and to inhibit cancer cell growth. **NC**

■ Take a good quality multi-vitamin and mineral. **S**

■ *Indole 3 Carbinol* (I3C) is a phytochemical supplement isolated from cruciferous vegetables (broccoli, cauliflower, Brussels sprouts, turnips, kale, green cabbage, mustard, bok choy, etc.) Among the most powerful anti-cancer substances in these vegetables is indole 3 Carbinol. (To ingest therapeutic quantities of this indole would require eating enormous amounts of raw vegetables as cooking tends to destroy these phytochemicals). Take one tablet two or three times a day. **NC**

Helpful Hints

■ Examine your breasts at least once a month. If you find even the hint of anything unusual or any type of lump, see your doctor immediately. Remember, the earlier any problems are detected the greater your chance of a complete cure.

■ Avoid wearing a bra for too much of the day. Women who wear a tight fitting bra for 14 hours or longer a day are 50% more likely to develop breast cancer. At the very least find yourself a comfortable loose fitting bra that doesn't block lymph drainage.

■ Exercise should be taken on a regular basis as this helps reduce stress and strengthens our immune system, making us less susceptible to disease.

■ Always use natural deodorants such as *Pit Rok* or a tea tree based deodorant. Remember your skin is your largest organ and chemicals in creams and deodorants are absorbed into the body.

■ Breast cancer is more common in people who are overweight and obese – control your weight. See also *Weight Problems*.

■ High stress levels are associated with breast cancer – make sure you get plenty of exercise, which reduces the tendency towards stress. Make some time for proper relaxation.

■ Read *The Breast Cancer Prevention and Recovery Diet* by Suzannah Olivier, Michael Joseph. Tel: 0117 983 8851.

■ **Bristol Cancer Help Centre**, Grove House, Cornwallis Grove, Bristol, BS8 4PG. Helpline: 0117 980 9505 or 0117 980 9000, 9.30am-5.00pm weekdays. Website: www.bristolcancerhelp.org Email: info@bristolcancerhelp.org

Learn to laugh at yourself.

CANDIDA

(see also *Allergies*)

Candida albicans is a yeast that is responsible for the condition known as thrush. Common symptoms include itching in the vaginal area, odour and discharge. Although commonly found in the vagina, candida can also occur in the throat, mouth and gut. Normally, relatively low levels of candida are present in the gut as they are balanced by large amounts of healthy bacteria which helps to keep the yeast in check. Problems arise when the yeast begins to overgrow in the gut which ultimately triggers a variety of symptoms including bloating, wind, constipation/and or diarrhoea, food cravings: especially for sugar and wheat-based foods, headaches, mental confusion, mood swings, skin rashes, persistent coughing, regular bouts of thrush, arthritis-type aching joints and chronic fatigue. Candida can irritate the gut lining which increases the risk of food sensitivities (see *Leaky Gut*).

It is crucial to kill the candida or keep it under control by using herbs, supplements and, most important, dietary changes. One of the primary triggers for candida is overuse of antibiotics, others are long-term use of the Pill, steroids, diabetes, HIV and pregnancy.

Many women believe that you cannot have candida if you don't have thrush, but the majority of women with candida do not have thrush. Men are also sufferers.

Dr Gwynne Davies, a clinical ecologist based in the UK, an expert on candida says 'Candida now affects up to 70% of the population. It can become a serious condition if left untreated and is little understood by many doctors.'

He is right. During my teens I was given dozens of antibiotics for my acne, thrush and ear infections. And every time the thrush returned, I would be given more antibiotics which in the long run made the vicious cycle worse. I strongly advise anyone tested postive for candida should consult a doctor who is also a nutritionist (See *Useful Information*).

Foods to Avoid

- Initially remove all yeast from the diet – this includes all aged or mouldy cheeses including Stilton, Brie, Camembert and so on. Avoid malt vinegar, tomato ketchup, gravy mixes (many contain brewer's yeast), soy sauce, miso, pickles, tempeh, mushrooms and alcohol – especially beer and wine.

- Avoid all white-flour products for at least one month, including crackers, pizza and pasta.

- Sugar in any form feeds the yeast – so for a month avoid sugar in any form including honey, maltose, dextrose or sucrose and really sweet fruit such as grapes, peaches, kiwi and melon. I know it will be hard as sugar is highly addictive but you also need to avoid dried fruits and canned drinks for this period as they are high in sugar.

- Avoid peanuts and peanut butter which tend to harbour moulds.

- Avoid cow's milk for one month.

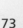

■ If you have really severe candida, for the first two weeks avoid courgettes, carrots, corn, cucumber or any of the squash family as they convert to sugars in the gut.

Friendly Foods

■ Eat fresh fish and shellfish, chicken, turkey and lean meats, eggs, tofu and pulses.

■ Include more artichokes, asparagus, aubergine, avocado, broccoli, cabbage, cauliflower, Brussels sprouts, celery, green beans, leeks, lettuce, garlic, onion, parsnips, spinach, tomatoes, and watercress. Fruits which I found OK during my detox were apples, pears, bananas, raspberries, blueberries and fresh figs.

■ Use organic rice or soya milk instead of cow's milk.

■ Live, plain unsweetened yoghurt which contains the healthy bacteria acidophilus and bifidus.

■ Try to eat more brown rice, plus lentils, corn or rice pastas, rye crisp bread, oat or rice cakes, soda bread, scones made with a little butter. As a wheat substitute, try yeast-free rye bread. It can take some getting used to but for a month it's acceptable.

■ Coriander is a great herb for helping control this infection, so use liberally in soups and stews.

Useful Remedies

■ *Vegidophilus* (healthy bacteria) will help, so begin by taking one daily and after 2 weeks increase to 2 daily for a further 6 weeks. **BC**

■ Take one yeast-free B complex. **BC**

■ Take a good multi-vitamin and mineral. **BC**

■ Take one *Candicidin* – a formula made specially to help eliminate the fungus. **BC**

■ Take *AD 206* – containing ginseng and pantothenic acid, to support adrenal function, which is often exhausted in candida patients. **BC**

■ To help cleanse the liver, take one *HEP 194* and 1 gram of vitamin C. **BC**

■ Take *Black Walnut and Calendula Tincture*, 2–4ml twice a day. **FSC**

■ Take *Kolorex* – a formula containing the powerful anti-fungal agents pseudowintera and milled aniseed, which are effective against resistant candida infection, particularly where it fails to respond to standard treatments. **NC**

■ *Arabinogalactan* (AG), is a fibre from the larch tree, and upon entering the colon, it reacts with the existing bacteria to produce short chain fatty acids (SCFAs). These are a good food source for the friendly bacteria in the gut and promote a lower pH in the colon. The beneficial bacteria crowd out the pathogenic yeast and support immune function. One capsule can be taken twice a day. **NC**

■ I realise I have suggested numerous supplements here – there is certainly no need to take them all, I am simply giving you plenty of choices!

C

Helpful Hints

■ Many women who suffer candida are very stressed and exhausted – the best thing you can do to help boost immune function is to go away for at least a week.

■ Avoid compost heaps, cut grass and staying too long in moist, humid atmospheres where moulds can thrive.

■ Women who wear nylon underwear are twice as likely to suffer with thrush as those who wear cotton underwear.

■ The *Clear from Candida* video offers a one-hour workshop lecture on what candida is and how to treat it, a one-hour cookery demonstration and a discussion on stress and the immune system, with questions from the floor. It comes with a free recipe book. To purchase contact *S.A.F.E. Ltd*, 10 Eveford by Dunbar, East Lothian, EH24 1RF, Tel: 01368 854 834. Fax: 01368 865773.

■ For further help contact the *National Candida Society*, PO Box 151, Orpington, Kent, BR5 1UJ. The helpline is open Thursday, Friday and Saturdays, Tel: 01689 813039. Website: www.candida-society.org.uk Email: info@candida-society.org.uk

■ Recent research indicates that people who have persistent and chronic candida may have intestinal parasites. Dr Hulda Clark from Canada has shown that a herbal combination containing wormwood, tincture of black walnut hull and cloves, plus the amino acids ornithine and arginine helps eliminate parasites successfully. For details of this candida cleansing formula call *G&G Food Supplies* on 01342 312811. Email: sales@gandgvitamins.com Website: www.gandgvitamins.com

CARPAL TUNNEL SYNDROME (CTS)

Carpal tunnel is caused by the compression of the median nerve that runs under tissues in the wrist. People who use keyboards and other machinery on an everyday basis are the most frequent sufferers; symptoms range from pain, numbness or tingling in the fingers. CTS is relatively common in pregnancy and more women suffer than men, it is also linked to an underactive thyroid, weight gain and arthritis. The single most successful supplement for this condition is vitamin B6.

Foods to Avoid

■ Because this problem is often associated with fluid retention, avoid adding too much sodium-based salt to food. Use a little magnesium-based sea salt for cooking.

■ Reduce your intake of salty foods, such as crisps, pre-packaged meals, pies, soy sauce etc.

■ Foods containing monosodium glutamate (MSG), often found in high amounts in Chinese takeaways and used in many Japanese restaurants, dehydrate the body. MSG depletes vitamin B6 from the body, as does the contraceptive pill.

■ In some people, foods such as oranges, tomatoes and wheat further exacerbate the problem.

Friendly Foods

- Foods rich in vitamin B6: liver, cereals, lean meat, green vegetables, nuts, fresh and dried fruits.
- Eat more brown rice, beans lentils, pulses, wholemeal pasta and breads.
- Eat oily fish such as salmon, tuna, mackerel, herrings and sardines which are rich in omega 3 fats that have anti-inflammatory properties.
- Use unrefined linseed oil, rich in omega 6 fats, with organic extra virgin olive oil for salad dressings.
- Eat pineapple before meals, which contains bromelain that helps to reduce inflammation.
- Bilberries and blueberries are rich in bio-flavonoids which have anti-inflammatory properties.
- Cook with more ginger, turmeric and cayenne.
- Drink at least 8 glasses of water a day.

Useful Remedies

- Take B6, 100mg, plus a B complex.
- Take magnesium, 200–600mg which nourishes nerve endings and relaxes muscles.
- Take a good quality multi-vitamin and mineral.
- Take 1–2 grams of *Evening Primrose Oil* or 500 mg of *Mega GLA*. **BC**
- The herbs white willow bark and *Devil's Claw* are highly anti-inflammatory.

Helpful Hints

- If you are a regular computer user, try to find an ergonomic keyboard which will be easier to use.
- If symptoms are severe, buy a wrist splint, which is available from good pharmacies.
- Sleeping heavily on your side, with your wrists under you, can also cause this. If you wake up with numb hands, immediately shake them and give them a massage to restore circulation.
- Acupuncture and daily massage with homeopathic *Rhus tox* ointment are also helpful.

If you keep looking for problems – you will surely find them.

CATARACTS

As we age the normally clear and transparent lens of the eye oxidises to become cloudy, which can severely impair vision. Many people who live in the Tropics develop cataracts and they are a major cause of blindness in developing countries. Cataracts are becoming more common in the West in those people who tend to take too much sun. A poor diet lacking in antioxidant nutrients, smoking, diabetes and overuse of steroids and other prescription drugs can all cause cataracts. As with so many other conditions, cataracts are much easier to prevent than to cure. Once you have cataracts, the normal approach is laser treatment, however, some individuals claim to have reversed their cataracts with a combination of herbs and nutrients.

Foods to Avoid

■ Smoking, fried foods and sugar speed up the oxidation process and make cataracts more likely to develop.

Friendly Foods

■ Bilberries and blueberries are very rich in bioflavonoids which help protect the eyes.

■ Leafy green vegetables, in particular spinach, contain lutein, the powerful antioxidant found in most green vegetables that has specific properties for protecting the eye.

■ Sweet potatoes have high levels of carotenes which convert to vitamin A within the body. Other good sources of carotenoids are carrots, green vegetables, tomatoes, apricots, cantaloupe melons and pumpkin.

■ Include plenty of oily fish in your diet, which is rich in vitamin A.

■ All foods high in vitamin C, E and selenium help to support the eyes. These include wheatgerm, avocado, sprouting seeds, sunflower, pumpkin and linseeds, eggs, nuts, lean meats, wholegrain cereals and fresh fruits, especially cherries and kiwi fruit and green peppers.

Useful Remedies

■ People who take vitamin C on a regular basis over a number of years are at a much lower risk of developing cataracts. Take 1 gram daily in an ascorbate form with food.

■ People with low levels of vitamin E are nearly four times more likely to form cataracts, so take 400iu of natural source vitamin E a day.

■ Take *Bilberry Eye Formula* 1–2 capsules a day. People who consume bilberry on a regular basis have a much lower risk of forming cataracts. FSC

Helpful Hints

■ Anyone concerned about developing cataracts should protect their eyes from bright sunlight with sunglasses which have been verified for UV filtering ability. If you work outside, wear a hat to protect your eyes. UV filtering contact lenses are also available, ask your optician for details.

Angry people tend to suffer more heart attacks – learn to lighten up.

CATARRH

Catarrh, or chronic congestion, can be caused by an allergic response to airborne allergens, such as the house dust mite or cat fur, but in most cases it is triggered by foods that you eat on an everyday basis, such as cow's milk, cheese or chocolate.

Many people assume that dairy products cause catarrh, but in reality this is only the case if you have an intolerance to these foods. Catarrh can just as easily be caused by wheat, eggs, citrus or any foods to which you have an intolerance.

It is important to get to the route cause of the problem, so if you are suffering with a lot of catarrh look at the foods you eat daily. Cut out one food at a time and keep a diary of the results. After a few weeks it is usually easy to find the culprit (see under *Allergies*).

Foods to Avoid

■ Avoid any foods to which you have an allergy or intolerance. Typically this might include cow's milk and produce, especially full-fat cheeses, yoghurts and chocolate plus caffeine, citrus fruits and juices, peanuts, wheat, and foods from the nightshade family that includes tomatoes, potatoes, aubergines and peppers.

■ I personally also find that goat's cheese and too much soya milk or yoghurts tend to leave me feeling very 'bunged up'. Also avoid rich, creamy sauces.

■ Avoid foods containing too much sugar which weaken the immune system making you more susceptible to food intolerances. And most foods high in sugar are high in saturated fats.

Friendly Foods

■ Garlic, ginger, horseradish, onion, cayenne pepper, pineapple and pears can help the body fight an infection if there is one and loosen up mucous so the body can expel it more easily.

■ The herbs thyme and fenugreek make great expectorants, which helps relieve congestion.

■ Keep the diet full of wholegrains, fruits, and fresh vegetables.

■ When people go on a cleansing diet, the catarrh usually disappears.

Useful Remedies

■ Take Garlic, Ginger and Horseradish Winter Formula, use 1ml of tincture 3–4 times a day. **FSC**

■ **New Era** make tissue salts specifically for catarrh.

■ Take *Muccolyte*, a complex containing bromelain, potassium plus vitamins A, C and D to help support the mucous membrane and loosening up existing mucous. **BC**

■ Take 1 gram of vitamin C with added bioflavonoids daily with meals.

Helpful Hints

■ Make a soup from 6 onions, a whole bulb of garlic, a small spoon of honey, 2.5cm of fresh root ginger and if you're brave a bit of cayenne pepper, in a vegetable or chicken stock. This will fight most infections and help clear catarrh.

■ Invest in a humidifier/air filter to help keep the air free of potential allergens.

■ Inhale a mixture of cooled boiled water, mixed with a small amount of olive oil and a pinch of salt to wash out the sinuses. I do this by simply splashing the mixture into the palm of my hand and inhaling it. Not pleasant – but very effective!

■ Many people have found that lime-flower tea is useful for reducing catarrh.

■ If your ears are blocked due to excess mucous, use warm 'hopi' ear candles, which gently remove excess wax and congestion. For details, call **Revital** Tel: 020 7976 6615 Email: enquire@revital.com Website: www.revital.com

What you find in your mind is what you put there.

Ron Rathbun.

CELLULITE

Cellulite is suffered by nearly nine times as many women as men. This is partly due to the different structure of the skin, and the fact that women have more underlying fat. Cellulite is mainly due to water retention plus an accumulation of toxins in the body, which have weakened the connective tissue just below the surface of the skin. It is much less common in female athletes who have very low body fat.

Foods to Avoid

- High-fat foods, refined carbohydrates such as mass-produced cakes and biscuits plus meat pies and pastries.
- Foods with a high salt content such as tinned foods, pre-packaged foods and takeaways, which also tend to contain a lot of saturated fats.
- Also avoid too much coffee and alcohol which place a strain on the liver which is already struggling to deal with the toxins from your diet. The more you take care of your liver, the more your skin will improve.

Friendly Foods

- Eat plenty of complex carbohydrates like beans, lentils, fruits, vegetables, and brown rice. These foods help increase the rate of metabolism, making fat deposits less likely and increase elimination of toxins from the body.
- Make sure you drink plenty of water and add organic seeds like sunflower, pumpkin and linseed to fruits salads and cereals.
- Pectin in apples helps to absorb and eliminate toxins – eat an organic apple daily.

Useful Remedies

- The herb *Gotu kola* is by far the best researched and most successful remedy for cellulite when taken orally. Try 500mg 3 times a day for 2–3 months.
- A multi-vitamin mineral daily.
- Horse chestnut cream, gel or lotion applied twice a day reduces some of the swelling and discomfort and helps to strengthen the connective tissues which tends to be damaged when you have cellulite. Available from all good health stores.

Helpful Hints

- Massage in any form is beneficial as it increases circulation and lymph drainage. If you are not able to treat yourself to a massage on a weekly basis, invest in a skin brush which increases circulation and helps eliminate toxins from the body. Skin brushes are available from all health shops and the Body Shop.

■ Begin taking more exercise to encourage circulation and elimination of toxins. Rebounding on a mini-trampoline and Yoga are great for reducing cellulite.

■ If you need to lose weight do it gradually, as losing weight too quickly can make the appearance of cellulite much worse.

■ Try the *Lashford 7-day detox* (see *Allergies*)

Drink at least 5 glasses of water daily if you want great skin.

CHILBLAINS
(see also *Circulation*)

Chilblains are caused by poor circulation and are characterised by red inflamed areas that affect the extremities. Chilblains can cause intense itching, swollen toes and sensitivity to heat and cold. Some unfortunate individuals suffer in both hands and feet. It is more common in cold weather, because the small blood vessels in the skin naturally constrict when it is cold. If you tend to suffer with chilblains every winter then you should improve your circulation. To prevent chilblains in the long term you should make sure your circulation is as efficient as possible.

Foods to Avoid

■ Anything that worsens circulation – this inevitably means foods which tend to encourage hardening of the arteries such as animal fats, full-fat dairy produce, low-fibre foods such as ice cream, jelly, fatty puddings and cakes. See diet under *Circulation*.

Friendly Foods

■ Oily fish, cayenne pepper, garlic, onion, ginger, soluble fibre like linseeds plus oat and rice bran. All of these foods can help either to improve circulation or help reduce levels of LDL (the 'bad' cholesterol) which in the long-term will help your circulation. (see *Fats You Need to Eat* and *General Health Hints*).

Useful Remedies

■ *Ginkgo biloba*, 120 mg of standardized extract twice a day or 1ml of tincture twice a day increases circulation to all extremities.

■ *Udo's Choice Oil* is a blend of omega 3 and 6 fats which help to keep one's blood healthy. Use 1 dessertspoon a day over cooked food. To find your nearest stockist, tel: 0845 0606070.

■ Vitamin E – 400iu a day helps to thin the blood naturally.

■ Take niacin (vitamin B3) 30mg–100mg daily which pumps blood into the minor capillaries. But beware if you are taking niacin for the first time, only take 30mg and slowly increase to 100mg daily. Niacin causes a flushing sensation in the skin. This is simply blood moving into the small capillaries, but it can make you look like a freshly cooked lobster for a few moments. As all the B vitamins work together, also take a B complex.

■ Include a multi-vitamin and mineral in this regimen plus 1 gram of vitamin C with bioflavonoids which helps to strengthen small capillaries. **S**

Helpful Hints

■ Smoking restricts circulation – so give it up.

■ Have a regular massage or reflexology. Essential oils such as black pepper or rosemary (do not use black pepper undiluted) can be rubbed into your feet every morning to improve circulation. Regular exercise such as walking, rebounding and skipping all increase microcirculation.

■ I used to suffer chilblains every winter, after having varicose veins removed years ago. The surgeon told me that I would still have plenty of veins left, but the legacy has been poor circulation. Obviously the key would have been for me to have avoided varicose veins in my youth! Keep this in mind and wear bed socks during winter months. Never wear tight-fitting shoes as this really aggravates chilblains by restricting circulation to the toes. Invest in fur-lined boots during cold weather.

■ Try massaging homeopathic *Tamus* cream into the chilblains. This cream is made from wild black bryony root, and has helped many people.

■ Homeopathic *Agaracus 3x* or *6x* can be taken 2 or 3 times daily. This is a classic homeopathic remedy for chilblains.

■ *Sixtus Anti Cold Foot Balm* is based on alpine herbs and herbal extracts to increase circulation. Available by mail order from JICA Beauty Products Ltd, 20 Island Farm Avenue, Molesey Trading Estate, West Molesey, Surrey, KT8 2UZ. Tel: 020 8979 7261 Email: beauty@jica.com

■ Magnets Increase circulation, which brings more oxygen to the affected areas. If like me you suffer cold feet, wear magnet insoles in your shoes and in the depths of winter wear bed socks with the inserts inside them. Call **Homedics**. Tel: 0161 798 5876, Helpline 0161 798 5885. Website: www.homedicsuk.com

Keep coffee to a minimum – more than 3 cups a day increases your chances of developing osteoporosis by as much as 82%

CHOLESTEROL, HIGH and LOW

Every year in Britain alone, more than 200,000 people die from a heart attack or stroke, and a high cholesterol count increases your chances of becoming one of these statistics by more than 60%. Cholesterol is a fatty substance manufactured by the liver and is a vital component of every cell. We don't need cholesterol from foods as the body makes all it needs, so generally a high count means you are ingesting too much saturated fat from your diet.

There are two types of cholesterol HDL (high density lipoproteins) and LDL (low density lipoproteins). The HDL are good for us – the easy way to remember this is H is for healthy. The LDL are generally bad for us – L stands for lethal.

A high LDL cholesterol level is one of the major risk factors for developing heart disease and stroke – whilst low cholesterol is associated with depression.

Ideally, 20%–40% of your total cholesterol should be HDL. There is also a type of cholesterol, VLDL (very low density lipoprotein) which is extremely bad for you. Ideally, your cholesterol reading should be between 3.0mmol/l and 5 mmol/l. As soon as your cholesterol reading goes above 5.2 you are at a higher risk of contracting heart disease. If, on the other hand, your cholesterol reading is below 3.0, it tends to indicate that your liver is not functioning properly and there may be an underlying problem such as undiagnosed food intolerances. When cholesterol is high your liver is not breaking down the LDL cholesterol properly, so it is important to keep your liver as healthy as possible. Low cholesterol can also denote an imbalance in the liver.

Some families seem genetically predisposed to manufacture more cholesterol, which means that they need dietary cholesterol even less. Then there are people who seem to live on fatty foods and still maintain a normal cholesterol level. There are always exceptions. From a dietary point of view it is very important to reduce saturated fats and increase soluble fibres. The former tend to increase the levels of LDL cholesterol and the latter reduce them. If you do have a high cholesterol level, the two of the most important supplements you can take are vitamin E, which helps to prevent the cholesterol oxidising, and B group vitamins including B12, B6, B3 and folic acid, all of which prevent the elevation of homocysteine levels (a toxic by product of protein metabolism) which again tends to oxidise cholesterol and leads to plaque formation in the arteries. Thanks to eating too much animal fat many children in the West now have raised cholesterol and arterial plaque by the age of 10.

If you have a persistently raised cholesterol level but eat a healthy diet, you may have an underactive thyroid.

Foods to Avoid

■ Reduce all foods containing saturated fats including pork, beef, sausages, meat pies, cheese, butter, chicken skin, ice cream and all dairy products except fully skimmed milk and products.

■ Eggs are a rich source of choline which is great for memory and in recent years eggs have been much maligned – but many scientists now believe that it's the frying that damages the cholesterol which triggers many health problems, not the cholesterol itself. Boiling an egg therefore does not damage cholesterol, the lesson being not to eat fried eggs.

■ Sugar, if not used up during exercise, turns to a hard fat within the body, therefore all foods and drinks containing high levels of sugar should be kept to a minimum.

■ Coffee, particularly percolated coffee or microwaved coffee, can increase cholesterol levels.

Friendly Foods

■ Most important are the foods high in soluble fibres like oat bran, psyllium husks, linseeds, hemp seeds and fruits with pectin such as apples. One study found that consuming two raw carrots a day was sufficient to lower cholesterol.

- Fish eaten on a regular basis helps elevate HDL cholesterol and when combined with garlic in a meal it is very effective at lowering LDL cholesterol. Oily fish contain essential fats that help to protect the heart.

- Vegans have the lowest cholesterol levels and people who switch from a normal meat based diet to either a vegetarian or vegan diet with the occasional fish meal have been able to reverse their cholesterol problems.

- Add more beans, especially red kidney beans plus lentils to your diet as they are good sources of soluble fibre and help to replace the protein you may be missing if you suddenly cut meat out of the diet.

- Boiled eggs are fine – use a little *Solo Salt* which is magnesium and potassium based. The kind of fat you find in an egg depends on what the chickens have been fed on. Some free range eggs such as *Columbus* are high in healthy omega 3 fats as the chickens have been fed seeds which are rich in essential fats.

- Try rice milk instead of full-fat cow's milk.

- Include low-fat, live yoghurt in the diet – these contain healthy bacteria that bind fat and cholesterol in the intestines, and remove them from the body.

- Replace spreads containing hydrogenated or trans fats with healthier versions such as *Biona* and *Vitaquell*.

- If you enjoy soya-based foods like tofu, tempeh, miso, soya yoghurt and milk there is plenty of evidence that soya can help lower LDL cholesterol. If you find soya-based foods unpalatable then try a GM-free soya protein powder and use about 30 grams a day, or add this dose to fruit juice and have it as a breakfast shake.

- Use extra virgin olive oil at every opportunity, whilst avoiding refined, mass-produced vegetable oils. Olive oil helps to lower the bad cholesterol.

- Many people on a cholesterol lowering diet drastically reduce their fat intake which can trigger depression, hormonal problems and the skin, hair and nails suffer (see *Fats You Need To Eat*).

- Healthy fats are found in oily fish, avocados, sunflower, pumpkin, linseeds and sesame seeds and their unrefined cold oils.

- Very low-fat diets can lower HDL, the healthy cholesterol, but this doesn't happen if you use olive oil. If you still insist on eating high-cholesterol foods then include plenty of garlic in your diet.

- Include almonds, walnuts, pistachios and macadamia nuts in your diet as they are a rich source of minerals, fibre and vitamin E and they help lower LDL cholesterol levels.

- Two minerals in particular, magnesium and potassium, are very protective of the heart. Green vegetables, cereals, honey, kelp, sunflower seeds, fresh and dried fruits are rich in these minerals.

- Artichokes and fenugreek eaten regularly can help keep cholesterol under control.

Useful Remedies
- Try taking vitamin B3 (**non-flush** niacin) supplied by **Country Life**, Tel: 0800 146215. Website: www.country-life.com. 1 gram daily until cholesterol goes down.

- Take *Inositol Hexaniacinate*, 500mg 3 times a day. This form of niacin has been shown to lower cholesterol without causing any toxicity. As the B group vitamins work together within the body, also take a B complex which also helps to lower homocysteine levels.

- Take 400iu of natural source vitamin E which protects the cholesterol from oxidising.

- Take 1 gram of vitamin C daily.

- The mineral chromium, taken 200mcg a day, helps elevate HDL levels whilst reducing cravings for high-sugar foods.

- Take 1000mg calcium and 500mg magnesium which may help to lower cholesterol.

- Lecithin granules derived from soya are a great way to lower LDL, and help control the growth of kidney and gall stones – I sprinkle a dessertspoon daily over my breakfast cereal or into fruit whips and yoghurts.

- If you don't like eating garlic, then take a garlic oil capsule daily which over several months will lower LDL. 900 mg a day provides 5000–6000mcg of allicin. If you are taking prescription blood-thinning drugs as well, these supplements add to the effect and you would need regular check-ups.

- One of the best ways I have found to lower cholesterol is taking grapefruit pectin fibre every day. This has been well-researched and shown to lower cholesterol even in people who refuse to change their high-fat diet. Known as *Profibe* this powdered fibre is available from all good health stores. **NC**

- A newly discovered extract of rice bran, called P25 has been shown to be 40 times more effective than vitamin E in this condition. **NC**

- Dandelion and milk thistle tincture, taken as 20 drops 3 times daily will help support the liver. **FSC**

Helpful Hints

- People who eat smaller meals regularly find it is easier to lower their cholesterol than people who eat three large meals.

- Try to find some way of relaxing. Type A individuals are those very stressed individuals who have to get everywhere in the next 5 minutes, want everything done yesterday, tend to feel aggressive and explode regularly, as well as those who are boiling on the inside and would like to explode but find it hard to say what they really mean! Stress thickens the blood.

- Regular exercise is absolutely vital for lowering cholesterol and keeping the heart healthy. If you do nothing else, begin walking for 30 minutes every day, increasing to one hour or more. Swimming, yoga and skipping are all excellent ways to stay fit.

CHRONIC FATIGUE

(see *Exhaustion* and *ME*)

Remember stress thickens your blood – learn to feel calm

CIRCULATION

(see also *Chilblains, Cholesterol* and *Raynaud's Disease*)

It is amazing how many conditions are linked to poor circulation. Common symptoms range from cold hands and feet to leg ulcers and varicose veins. Hair loss can be triggered by poor circulation to the head – hence why Uri Geller practises a yoga head stand daily to keep his thick hair in tip-top condition.

Poor circulation to the brain can lead to memory loss and eventually dementia. Poor circulation is generally due to constricted arteries which can become blocked with a sticky plaque-like substance. Conditions such as chilblains and Raynaud's are due to arterial constriction, while conditions like angina and dementia are usually due to a hardening of the arteries. Out of the 60,000 letters I have answered on health issues, a good 25% are related to poor circulation. We definitely need to get off our backsides more if and when we can.

Foods to Avoid
- I'm afraid this becomes like a long-playing record – but reduce all animal fats and full-fats milks, cheeses and chocolates.
- See *General Health Hints*.

Friendly Foods
- Essential fats are vital for healthy blood, so eat more oily fish, nuts and seeds. Avocados are a rich source of mono-unsaturated fats – eat one every week. Choose low-fat or cottage cheeses and use rice or oat milks that are lower in unhealthy fats than dairy milks.
- Make an effort to eat more crisp, lightly cooked vegetables and include at least four pieces of whole fresh fruit in your every day regimen.

Useful Remedies
- Vitamin E helps to reduce stickiness in the blood – take 200iu daily.
- Vitamin C with bioflavonoids helps to strengthen capillaries – take 1 gram daily.
- *Ginkgo biloba* is a great herb for increasing circulation. In one in a million people this herb can cause a rash – I am one such person. It won't harm you but as the rash is unsightly you should obviously stop taking it.
- Niacin (vitamin B3). It causes a reddening of the skin and increases circulation – begin at 30mg and work up to 100mg daily.
- A vitamin B complex will help.
- The herbs *butchers broom* and *gota kola* help to increase circulation in the lower limbs. Take 500mg of each twice a day.

Helpful Hints

■ Exercise is great for stimulating the circulation. Take a brisk walk every day for at least 30 minutes. Any exercise that gently pounds the feet will help improve circulation; like dancing, skipping and rebounding.

■ Add half a teaspoon of powdered mustard to a bowl of warm water and soak your feet to stimulate circulation. Essential oil of black pepper can also be used.

■ Reflexology and massage are excellent for people who, for health reasons, cannot manage much exercise (see *Useful Information*).

■ Alternatively, you could try an energy roller which works on the same principle as reflexology – roll bare feet for two minutes daily on the roller; it hurts initially but it gets easier! Send a SAE to **Shakti Chakra Ltd**. 106, West Street, Erith, Kent, DA8 1AQ. Tel: 01322 447610. Fax: 01322 405994.

■ Magnets increase circulation which will bring more oxygen to the affected areas. If like me you suffer cold feet, wear magnet insoles in your shoes and in the depth of winter wear bed socks with the inserts inside them. Contact **Homedics**, Tel: 0161 798 5876, Helpline 0161 798 5885. Website: www.homedicsuk.com

When you lose at something – don't lose the lesson.

The Dalai Lama

COELIAC DISEASE

Coeliac sufferers cannot break down a protein called gluten which is present in wheat, rye, barley and oats. However, most coeliacs appear to be able to tolerate a small amount of oats. This condition often goes undiagnosed for several years. Symptoms include frequent indigestion, abdominal pain, loss of weight and depression. Because fat is poorly absorbed, the stools can be pale, frothy and foul smelling. It is very important that if you suffer with any or some of these symptoms over a period of several months that you see a doctor. The longer you suffer with coeliac disease, particularly if it goes undiagnosed, the more likely you are to do more damage to the gut lining. This greatly reduces the body's ability to absorb adequate levels of nutrients which can even lead to malnutrition (see also *Leaky Gut*).

Foods to Avoid

■ Any foods containing wheat, rye and barley are absolutely crucial to avoid. Quite a few people with coeliac disease also have a problem with cow's milk and dairy products or soya foods.

■ You will also need to avoid mass-produced cakes and desserts.

■ Until the condition is under control also avoid fatty meats, sausages, pies and processed meat products.

Friendly Foods

- Fortunately, these days, there are plenty of gluten-free foods available, most of them fairly palatable. Some will be high in sugar so be sure to read labels carefully – sugar turns to a hard fat in the body if not burned up during exercise and in coeliac sufferers, fat is poorly absorbed. Look out for the *Trufree* range of products, as they are all free from the common allergens of wheat, dairy, soya and egg.

- Look for breads, instant foods and flours made from grain alternatives like quinoa, amaranth, millet, corn, rice, buckwheat and lentils.

- Dairy alternatives to cow's milk include rice, oat, pea and even almond and hazelnut milk.

- Eat plenty of leafy greens, which are rich sources of magnesium and calcium. Cabbage is rich in the amino acid L-glutamine which helps to heal the gut – try making fresh vegetable juices that include raw cabbage, a little root ginger which is very soothing plus any vegetables you have to hand. If you cook cabbage in water, save the water and make gravy with it. Or add cabbage to stews and soups.

- Try to eat more fish to provide vitamin D, which is often deficient in coeliac sufferers.

- Eat plenty of nuts, seeds, fish, free-range low-fat meats such as venison and turkey to keep up zinc intake often deficient in coeliacs.

- Essential fats are needed to heal the gut, so use a little organic sunflower, sesame, olive or walnut oil for salad dressings.

- Eat an avocado once a week as they are rich in vitamin E.

Useful Remedies

- All of the supplements suggested will not cure coeliac disease, it's just that the vast majority of nutrients are often deficient in coeliac sufferers. It is very important to increase your intake of these nutrients to prevent deficiency.

- Calcium 500mg and magnesium 250mg are vital minerals, as many coeliac sufferers have a low bone density.

- Folic acid, 400–800mcg and vitamin B6, 50–100mg.

- Vitamin A 20,000–30,000iu, (if you are pregnant no more than 5000iu) vitamin D 400–1200iu.

- A high-strength multi-vitamin and mineral to make up for any other nutritional deficiencies.

- Essential fatty acids, 1–3 grams a day of *Efalex* or 10–20mls of *Udo's Choice Oil* (before taking any fats and oils see *Fats You Need To Eat*).

Helpful Hints

- Breast-fed children are much less likely to develop coeliac disease than those fed on cow's or soya milk formulas. Formula milks are harder to digest and potentially can cause health problems later on.

- **The Village Bakery** in Cumbria make great wheat-, rye- and barley-free breads and cakes. Sold at most health stores. Tel: 01768 881515. Fax: 01768 881848.

■ Research from Finland shows that small amounts (50–70 grams) of oat-based products can be tolerated by coeliacs without damaging intestinal absorption.

■ *Slippery Elm* tablets help to reduce the irritation. Take one tablet with each meal.

*It's often the foods you crave and eat the most that are
doing the greatest harm.*

COLDS and FLU

Colds and flu are caused by viruses and the secret to avoiding them is to keep your immune system in great shape. See also *Immune Function*.

Flu symptoms are usually far more severe and symptoms include a fever, aching joints and dreadful headaches. With colds there is plenty of congestion, often accompanied by a headache. With heavier bouts of flu your joints ache, and all you want is bed rest, which is one of the fastest routes to recovery. If you have a temperature, take paracetamol every four to six hours to help bring it down. Only if you contract a secondary bacterial infection – meaning if it hurts to breathe and you are wheezing – then antibiotics may be warranted.

We become more susceptible to colds and flu if we overwork, over-train or consistently eat a poor diet high in saturated fats and sugars. For instance, if you eat a sugar rich pudding and a bar of chocolate, and are then immediately in contact with someone suffering with a cold or flu – you have doubled your chances of picking it up.

Foods to Avoid

■ All sugars plus refined carbohydrates such as white bread, cakes pies and biscuits plus high fat foods, alcohol and caffeine. All of these can weaken the immune system and make us more susceptible to infection.

■ Generally while you have a cold reduce your intake of mucous-forming foods such as cheese, chocolate and full-fat dairy produce.

Friendly Foods

■ Garlic and onions are great foods as they are anti-bacterial and have antiseptic properties. A traditional remedy for colds and flu is a soup made with 6 onions, a whole garlic, 2.5cm of grated fresh ginger, and some cayenne pepper mixed in a vegetable or chicken stock. You could also add lemongrass. For children it is probably preferable to leave out the cayenne pepper – although it does make the other herbs more effective, it is often too hot.

■ Liquorice is a pleasant tasting food which you can make into tea and eat as confectionery if it is sugar free. It has both anti-viral and anti-bacterial properties and will soothe the throat when it's inflamed.

■ Whilst you have a cold or flu try to base your diet on fruits, vegetables and brown rice with a little fish, chicken or pulses. Keep your diet clean. See *General Health Hints*.

- Drink plenty of lemon and ginger herbal tea or make your own by finely chopping a 2.5cm piece of fresh ginger, stand it in boiling water for 15 minutes with a squeeze of lemon juice and freshly chopped spring onions; strain and sip.

- Keep up your fluid intake – tea and coffee dehydrate the body, so drink plenty of water and herbal teas.

Useful Remedies

- *Echinacea*, taken either as tincture or tablets every couple of hours, fights a cold or flu. Echinacea has been shown in a number of studies to shorten the length of a cold from 7 days down to 3–4 if taken regularly, generally 1–2mls every 2–3 hours. **FSC**

- I tend to take herbs like *Echinacea* in the winter when we are more susceptible to colds. It is more effective when taken cyclically. Take for a month, then stop taking for a week. Continue throughout the winter.

- Vitamin C is strongly anti-viral and research has shown that it can shorten the severity and duration of most colds and flu if taken in sufficient amounts. During the winter, take 1 gram daily, but if you feel a cold coming on, increase your intake to 1gram – 3 times daily with meals in an ascorbate form until the cold has gone.

- Take a multi-vitamin and mineral that contains at least 30–60mg of zinc to boost the immune system while fighting an infection. **BC**

- If you are suffering from a sore throat try zinc gluconate lozenges that contain 15–25mg of zinc. Take 1 every 3–4 hours. The zinc lozenges help to kill bacteria in the throat.

- *Olive Leaf Extract* acts like nature's antibiotic. I take 2 daily to help keep my immune system in shape when I am feeling run down. **NC**

- *Sambucol* is an extract of the European black elderberry plant which has potent anti-viral properties. If taken at the onset of a cold or flu it can help reduce the severity and length of the illness. Available from all health stores or call 01782 794300 for your nearest stockist.

Helpful Hints

- Homeopathic *Aconite 30c* can be taken two or three times daily at the onset of a cold to help stop the cold from developing.

- **Ainsworth's** famous *Anti Cold and Flu* remedy is a homeopathic preventative for colds and flu symptoms, which is tailored to the current strains each year. They also supply a remedy called *Anas Barb Co*, which is for use at the onset of a cold or flu to prevent symptoms from developing further. Contact **Ainsworth Homeopathic Pharmacy** at 36 New Cavendish Street, London, W1M 7LH. Tel: 020 7935 5330. Website: www.ainsworths.com Email: ainshom@msn.com

- Keep warm and avoid changes in the temperature of your surroundings for at least 48 hours until symptoms subside. Rest is essential if you have a temperature.

- Do not struggle into work if you have a really bad cold – all you do is make it last longer and you pass it on to your colleagues.

■ Wash your hands regularly if you are in contact with people who have a cold as viruses can easily permeate the soft skin on the palms of the hands. Viruses are airborne and spread quickly at large gatherings. Avoid being in stuffy, smoky rooms for too long. Get plenty of exercise and fresh air.

An organic alfalfa salad sandwich provides more nutrients that a cheap multi-vitamin pill.

COLD SORES

(see also *Herpes*)

Cold sores are caused by the herpes simplex virus. Once contracted the virus lies dormant in the body and tends to re-activate if you become run down, stressed or after sudden exposure to very hot or cold weather. Some women suffer an attack during menstruation. Others find that if they eat large amounts of nuts or chocolate that contain the amino acid arginine on which the virus thrives, this can also trigger an attack. There have been a number of studies showing that you can reduce the frequency of attacks by taking vitamin C and the amino acid Lysine on a regular basis.

Foods to Avoid

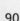

■ Foods which are very rich in arginine, an amino acid found commonly in chocolate, lentils, beans and nuts.

■ Avoid sugar, refined foods made with white flour and high saturated-fat foods which again have a negative effect on the immune system.

■ Certain people notice when they eat too much dairy produce from cows they suffer an attack.

Friendly Foods

■ Eat good quality protein such as lean meats including turkey, duck, lean pork plus fish, corn and soya, all of which are rich in Lysine, an amino acid that has been shown to interfere with replication of the virus.

■ See *General Health Hints*.

Useful Remedies

■ At the onset of symptoms begin taking 500–1000mg of lysine daily.

■ If you already have an attack take up to 4 grams daily.

■ To help prevent attacks take 1 gram of vitamin C daily and up to 3 grams daily when cold sores are acute. Take with food and if you are taking higher doses take in an ascorbate formula.

■ Also apply pure vitamin C cream topically as soon as the sores begin to form – but not if the skin is broken. **BC**

■ Natural source vitamin E applied topically helps reduce the pain and irritation. Pierce a 400iu capsule and apply directly to the sores. Leave it on for about 15 minutes and generally within 8 hours the pain disappears.

■ Lemon balm as a tincture or as a cream applied directly to the cold sores helps kill the virus.

■ Liquorice as a tincture or cream applied to the cold sore again helps to fight the virus and often makes it a lot more comfortable.

■ Zinc cream applied regularly can help fight the virus. Also take 30mg daily internally.

■ If you find you or your children regularly suffer cold sores you definitely need to include a good quality multi-vitamin and mineral in your regimen. There are now plenty of sugar- and additive-free chewable vitamins for children or add liquid vitamins and minerals to their food. **NC**

■ A new extract of the larrea bush has had a 97% success rate in treating all types of herpes. It is available in capsules or a lotion. Take one capsule up to 3 times daily and apply the lotion topically. Sold as *Larreastat*. **NC**

Helpful Hints

■ Make sure you change your toothbrush and face towels regularly as these can harbour the virus.

■ Calendula tincture can be dabbed directly on to the sores.

■ Homeopathic *Rhus Tox 30c* helps to eliminate the eruptions. Take as soon as the tingling starts. Take twice daily for three days.

■ Several people have told me that when they take *Bach Rescue Remedy* internally and dab it externally onto the cold sores it prevents the cold sore from developing. As *Rescue Remedy* is also available in a cream this is certainly worth a try.

Men who eat organic foods have a higher sperm count.

CONJUNCTIVITIS

Conjunctivitis is an inflammation of the outer surface membrane which lines the eye. This can be triggered by an external allergen such as perfume or insect sprays in which case the eyes are usually very red, itchy and irritated. When caused by a bacteria or a virus this can be accompanied by a yellow or white mucous-type discharge and it should be treated by a doctor. People who suffer chronic conjunctivitis are often deficient in vitamin A.

Foods to Avoid

■ All foods and drinks containing sugar which reduces the body's ability to fight an infection.

■ Reduce your intake of animal fats, white-flour-based cakes, breads and biscuits, all of which weaken the immune system.

■ See *General Health Hints*.

Friendly Foods

■ Bilberries, blueberries, blackberries and all blue and purple coloured fruits are rich in antioxidant nutrients that nourish the eyes.

■ Foods rich in vitamin A such as leafy green vegetables, calf or lamb's liver, cod liver oil, carrots and fish help encourage healthy eyes.

■ Natural carotenes found in tomatoes, sweet potatoes, dried apricots, mangos and raw parsley are all great foods for the eyes.

■ Eat more pineapple – rich in the enzyme bromelain which has anti-inflammatory properties.

Useful Remedies

■ *Echinacea, Eyebright and Bilberry* tincture, 1–4ml a day.

■ Bromelain, 1,000–3,000mcu a day. **FSC**

■ When the infection is acute take 20,000iu of vitamin A daily for 14–21 days as some people with conjunctivitis are deficient in vitamin A. If you are pregnant take no more than 5000iu of vitamin A per day.

Helpful Hints

■ Try using a few drops of liquid *Colloidal Silver* solution directly into the eyes to help kill any bacteria or viruses. **HN**

■ Conjunctivitis is highly contagious when caused by a viral infection. Be really careful not to use the same handkerchief or tissue to wipe both eyes. Be scrupulous with hygiene and make sure no one else uses your towels or make up.

■ Eyebright tincture plus goldenseal tincture, take 2 drops of each and add to an eye bath full of purified or boiled water and use when cool. Use twice daily.

■ Dilute homeopathic *Euphrasia* mother tincture in an egg cup full of cooled boiled water and use as an eye bath.

Gentlemen – to help avoid heart attacks and strokes –
avoid a waist measurement of more than 39 inches. For ladies it's 35 and a half inches.

Colin Sutherland Ph.D

CONSTIPATION and BLOATING

(see also *Flatulence*)

In Britain we spend more money on laxatives than any other country in Europe and still manage to suffer chronic constipation. Infrequent bowel movements can have a number of causes. The vast majority of people who complain of constipation could find relief if they were to take more exercise and change their diet. Regular stomach exercises are very useful as they encourage waste matter to move through the bowel more quickly. In the West we tend to eat far too many foods based on flour. If you mix any flour and water together you get a thick glue like paste which tends to block the bowel rather like a cork in a wine bottle. Melted cheese has a similar affect. Lack of water is a major cause of constipation. Far too many people drink caffeinated beverages, alcoholic drinks and fizzy canned drinks which all dehydrate the bowel – you need more water.

It is crucial not to become dependent on laxatives as they have a tendency to make the bowel lazy in the long term and deplete the body of vital nutrients.

Constipation can also denote irritable bowel syndrome especially if it alternates with diarrhoea, gas, bloating and general discomfort. Foods like meat tend to progress more slowly through the bowel so it is important when you do eat meat that you accompany it with plenty of vegetables or brown rice, which are rich in fibre. Also when food is inadequately digested, it often stays in the bowel too long. If you then eat a large portion of fruit after a heavy meal this can trigger fermentation which further aggravates the situation. Candida and food sensitivities can also cause constipation – see also *Candida*. Antibiotics and pain killers can add to the problem.

Foods to Avoid

■ Low-fibre foods such as jelly, ice cream and soft desserts, all white flour products and refined breakfast cereals which contain virtually no fibre.

■ Reduce your intake of meat, coffee, tea, alcohol and fizzy drinks.

■ Also avoid foods to which you have an intolerance, for instance cow's milk has been found to be responsible for a lot of infant constipation.

■ Cut down on full-fat cheeses and don't eat melted cheese over food – it sets like plastic in the bowel.

Friendly Foods

■ Bran as it is an insoluble fibre derived from rice, soya or oats. The insoluble fibre is needed to stimulate the bowel to work properly. Wheat bran is fine so long as you don't have an intolerance to wheat, otherwise this can actually aggravate the problem.

■ Try eating more brown rice and beans like black-eyed beans, kidney, haricot, butter and cannellini beans.

■ Linseeds are a blend of insoluble and soluble fibres which bulk the stool, encouraging it to move gently through the bowel.

■ Whole wheat rye bread, *Ryvita*-type crispbreads or amaranth crackers can be eaten as an alternative to wheat bread.

■ Other high fibre foods are fresh and dried figs, blackcurrants, ready to eat dried apricots and prunes, almonds, hazelnuts, fresh coconut and all mixed nuts.

■ All lightly cooked or raw vegetables and salads will add more fibre to your diet.

■ Eat more, live, low-fat yoghurts which contain healthy bacteria – a lack of which can exacerbate constipation.

■ Drink at least 8 glasses of water daily.

Useful Remedies

- Dr Gillian McKeith's *Living Food Energy*, 1–2 teaspoons a day. This blend of fibres and nutrients helps improve bowel function and digestion. Available from all health shops.

- Acidophilus and bifidus are healthy bacteria which can be taken after a meal particularly if constipation has started after antibiotics.

- Add a heaped dessertspoon of linseeds to any breakfast cereal, yoghurt or over salads to ensure a good supply of both insoluble and soluble fibres.

- Vitamin C powder with added calcium and magnesium, 1 level teaspoon 2–3 times a day for a few days, can help soften the stool and increase the frequency of bowel movement. Magnesium helps to tone the bowel muscles.

- One of the best ways I have found to eliminate constipation is to replace one meal a day with a fruit and vegetable blend whilst eliminating all flour from any source for at least 2 days. I put half a cup of aloe vera juice, a banana, an apple, blueberries and any fruit I have to hand, plus a teaspoon of any good green food mix, a teaspoon of sunflower seeds, a dessertspoon of linseeds and a teaspoon of olive oil into my blender. To this I add half a cup of organic rice milk and blend. It's delicious and packed with fibre. On alternate days I make a vegetable juice to which I still add the aloe vera juice but not the rice milk.

- Arabinogalactan (AG), a fibre from the larch tree, is very useful in the treatment of constipation. It acts as a stool softener which helps to normalise bowel movements. Also when AG enters the colon, it reacts with existing bacteria to produce short chain fatty acids (SCFAs). These are a good food source of friendly bacteria in the gut and promote a lower pH in the colon, which in turn promotes peristaltic movement. Try one capsule twice daily. **NC**

- Add 2 teaspoons of psyllium husks to cereal and drink two glasses of water immediately.

Helpful Hints

- It is very important that you eliminate any underlying causes for your constipation. Visit your GP and make sure there is nothing more serious going on.

- Do not strain when you have a bowel movement as this places a strain on the vascular system and can, over time, lead to varicose veins or piles. Remember rather than fall asleep after every meal, go for a leisurely walk. This will make you feel better, aid digestion and encourage healthier bowels.

- When you feel the need to pass a motion, be sure not to ignore the signal; take the time to read a magazine on the loo!

- For healthy bowel movements you need about a pint of fluid in between each meal to get waste moving through successfully.

- See also *Allergies* for *The Lashford technique* which helps eliminate constipation.

- Stress is a major factor.

- When you add more fibre to your diet and you're not used to it, it is essential that you drink more water. Adding fibre without more fluid can actually aggravate the problem.

- In the elderly, a lack of folic acid has sometimes been found to be the cause of constipation, therefore, supplementing with folic acid in the form of a good quality multi-vitamin and mineral should help.

- In infants, there is a common link with cow's milk and constipation. Infants on formula rather than breast milk will benefit from a children's acidophilus powder. In adults it isn't just milk, but a number of foods that can cause constipation if you are intolerant to them. Identifying them is a very worthwhile exercise. **BC**

- For severe constipation especially after surgery – and with your doctor's permission – try colonic irrigation. I have a colonic two or three times a year as a thorough cleanse especially if I am forced to take antibiotics which cause me real problems! (see *Useful Information*). You can also give yourself a home colonic. It helps to re-educate the peristaltic movements and is called the *Clysmatic*, which is easy to use. Call Penny Davenport on 01424 774103.

CONTRACEPTIVE PILL

(see *Pill*)

If you are juicing fresh apples remove the pips as they contain cyanide.

COUGHS

Coughs are often due to an infection such as a cold or flu and sometimes asthma. Many people who smoke develop a persistent cough. Sometimes the cough can lead to production of phlegm. If this is yellow or green in colour it is indicates a bacterial infection, in which case you would need to see a doctor. If you have a cough that lasts longer than two weeks or produces blood at any stage, it is very important to seek medical attention. Coughs which produce a lot of catarrh are often helped by mullein and other expectorant herbs. If the cough is dry and tickly, cherry bark is more useful. A persistent cough, especially after eating foods containing wheat or sugar could be linked to candida (see *Candida*).

Foods to Avoid

- For a few days, eliminate all cow's dairy products – even skimmed milk. I also find that if I have a cold I also need to avoid soya milk which can increase mucous production.

- Cakes, biscuits, sausage rolls, meat pies, burgers etc. should all be avoided for at least 14 days to give your sinuses and throat time to clear all mucous. Also avoid white bread and pasta.

- Most foods containing sugar tend to be high in fat and sugar lowers immune functioning.

Friendly Foods

- Drink plenty of water to keep the throat well lubricated.

- Pineapples help loosen up mucous and make breathing easier. Fresh pear juice is good for easing coughs.

- If the cough is making you feel tight chested and congested try adding horseradish, cayenne or ginger to meals.
- Liquorice either as a tea or sucked as a pure liquorice juice stick can be very soothing.
- Tea made from fresh thyme can ease the cough and has historically been used for whooping cough.
- Eat plenty of fresh vegetables, chicken, fish, pulses, grains and fresh fruit.
- Drink herbal teas such as lemon and ginger and try organic rice milk as a dairy substitute.
- Live, low-fat plain yoghurts are usually well tolerated and they help to boost friendly bacteria in the gut.

Useful Remedies

- *Mullein Formula* 1–3ml a day. Expectorant and antiviral herbs combine to make a wonderful cough mixture. **FSC**
- *Bioforce Thyme* tincture taken as directed.
- Zinc lozenges. Suck one every 3–4 hours to ease discomfort of sore throats and reduce the tickling of the cough. **FSC**
- *Olive Leaf Extract* acts like a natural antibiotic and has been found especially useful for respiratory problems. Take 3 capsules daily while symptoms last.
- Include a multi-vitamin and mineral in your regimen.

Helpful Hints

- If you begin wheezing after food or when stressed, you may have developed a touch of asthma – see under *Asthma* and see a doctor.
- If you find you get tight chested after exercise, 2 grams of vitamin C can often be very helpful.
- Taken at the first sign of a cough, homeopathic *Aconite 6c* can help prevent the cough developing.
- Keep a food diary and note when symptoms are worse. For instance if your nose runs within a few minutes of eating certain foods, especially cow's milk, wheat- and sugar-based foods, then you may be sensitive to those foods. High-sugar fruits such as grapes can even be a problem for some people.
- Dilute a few drops of essential oil of sweet majoram and frankincense in a grapeseed oil base and massage into your chest and back to encourage deeper breathing.
- *Culpeper's Herbal Cough Mixture* has given relief to many readers with chronic coughs. For further information or to find your nearest stockist call **Culpeper Ltd** on 01223 894054. Website: www.culpeper.co.uk Email: info@culpeper.co.uk
- Take two tablespoons of aloe vera juice every day to soothe your throat and boost your immune system.
- Stop smoking.

40,000 people die annually in Britain from orthodox medical errors.

CRAMPS

Most people will experience cramp at some time or other and it's a painful muscular spasm or contraction, often caused by a poor blood supply to the muscles (see also *Circulation*). It can also be triggered by extreme exercise. Unless you live in a very hot country where you are sweating profusely, it is unlikely to be due to a lack of sodium (salt). Cramp is most commonly caused by poor circulation and lack of magnesium, calcium or potassium.

Foods to Avoid
- Cut down on white-flour-based foods like white rice, biscuits, cakes, pizza and pasta, all forms of sugar and coffee. All of these foods deplete magnesium and potassium from the body. Some breads now have added calcium – check the labels.

Friendly Foods
- Plenty of fresh fruits and vegetables, especially bananas, raw cauliflower and jacket potatoes, fresh fruit juices, dried apricots and dates, seafood, leafy greens, avocado, lean steak, mackerel and beans in particular are all good sources of magnesium and potassium.
- Snack on almonds, sesame seeds and Brazil nuts all rich in these 3 minerals. Calcium foods are dried skimmed milk, sesame seeds, sardines, muesli, Parmesan cheese and curry powder.

Useful Remedies
- *Black Cohosh and Cramp Bark*, 1–2mls as needed. **FSC**
- Take *Ginkgo biloba*, 120mg of standardised extract 1–2 times a day, which is useful for increasing circulation.
- A liquid multi-mineral supplement taken in water daily can help reduce cramps. **Trace Mineral** Tel: 01342 824684.
- Take 500mg of extra magnesium which is often lacking in people who suffer cramps.

Helpful Hints
- If you tend to get cramps at night, try stretching out your calves before going to bed. If you have a friend you can walk with – have a regular evening walk.
- Exercise regularly, but not to excess and indulge yourself with a massage on a regular basis. Use geranium, ginger and cypress oils in your mix of oils.
- Reflexology helps to improve circulation and reduce cramps if undertaken on a regular basis (see *Useful Information*).

In America 180,000 people die every year due to orthodox medical errors.

CROHN'S DISEASE

Crohn's is an inflammatory disease of the bowel and tends to affect the small intestine and the colon but can also affect the stomach, duodenum and mouth. Blood in the stool, weight loss, loss of appetite, nausea, severe abdominal pain, diarrhoea, fever, chills and weakness are all common symptoms of this disease. Malabsorption of nutrients from the diet is one of the biggest problems in Crohn's and most nutrients particularly the fat-soluble nutrients are poorly absorbed. Crohn's has been labelled a modern disease as in 'primitive' cultures Crohn's is virtually unknown.

Around 40,000 people in Britain suffer this painful condition most of whom were born after 1950 when we really began eating a more refined diet. Over consumption of antibiotics and ingesting residues from meats plus cow's milk and vaccinations are all suggested as possible triggers. Children who are breast fed are less likely to contract Crohn's. Candida is also linked to this disease (see *Candida*).

Foods to Avoid
- Sugar has been strongly linked with the development of Crohn's and some people find that avoidance of sugar slows down the rate of progression. Sensitivities to certain foods aggravate the problem.
- Tomatoes, raw fruit and nuts are often problematic for some people.
- Yeast and dairy are two food groups which many people find difficult to digest and avoidance of them has helped many sufferers.
- Gluten-rich foods such as barley, wheat, rye and oats are often a problem.

Friendly Foods
- Oily fish which is a rich source of EPA and DHA, two essential fatty acids, have been found to reduce the severity of Crohn's and the frequency of attacks.
- It is important to eat unprocessed foods in their fresh state.
- Most sufferers can tolerate meat once or twice a week with plenty of lightly cooked vegetables. If raw fruit is a problem – lightly stew or grill fruits which makes them easier to digest.
- A couple of teaspoons of apple cider vinegar in a little warm water sipped throughout the morning helps to correct the pH level within the bowel and aid liver function.

Useful Remedies
- Liquid amino acids aid digestion and healing. Contact **Twinlab** Tel: 01332 638005 Website: www.twinlab.com
- As malabsorption is a big problem, liquid vitamins and minerals are more easily absorbed. **BC**
- Make sure you take a high potency B complex tablet every day as low levels of folic acid and B12 are often lacking in Crohn's patients. **BLK**

■ Zinc, 30mg a day, to aid tissue healing.

■ Vitamin A 25,000–30,000iu (only 5000iu if you're pregnant or wanting to become pregnant).

■ Cod liver oil 1–3 capsules a day or 1 teaspoon a day as this contains EPA, DHA and vitamin D. EPA and DHA are anti-inflammatory and the vitamin D is needed to maintain healthy bones.

■ Take *Lipase*, a digestive enzyme needed to help absorption of nutrients, with meals. **BC**

■ Make sure you take friendly bacteria daily – acidophilus and bifidus are available at all good health stores and should be taken after meals and the capsules should be kept in the fridge.

Helpful Hints

■ Smoking has been linked with the development of Crohn's disease.

■ Lymph drainage massage and skin brushing helps to eliminate toxins from the body.

■ Buy foods as fresh as possible. Everything tastes better and you'll appreciate the effort in the long run.

■ Crohn's disease is exacerbated by stress, therefore any techniques known to reduce stress such as yoga, t'ai chi, meditation, massage or hypnotherapy will help. Spiritual healing has helped many sufferers (see *Healing*).

■ Adequate rest is essential for any Crohn's sufferer and gentle exercise is also beneficial.

■ To re-balance your diet and make sure you are taking the right supplements and herbs in the correct amount for your case, I strongly suggest you consult a doctor who is also a nutritionist (see *Useful Information*).

■ For further help, contact **The National Association for Colitis and Crohn's Disease** (NACC), 4 Beaumont House, Sutton Road, St Albans, Hertfordshire, AL1 5HH. Information Line: 01727 844296, weekdays 10.00am-1.00pm. Website: www.nacc.org.uk Email: nacc@nacc.org.uk

■ **Crohn's in Childhood Research Association** (CICRA), Parkgate House, 356 West Barnes Lane, Motspur Park, Surrey, KT3 6NB. Tel: 020 8949 6209. Website: www.cicra.org Email: support@cicra.org

84% of doctors agree that exercising a dog daily greatly reduces the risk of heart disease.

CYSTITIS

(see also *Candida* and *Thrush*)

Cystitis is more common in women than men and can also affect children. It is caused by a bacterial infection in the bladder and symptoms include a frequent urge to urinate plus a burning sensation when passing urine.

With cystitis or thrush there can be a whitish/ yellow discharge – but this is more common with thrush which is a yeast overgrowth. Whatever the cause, the entire outer area can swell which makes sitting extremely uncomfortable indeed. If the lymph nodes in the groin begin to swell (near the bikini line) or if you have pain in the loins, blood in your urine, or a fever, this denotes a kidney infection and you must see a doctor. A urine test can confirm which bug is responsible and usually antibiotics are then prescribed. Women who suffer candida and food intolerances regularly suffer thrush or cystitis (see also *Candida*).

These types of infections are more likely to occur in warm, moist, humid atmospheres. If you are run down, you are more prone to an attack. If you suffer thrush regularly you may be diabetic. Have a urine test to eliminate this possibility.

Foods to Avoid
- While symptoms are acute avoid as much as possible all foods and drinks containing sugar and yeast – especially cheeses, malt vinegar, ketchups, soy sauce, miso, pickled foods, breads containing yeast, mushrooms and alcohol.
- Sugar in any form including honey, maltose and so on feeds the yeast – for the first week avoid all cakes, biscuits, pizza or fizzy cola type drinks.
- Avoid junk-type burgers and fried foods which are all hard to digest and add to the toxic load.
- Avoid high-sugar fruits such as grapes and mango for the first few days.

Friendly foods

- Eat plenty of live, low-fat yoghurt that contain the friendly bacteria acidophilus and bifidus.
- Cranberry juice without sugar or eat fresh or frozen cranberries – they are rich in hippuric acid which helps prevent bacteria clinging to the bladder walls.
- Drink 8–10 glasses of water every day.
- To re-alkalise your system, eat plenty of salads and green vegetables.
- Include bananas, apples, pineapples, papaya and pears for fruit
- Eat lots more garlic and onions which are antiseptic.
- See also *Candida*.

Useful Remedies
- Bromelain 1000–3000mcu for its anti-inflammatory properties.
- Vitamin A 10,000–25,000iu (only up to 5000iu if you are pregnant).
- Vitamin C and flavonoids help to fight the infection. Take up to 4 grams daily with food for the first week and then reduce to 1 gram daily. When you take large doses of vitamin C make sure it's in an ascorbate form that does not irritate the stomach.
- Buchu and Uva Ursi are two herbs that are particularly helpful for urinary tract infections as they are anti-bacterial. 10 drops of each every 3 hours when symptoms are acute. **NC**
- Take 2 acidophilis/bifidus capsules daily with food for at least 6 weeks.
- Include a high strength multi-vitamin and mineral in this programme **S**

■ *Cran-Max* is a supplement made from 100% cranberry fruit solids and is sugar and preservative free. One capsule 500mg will help to fight and prevent urinary tract infections. Available from health stores. Tel: 0800 085 2370.

Helpful Hints

■ Consuming live yoghurt on a daily basis can reduce the incidence of developing cystitis or thrush.

■ Drink organic *Aloe Vera Juice* that contains extract of cranberry and cherries. **HN**

■ Drink three to four cups of nettle tea daily.

■ Some women use a bruised clove of garlic as a pessary – but if this burns or stings too much then remove it after a few minutes.

■ Drink plenty of water each day to help flush out unhealthy organisms from the bladder.

■ Urinate as soon as possible after having sexual intercourse to stop transmission of bacteria into the bladder. If symptoms are acute, avoid intercourse for at least one week, as you can pass the bacteria from one partner to another.

■ Avoid perfumed soaps and vaginal deodorants at all times.

■ Wear cotton underwear. Avoid tightly fitted jeans, especially in hot weather.

■ As much as possible when you are at home wear a skirt and no underwear to keep the vaginal area cool.

■ If you have to sit all day, get up and walk around regularly.

■ Get plenty of rest.

■ Use a pH balanced soap.

■ Douche daily with diluted tea tree oil, crushed garlic and lavender oil or add a few drops to your bath.

■ Acupuncture and homeopathic remedies like *Cantharis 30c* (reduces the burning sensation) have helped many sufferers (see *Useful Information*).

Cats purr in Alpha waves – the brain waves produced during meditation –
hence why stroking a cat calms you down.

DANDRUFF

(see *Scalp Problems*)

DEPRESSION

Currently, 3 million people in Britain alone are diagnosed with depression, which in varying degrees affects most people at some stage in their lives. It is common in anyone who has undergone a trauma such as the death of a loved one, an illness, accident or the loss of a valued job. But for the huge majority, the basis of their depression often remains a mystery. Persistent depression can result in loss of sex drive, inability to sleep or excessive sleep, headaches, irritability and an extreme sense of negativity and lethargy. A feeling like 'I'm in a black pit and I can't seem to climb out of it' or 'I just cannot be bothered with anything or anybody.'

Poor thyroid function can lead to depression, as can blood sugar imbalances (associated with excessive intake of refined sugar and stimulants) and our modern lifestyle and diet, which is low in nutrients and high in stress, triggers many people into mild bouts of depression. All of these factors contribute to a biochemical imbalance which adds to the problem.

If you are under a lot of stress and cannot sleep, this feeling of sheer exhaustion can take you into a very depressive state. The current view on the main cause of depression is an imbalance in neurotransmitters, the molecules of emotion, which include serotonin and dopamine which affect mood, plus adrenalin and noradrenalin, which affect motivation. Anti-depressant drugs like *Prozac* work by stopping the body breaking down the neurotransmitter serotonin, therefore keeping more in the brain. But by taking the right supplements and foods, you can increase levels of serotonin naturally.

Foods to Avoid
■ Caffeine and sugar in any form deplete the body of vitamins C and B and minerals such as chromium can worsen depression.
■ Cut out any foods to which you know you are sensitive. The most common being chocolate, coffee, tea and wheat. Which foods do you eat every day and crave regularly? These are the foods that are usually doing the most damage (see *Allergies*).

Friendly Foods
■ Eat whole foods like brown rice, lentils, barley, oily fish, sunflower seeds, pumpkin seeds, linseed, pecan nuts, brazil nuts and hazelnuts. All of these contain essential fatty acids and nutrients that are usually low in depressive people. Remember, the brain is 60% fat.

- Eat oily fish such as mackerel, herring or salmon at least twice weekly.

- Make sure your overall fat intake doesn't drop too low. Use unrefined extra virgin olive, walnut, sunflower and sesame oils in your salad dressings. Or try *Udo's Choice Oil* – a perfect blend of omega 3 and 6 fats, available from health stores worldwide. Tel: 0845 0606070 for your nearest stockist.

- Serotonin is made from a constituent of protein called tryptophan, therefore include more foods such as fish, turkey, chicken, cottage cheese, beans, avocados, bananas and wheat germ in your diet.

- Sprinkle wheat germ over breakfast cereal, my favourite is **Nature's Path** who make great cereals from amaranth, quinoa and kamut, that are sweetened with a little apple juice.

- Hot spicy foods, that include cayenne pepper produce endorphins that help raise mood.

- Include plenty of fresh vegetables and fruits in your diet.

- Drink 6 glasses of water daily.

Useful Remedies

- Take a strong B complex such as *Blackmores Executive B*, as deficiency in most of the B vitamins can lead to depression, particularly B3, B6, B12 and folic acid. **BLK**

- Also take 50mg of B6 as well as the above if it is pre-menstrual depression which can be made worse by the contraceptive pill.

- 5 hydroxytryptophan derived from the plant griffonia (5-HTP). Take 100mg twice daily to help boost serotonin levels naturally.

- This works even better when combined with L-tyrosine, an amino acid 500mg twice a day.

- Take 1 gram of vitamin C daily with food.

- A high potency multi-vitamin and mineral – All the companies under *Codes, How to Use this Book* sell good multis.

- The herb St John's Wort is the best researched herb proven to be effective for mild to moderate and, in a few cases, severe depression. 300mg two or three times a day should help mild depression and twice this amount for severe depression. If taken in the long term this herb can make you sensitive to prolonged sunshine. Also contraindicated if you are taking blood-thinning drugs. Check with your doctor.

- *Ginkgo biloba*, 120mg 1–2 times a day, this has been found to be effective for elderly people not responding to conventional anti-depressant drugs.

- *SAMe* (s-adenosyl L methionine) is an effective natural anti depressant that helps to increase dopamine levels. In one study, 66% of depressed subjects responded versus only 22% given the prescription anti-depressant, *Imipramine*. It works on all kinds of depression and response time varies from 1 day to 5 weeks. One tablet daily. **NC**

- **Bach** remedies gorse and sweet chestnut are useful.

Helpful Hints

■ It is vital that you take regular exercise, especially in daylight, which releases endorphins the body's own mood elevators. It also reduces levels of the stress hormone cortisol in the blood and increases serotonin levels.

■ Stop smoking as this is another stimulant.

■ Studies show that counselling and problem-solving sessions often prove more useful than anti-depressant drugs. By talking your problems through with someone – you get a better perspective. Tell your loved ones how you are feeling – they are not psychic. Ask your doctor to refer you for counselling. For details of a counsellor in your area, contact the *British Association for Counselling* (BAC), 1 Regent Place, Rugby, Warwickshire, CV21 2PJ. Tel: 01788 550899. Website: www.counselling.co.uk Email: bacp@bacp.co.uk

■ Some depressions can be due to an iron deficiency but don't take iron without having your blood levels checked first.

■ I recommend that anyone suffering from depression to read *Natural Highs* by nutritionist Patrick Holford with Dr Hyla Cass (Piatkus, £14.99). To order call 0207 323 2382.

■ Have a regular aromatherapy massage using oils like bergamot, geranium, lavender, rose, clary sage and sandalwood, which all help to lift one's spirits.

■ Many readers have found hypnotherapy and neuro-linguistic-programming very helpful for cases of chronic depression (see *Useful Information*).

People who suffer chronic conjunctivitis are often deficient in vitamin A.

DERMATITIS
Seborrheic dermatitis (Cradle cap)

Seborrheic dermatitis is a common inflammatory condition of the skin which most frequently occurs in children. This is why it's often known as cradle cap. In most infants it tends to clear up in the first year or so. Symptoms are thick scaly tissue on the scalp in particular and sometimes around the eyes and ears. The problem is linked to a deficiency in fatty acids and one of the B vitamins, biotin. Eliminating allergens from the diet usually helps clear cradle cap.

Foods to Avoid

■ The most common offending foods for causing cradle cap are cow's milk and produce, wheat and eggs. As with any problem which may be influenced by food intolerances, it is important to identify which are the problematic foods. Generally the child's diet needs to be as clean as possible (*see* General Health Hints).

■ Avoid mass-produced refined white flour based foods and any foods and drinks that are high in sugar.

Friendly Foods

■ Make your child nutrient-rich fruit blends – add any fruit you have to hand such as bananas, kiwi, raspberries etc. and put them in a blender with a tablespoon of sunflower seeds and linseeds (rich in essential fats). Add a low-fat, live fruit yoghurt such as Rachel's (available from all supermarkets) and whizz for 30–40 seconds. This makes a healthy dessert.

■ Oils such as *Udo's Choice* which is a perfect blend of omega 3 and 6 fats can be added to food once cooked – a teaspoon a day should be fine. I find that if you cook some sweet potatoes and mash them with a little skimmed milk and then add the oil as they are cooling, the child cannot taste the oil. Otherwise add to thick vegetable soups and stews before serving. To find your nearest stockist of *Udo's Choice* call 0845 0606070.

■ For adults with dermatitis, eat plenty of fruits, vegetables, whole grains such as brown rice or quinoa, barley and oily fish. See *General Health Hints*.

Useful Remedies

■ Many companies make liquid multi-vitamins and minerals for children which you can add to cold dishes to make sure your child is not malnourished. **NC**

■ Alternatively you can add green food powders rich in vitamins, minerals and essential fats to breakfast cereals or desserts.

■ Biotin, a B vitamin which is often lacking – 6mg daily.

■ If the child is being breast fed it is useful for the mother to take 10mg of biotin – which will in turn be delivered through the milk.

■ Fatty acids in the forms of oils can be applied directly to the affected areas. It should be applied twice a day for 2–4 weeks. Use either evening primrose or borage oil. You can also take 2000 mg of evening primrose oil daily.

■ As all the B vitamins work together in the body, if you are breast feeding or an adult with this condition, also take a high strength B complex. **BLK**

■ Adults should take a high strength multi-vitamin and mineral plus an essential fatty acid formula daily. **BC**

Helpful Hints

■ Note that many toothpastes, shampoos, soaps, detergents, perfumes etc. contain a myriad of chemicals. I have met several dozen hairdressers who suffer this condition caused by all the chemicals they are in contact with daily.

■ Buy products in their most natural and unadulterated state which are gentler on a child's delicate skin. For anyone who suffers dermatitis or skin allergies, **The Green People Company** make organic skin, hair, body lotions, sun screens, and toothpaste and also have an advice line. Tel: 01444 401444. E mail; organic@greenpeople.co.uk Website: www.greenpeople.co.uk

■ Use aloe vera gel topically to help calm the itching.

If you suffer from thrush regularly you may be diabetic – have a urine test.

DIABETES (*Diabetes mellitus*)

Commonly known as sugar diabetes, this is a condition in which the body's ability to handle sugar is impaired and blood sugar levels become too high.

There are two main forms of diabetes, juvenile and adult onset. Juvenile is due to a deficiency of the hormone insulin, which helps keep blood sugar levels in check. Adult onset usually starts in middle age or as we get older. Quite often adequate amounts of insulin are produced but the body becomes resistant to its effects. Adult onset diabetes is associated with a diet that is too high in sugar, alcohol and saturated fat. Early signs of diabetes include fatigue, poor wound healing, excessive thirst, fungal infections, blurred vision and frequent urination. As diabetes is a potentially life threatening disease, it is very important that you have it properly diagnosed by your doctor. Excess weight and stress are also contributing factors to the onset of diabetes. Finland has one of the world's highest incidences of diabetes and the highest dairy intake.

Foods to Avoid

- Sugar, alcohol and refined carbohydrates such as white rice, breads, cakes, biscuits, pasta and pizza which release sugar too quickly into the bloodstream.

- It is important to remember that high-fat foods can have an equally adverse effect on insulin levels as well as sugar. Avoid full-fat or semi-skimmed dairy products as the high fat content can be problematic.

- Greatly cut down on your use of sodium-based salt, use a little sea salt that is higher in magnesium.

- Cut out all red meat or eat only occasional lean steak or lamb.

Friendly Foods

- Eat more quality protein/ low-fat foods like lean fish, beans, pulses and lentils. You need to include more whole grains like brown rice, buckwheat, oats – especially porridge, and fresh fruit and vegetables which all release their natural sugars more slowly into the bloodstream.

- Add a soluble fibre such as psyllium husks, oat or rice bran or linseeds to a high-fibre cereal such as *Nature's Path* – made from amaranth, quinoa and spelt – all healthy ancient grains.

- Try to eat whole, fresh fruit rather than drinking fruit juice.

- Use extra virgin, organic olive or walnut oil for salad dressings.

- Eating fish on a regular basis seems to lower the risk of developing diabetes. Vegetarians, particularly vegans, have a much lower risk of developing diabetes, in fact when people switch to a vegan diet for at least four weeks, symptoms of diabetes and insulin control improve. One of the other benefits of following a vegetarian diet and avoiding animal proteins is that diabetics are less likely to develop kidney disease.

- Eat 100–200 grams a day of bilberries or find a sugar-free jam and use a modest amount as it helps reduce the risk of diabetic cataracts.

- Try non-dairy organic rice milk or soya light milk which make a healthier alternative to full-fat cow's milk.
- Sprinkle GM free lecithin granules over breakfast cereals and low-fat yoghurts which help to lower LDL – the bad type of cholesterol.

Useful Remedies

- Take 600–1000 iu of natural source vitamin E daily. Vitamin E is an antioxidant which also helps to lower the risk of other diseases associated with diabetes such as circulation and eye problems.
- Vitamin C – 1 gram daily with food.
- Vitamin B6, 100mg a day, as most diabetics tend to have lower levels of B6 and this has been associated with peripheral neuropathy.
- Vitamin B12, 500–1000mcg a day helps maintain normal healthy nerve cells and has been shown to help reduce nerve pain.
- Biotin 10–20mg which is essential to process glucose.
- Vitamin D 800–1200iu per day as it's required for adequate blood levels of insulin.
- The mineral chromium is vital for controlling blood sugar and recent studies from America and several other countries show that when people take 200mcg of chromium daily, incidence of late onset diabetes was reduced by half. Chromium also helps to reduce cravings for sweet foods. It is very important to note that if you are insulin dependent you need to tell your doctor before taking chromium as your medication could then be reduced over time.
- The mineral magnesium which is needed to process insulin is usually lacking in diabetics . Take a multi-mineral that contains 200mg of magnesium, 30mg of zinc and a trace of copper. **NC**
- *Co Enzyme Q10,* 60–120mg is needed for adequate carbohydrate metabolism. Most diabetics don't process carbohydrates properly.
- When 4 grams is taken daily for at least 6 months, evening primrose oil has been shown to reduce diabetic neuropathy. EPO is available on prescription in the UK.
- Alpha lipoic acid is an antioxidant. Take 200mg a day. Research has shown it also reduces diabetic neuropathy.
- *Gymnena sylvestre* is a herb from the Ayurvedic tradition in India. It has been used for centuries in India to treat diabetes. In studies, extracts of the plant decreased fasting blood sugar levels, lowered insulin requirements and enhanced insulin production. It helps to repair and regenerate the insulin producing cells in the pancreas. Two capsules daily. **NC**
- Aloe vera helps to lower blood-sugar levels in non-insulin dependent diabetes.

Helpful Hints

- Remember honey, maltose and dextrose are all sugars and can cause as much disruption to insulin as refined, grain sugar.

d

- Always let practitioners know you are diabetic. Regular eye checks and foot care are also recommended as both can be affected in diabetes.

- Many people who have diabetic problems suffer with poor circulation in their feet. Reflexology has proved very helpful for circulation (see *Useful Information*). Alternatively, you could try an energy roller which works on the same principle as reflexology – roll bare feet for two minutes daily on the roller; this hurts initially but it gets easier! Send a SAE to **Shakti Chakra Ltd**. 106, West Street, Erith, Kent.. DA8 1AQ Tel: 01322 447610, Fax 01322 405994.

- Regular exercise is vital when treating diabetes as it can reduce the need for insulin. Try walking for at least 15 minutes, increasing to 30 minutes daily or more.

- If you suffer from stress on a regular basis it is vital that you change your lifestyle.

- The actor, Terence Stamp, has developed a range of organic foods, which are sugar and dairy free. *Stamp Collection* foods are available from most health food stores, or contact Buxton Foods Ltd, 12 Harley Street, London, W1G 9PG. Tel: 020 7637 5505, Website: www.stamp-collection.co.uk Email: customerservices@stamp-collection.co.uk

Health is our Heritage.
Edward Bach

DIARRHOEA

Diarrhoea can have several causes including infectious bacteria, food poisoning, food allergy or intolerance, IBS or yeast overgrowth (see also *Candida*). It may also be associated with more serious conditions like Crohn's disease and ulcerative colitis. If it is a chronic problem it is more likely to be associated with a food intolerance.

Severe diarrhoea must be treated quickly, as the body can rapidly become dehydrated and the person can eventually lose consciousness. Adequate intake of fluids, particularly water, and electrolyte sachet drinks should be given hourly to prevent severe dehydration.

Foods to Avoid

- Certain foods can aggravate the problem on their own, for instance, apple and other fruit juices because of the fructose.

- Avoid sorbitol, which is used as a sweetening agent.

- Lactose, the sugar in milk, is a common cause of chronic diarrhoea.

- If you are a regular coffee drinker, it's worth giving it up for a few days and seeing if this helps.

- Many people who have a sensitivity to wheat and gluten suffer chronic diarrhoea. See also *Leaky Gut*.

Friendly Foods

- Although we tend to associate fibre with ensuring adequate bowel movement and frequency, it can also help to control diarrhoea as the fibre will give bulk to the stool. Try soluble fibres like oat or rice bran, linseeds, psyllium husks and plenty of water or electrolyte drinks.

- Drinking three to four cups of camomile or black tea a day has been used for many centuries as a gentle way of dealing with diarrhoea.

- Eating either dried bilberries or bilberry juice can also help (but not fresh bilberries as they can actually aggravate the problem).

- Fresh vegetable soups with a little root ginger, or a small portion of poached fish and brown rice are usually well tolerated. Move onto solids only when symptoms begin to ease as sometimes diarrhoea is your body's digestive system telling you it needs a rest.

- Eat plenty of low-fat, live yoghurt to replenish healthy bacteria in the bowel.

- Drink plenty of cooled, boiled water.

- For acute diarrhoea, grate an apple, let it go brown and then eat it. Greenish bananas are very binding. *Slippery Elm Powder* can be mashed into a paste with banana and honey.

Useful Remedies

- Whilst symptoms last take 7500iu of vitamin A and 30mg of zinc, as lack of zinc has been shown to trigger diarrhoea.

- Thereafter, take a good quality vitamin/mineral to help prevent malnutrition.

- The herb Pau D'Arco kills many harmful organisms. Take 2–3ml of tincture 2 or 3 times a day, or 1 gram of capsules 2–3 times a day.

- If you are susceptible to diarrhoea when you travel abroad, taking acidophilus for two weeks prior to your trip can help increase the number of healthy bacteria in the gut which reduces the risk of picking up a tummy bug.

- *Culturelle* contains a strain of bacteria called *Lactobacillus Acidophillus GG* (LAGG). Extensive research in developing countries has shown this supplement treats and in some cases prevent dangerous forms of childhood diarrhoea. It is also effective against traveller's diarrhoea, antibiotic-associated diarrhoea, and colitis, in both children and adults. Take 2 capsules daily. **NC**

Helpful Hints

- Drink water from cooked brown rice or mix 15 grams of carob powder with some apple puree to make it palatable.

- *Bee Propolis*, *Grapefruit Seed Extract* and *Olive Leaf Extract* are all natural antibiotics.

- **Potter's** make a *Spanish Tummy Mixture* containing herbs and tinctures to heal the gut. Available from all good health stores. To find your nearest stockist call *Potter's (Herbal Supplies) Ltd*. Tel: 01942 405100. Website: www.pottersherbal.co.uk

- Stabilised liquid oxygen helps to re-alkalise the body, encourages healthy bacteria in the gut and has been shown to kill bacteria such as E coli, some viruses, parasites and fungi. Available from all good health stores or call 0208 886 6555.

- Never drink tap water unless you are sure it is safe to do so and avoid salads and fruit washed in local tap water in countries like India and Africa. Avoid ice cubes made from local tap water. Eat only thoroughly cooked foods if you are worried about getting a bad tummy upset. Use bottled water and fizzy drinks but only if they have sealed tops.

- If the diarrhoea resembles water coming out of a hose try homeopathic *Podophyllum 30c* every few hours for a day. Charcoal tablets are also useful for stopping diaorrhea.

- For teething children who have this problem use homeopathic *Chamomila 30c*, 3 times daily.

- If you suffer persistent diarrhoea, you must see a doctor.

DIVERTICULAR DISEASE OR DIVERTICULITIS

This occurs when the mucus membranes lining the colon form small finger-like pouches known as diverticula. If they become inflamed Diverticulitis results. Generally these pouches do not cause problems but if one or more become infected, extreme pain can result, primarily in the descending colon which is situated on the left hand side of the abdomen. Symptoms range from extreme pain, bleeding, diarrhoea and fever. Chronic constipation is the most common underlying cause of this condition and most sufferers tend not to drink sufficient water and ingest insufficient fibre (see also *Constipation*). Occasionally, a pouch may burst which requires urgent medical attention.

Foods to Avoid

- Foods containing seeds like tomatoes or grapes, as the seeds can lodge in the pockets and cause a lot of pain.

- Although fibre is necessary for a normal bowel movement the abrasive fibres in wheat bran or high-fibre breakfast cereals such as *All Bran* can temporarily aggravate the problem.

- Don't eat any fried or spicy foods.

- Reduce saturated fats such as full-fat milk, cheese and chocolates.

- Avoid as much as possible white bread and pasta, white rice, cakes, biscuits, take-aways and mass-produced burger-type foods.

- Greatly reduce your intake of red meat which takes a long time to pass through the bowel.

- Whilst symptoms are acute also avoid all yeast-based foods including *Marmite*, *Bovril*, cheese, soy sauce, vinegar etc.

- Avoid all sweeteners containing fructose, sorbitol and aspartame.

- Carageenan is a milk protein stabilizer often used in ice cream, that causes problems for people with digestive/bowel problems.

- Tea, coffee, fizzy drinks and alcohol all dehydrate the bowel.

Friendly Foods

- When the bowel is inflamed, eat soothing foods such as vegetable soups with added cabbage, celery and ginger plus lightly stewed apples, apricots, prunes, papaya and porridge made with non-dairy light soya or rice milk.

■ Once the inflammation is under control introduce a little steamed or grilled fish and low-fat meat such as skinless poultry.

■ Gradually increase your intake of high-fibre foods such as brown rice, bread and pasta, fresh vegetables, pulses, oat-based cereals and fruit (especially figs). There are many excellent organic high-fibre mueslis and cereals made from ancient grains such as amaranth, kamut and quinoa. **Nature's Path** make a good range available from health shops and supermarkets worldwide.

■ Live, low-fat yoghurt containing acidophilus and bifidus helps maintain the level of bacteria in the bowel and stool which encourages regular bowel movement.

■ Drink at least 8 glasses of water daily to make sure there is adequate fluid in the bowel.

■ Use extra virgin unrefined olive or sunflower oils for your salad dressings and eat plenty of garlic for its antiseptic qualities.

■ Add ginger which soothes and heals the gut.

■ If you cook cabbage, leave the cooking water to cool and then drink. This is rich in glutamine, a nutrient that helps to heal the bowel.

Useful Remedies
■ 2–5 grams of psyllium husks with plenty of water.

■ Add half a cup of aloe vera juice to fresh vegetable juices daily to help heal the gut and increase bowel movements.

■ *Slippery Elm* helps to heal the digestive tract. Chew 2–3 tablets before meals. **BLK**

■ For 6 weeks, take 2 acidophilus/bifidus capsules daily after food.

■ Vitamin A heals tissue. Take 10,000iu daily for three weeks (if pregnant only 5,000iu)

■ Liquid vitamins and minerals are more easily absorbed when the gut is irritated – take a good quality multi that contains plenty of the B group vitamins along with a gram of vitamin C. **FSC**

■ Calcium fluoride tissue salts helps to strengthen the intestinal walls. Take 4 daily.

■ *Seacure* is a protein supplement extracted from lean white fish which helps to heal the gut wall. Take 6 capsules daily. **NC**

Helpful Hints
■ Exercise regularly which helps to encourage bowel movement.

■ Remember to drink plenty of water.

■ Stress makes any digestive, gut or bowel problem worse. Look at your lifestyle and take time out to practise yoga or t'ai chi.

DIZZY SPELLS

(see *Low Blood Sugar, Low Blood Pressure* and *Vertigo*)

Stop looking for someone or something to blame for a problem –
start looking instead for solutions.

EARACHE

(see also *Glue Ear, Tinitus* and *Vertigo*)

Most earaches are caused by the build-up of fluid in the middle ear which can lead to an infection causing pain, fever or loss of hearing. Children under the age of 5 are particularly prone to ear infections, usually triggered by a sensitivity to foods such as corn, eggs, peanuts, cow's milk and wheat. Cow's milk and milk products are without doubt the most likely culprit. I have vivid memories as a child screaming with chronic earache until eventually both my ear drums burst. My poor mother had no idea that it was our diet of milk, cream trifles, cheese, chocolate treats and lots of lard and dripping (solidified beef, lamb and pork fat) sandwiches that caused the problem. I was prescribed almost continuous antibiotics which undoubtedly contributed to my acne, thrush and chronic fatigue during my teens. So if you have young children, try as much as possible to avoid antibiotics by changing your child's diet and give supplements to boost their immune function. Cutting sugar also helps – as most foods containing saturated fats also contain sugar, which turns to a hard fat within the body if not used up during exercise. Note that many yoghurts and 'low-fat' foods are high in sugar!

If the earache is persistent, many doctors suggest insertion of grommets through minor surgery but in the majority of cases this procedure can be avoided. To make sure your child does not become malnourished I suggest you consult a qualified nutritionist. (See *Useful Information*).

Foods to Avoid

- Any foods to which there is a sensitivity, particularly dairy from cows plus wheat based foods and eggs.

- Avoid sugar as it tends to weaken the immune system and leave children more susceptible to infections.

- Excessive amounts of fruit juice as these are often citrus-based which sometimes add to the problem. Remember that most canned fizzy drinks contain up to 10 teaspoons of sugar and never use drinks containing aspartame as they place too much of a strain on the liver which can further exacerbate the problem.

Friendly Foods

- Once you have identified an allergen such as cow's milk, look for alternatives such as oat, rice, pea and light soya milk. However, I would not recommend soya milk and foods for any child under the age of 5 years.

- There are plenty of wheat-free pastas now available based on lentils, rice, corn and vegetables.

- Bread can be replaced by rye or rice bread, or rice, rye or amaranth crackers, cakes and oatcakes.

■ Eat plenty of fruit and vegetables to keep the immune system in good shape, particularly those rich in the carotenoids like sweet potatoes, carrots and spinach. Other useful foods for the immune system are cauliflower, broccoli and Brussels sprouts.

Useful Remedies

■ The herb *Echinacea*, if used as a tincture use one drop per 6 kilos of body weight. Take 3–4 times a day for up to three weeks at any one time.

■ To help fight infection and boost immunity, take up to 1 gram of vitamin C with food daily, preferably as a powder dissolved in diluted low-sugar apple juice.

■ Children's multi-vitamin and minerals to make sure children are not deficient in any nutrients which can impair their immune system. **HN**

■ As antibiotics destroy healthy bacteria, encourage your children to eat non-dairy low-fat yoghurts after each meal that contain the friendly bacteria acidophilus. If they hate the taste of plain yoghurt, add any fresh fruit you have to hand and whizz in the blender for a few seconds. Make low-sugar jellies with fresh fruit juices and serve with low-fat yoghurt instead of ice cream.

Helpful Hints

■ If parents smoke, it is definitely worth them trying to cut back or not smoking near the children as this has been strongly linked to the development of ear infections.

■ A warm hot water bottle wrapped in a towel can be placed by the ear.

■ Two drops of warm garlic oil placed in the child's ear helps to reduce the pain.

■ Warm an onion and place the core of the onion just inside the poorly ear wrapped in muslin, or squeeze a little onion water into the ear. Onion and garlic are natural decongestants.

■ For irritations in the ears and sinuses, mucous and catarrh, use ear candles which gently remove excess ear wax without pain. Excellent for children as they are fun to use and not painful. Available from all good health stores, or for details call 020 7976 6615 or 01895 629950.

■ Homeopathic *Pulsatilla 30c* or *Belladonna 30c* – every 3–4 hours helps if the earache is in the right ear.

■ If in the left ear try *Hepar Sulph 30c*

■ If there is a sticky discharge try *Kali Bic 6x*

■ Do not let a child swim underwater if their ears become infected.

■ Children who are given dummies are more prone to ear infections.

■ Consult an allergy specialist who can test for food intolerances which can exacerbate and trigger this problem.

■ See a cranial osteopath or chiropractor to check the alignment of the head and neck, as misalignment and poor drainage can cause earache (see *Useful Information*).

Walking for 15 minutes after food really aids digestion and helps you to avoid indigestion and bloating.

ECZEMA
(see also *Leaky Gut*)

Eczema is a very distressing condition when the skin becomes very inflamed, itchy and sometimes develops into open bleeding sores. It is sometimes caused by an external irritant such as perfumes, washing powders, shampoos (how many hairdressers have you seen with eczema on their hands and arms?) paint or cat hairs, but most commonly it is linked to a food intolerance or a leaky gut.

Eczema can appear at any age seemingly from nowhere. It tends to be aggravated by stress, exhaustion, sometimes by heat and frequently by exercise. Eczema does tend to come and go and people find it difficult to track down the trigger. For most people, symptoms worsen when they are under stress, but others notice that it is aggravated by certain foods or drinking too much tea or coffee. If it starts in early childhood, the most likely culprit is cow's milk and products. Either the child has been fed formula milk or the residues are ingested via the mother's breast milk. The commonest triggers for eczema in babies are dairy products, eggs, citrus and wheat. Avoidance of the offending food often resolves the problem.

The traditional response to eczema is some sort of cream or emollient, partly to relieve the itching and to suppress the symptoms of the skin disorder. It is very important to remember that by the time the eczema shows up on the skin it has worked its way through the body and you really need to address the root cause of the problem.

With any skin condition it is a good idea to support the liver which is the most important cleansing organ of the body. If the liver becomes overloaded with toxins it tends to start dumping them into the skin, so anything you can do to keep your liver functioning more efficiently will in the long term help your skin. Drugs such as *Ibuprofen* have been known to trigger an attack in some people.

Foods to Avoid
- Avoid all dairy products from cows, coffee, tea, chocolate, beef, citrus fruits, eggs, wheat, alcohol, tomatoes and peanuts. This is a long list of foods, but if you have eczema and cut out all of these foods, the eczema is guaranteed to improve.

- It is important to note that even decaffeinated coffee causes problems in people who are sensitive to coffee – it's not just the caffeine.

- As much as possible, avoid preservatives, additives, pesticides, food colourings (such as in the bright red glacé cherries on fancy cakes) and refined mass-produced cakes, biscuits and pies (see also *Allergies*).

Friendly Foods
- Eat plenty of fresh fruits and vegetables and whenever possible make them organic.

- Include plenty of cabbage in your diet – and drink any water the cabbage has been cooked in. It contains L-glutamine which helps to heal a leaky gut.

- Beetroot, artichokes, celeriac, celery and radiccio are foods which cleanse the liver. If you cannot bear to eat freshly picked dandelions from your local fields then it is easily available in a tincture.

- Pear juice is a good alternative to orange juice.

- If you react to cow's milk, there are plenty of alternatives such as low-fat soya, rice, oat and buffalo milk all of which have a much lower incidence of reaction, taste good and mostly work fine in cooking.

- If you do not react to fish, then oily fish can be particularly beneficial as the essential fatty acids in fish are anti-inflammatory and have been shown to improve eczema conditions.

- Try eating plenty of seeds – sunflower, sesame, linseeds (flax) and pumpkin seeds – and nuts with the exception of peanuts. The fatty acids and the high level of zinc and protein in these foods will help nourish the skin and speed up the healing process.

- Wheat germ (not the same as refined wheat) and avocados are rich in vitamin E which also aids healing.

- Use extra virgin olive oil, plus unrefined walnut and sunflower oil in salad dressings.

- Use non-hydrogenated spreads such as *Biona* and *Vitaquell* in preference to mass-produced hard fats (see also *Fats You Need to Eat*).

Useful Remedies

- Evening primrose oil 1–4 grams a day. This is the one supplement with the most research showing benefits in eczema – it is also available on prescription.

- The mineral zinc is needed to ensure adequate absorption of fatty acids, it's invariably deficient in eczema sufferers. It also speeds skin healing – 30mg twice daily.

- Also take 500iu of natural source vitamin E daily. This is of crucial importance whenever you take a fatty acid. Do not include the vitamin E that is in the *Evening Primrose Oil* capsules, that's just to keep the oil in the capsules fresh. You actually have a greater requirement in the body once you start taking supplemental fatty acids. The vitamin E will help prevent scarring and itching.

- Include a high-strength multi-vitamin and mineral plus a B complex. B vitamins help reduce stress, improve digestion and the absorption of fatty acids. **S**

- Burdock and nettle tincture, take 10–20 drops, 3–4 times a day. This tincture should help to reduce the itching and cleanse the liver. Burdock is what is known as an alterative herb which means it could appear initially to make the condition worse as it encourages the eczema to leave the body. If this happens, reduce the dose dramatically and start gently, maybe just taking it once a day and gradually pick it up until you are comfortable with the rate of progress. **FSC**.

- Nettle works as a mild antihistamine which can reduce the itching. This tincture can be applied both externally and taken internally. Ideally, do not apply to broken skin as the small amount of alcohol would sting the skin.

- For young children use one drop per 6 kilos of body weight – this will ensure you don't give them too much. *Allergenics* cream, available from **Health Imports**, this cream soothes the majority of cases and some people have said it has actually cleared their eczema up. For details call 0870 7479131.

- To help the liver reduce alcohol, saturated fats and take 500mg of milk thistle 3 times a day. **BLK**

Helpful Hints

- To reduce the stress that may be aggravating the eczema, try meditation, yoga, t'ai chi or some other means of relaxation.

- If you have access to and can afford a reflexology treatment or aromatherapy massage, not only will the oils improve the condition but they are also incredibly relaxing. A few drops of essential oils of lavender, Roman camomile, geranium, rose and cedarwood mixed in a good base carrier oil such as calendula can be applied to the affected areas.

- Exercise is generally beneficial for both reducing stress and improving the condition, however, wear lightweight, cotton, loose fitting clothing, as if you get too hot and sweaty this tends to aggravate the condition.

- Many people have found that aloe vera juice taken internally and the gel used topically has proved helpful for eczema.

- Constipation and a liver under stress are also associated with eczema (see also *Constipation*).

- If an allergy to some food is suspected, then avoid the offending food (see *Allergies*).

- Avoid soaps and soap powders; use soap substitutes or **Dead Sea** soaps available from good pharmacies and health stores.

- Chinese herbs have proved helpful in many cases but you need to see a qualified Chinese herbalist and may need to have liver function checked before and during treatment. Others report great success through homeopathy (see *Useful Information*).

- For further help, contact the **National Eczema Society**, 163 Eversholt Street, London, NW1 1BU. Tel: 020 7281 3553. Helpline: 0870 241 3604, Monday to Friday, 1.00pm-4.00pm. Website: www.eczema.org

In 1999, in the UK alone, 656 million prescriptions were issued.

ELECTRICAL POLLUTION and ELECTRICAL HEALING

Roger Coghill, a bio-electromagnetics research scientist who is one of the world's leading authorities on this subject, based in Gwent in the UK says 'Every cell in the human body emits its own unique frequency. This frequency is as unique to us as our DNA. We are electrical beings in a physical shell and electricity can be used to harm or to heal us. When functioning properly, our cells or groups of cells such as our liver or kidneys emit a healthy, harmonic signal which can clearly be seen through specialist photography or by measurements using electronic equipment.

When we become ill, cells then emit a disharmonic frequency, which again can be detected. Every food you eat also emits a frequency as does every nutrient and everything on the planet – even rocks. This is how scientists measure what other planets and stars are made of by measuring the spectral frequencies.

Conversely, electrical pollution is now thought to be a major contributing factor to many illnesses. People who live near power lines and substations and whose homes are packed with electrical equipment would appear to be more prone to illnesses such as ME (chronic fatigue), cancers, depression, migraines and insomnia. Research has shown that telephone engineers are several times more likely to commit suicide.

Sixty years or so ago a few households enjoyed the luxury of a radio set but today we are all being bombarded by a dangerous enemy. As I write (December 2000) there are more than 31 million mobile phone subscribers in the UK alone and 500 million worldwide. Studies show that excessive use of mobile phones trigger solid cancerous tumours. The hand free kits are also linked with health problems and if you use these phones for more than 20 minutes at a time you are at a much greater risk. We are living in a sea of artificial frequencies and because animals, especially whales, dolphins, insects and birds, are more sensitive to these man-made emissions, their sensory abilities are being greatly affected – hence why so many whales are beaching themselves. Humans are also becoming more electro-sensitive and there are even societies which help people who are either affected by, or whose fields affect electrical equipment.

Also if you have subterranean flowing water under your home or office, this often compounds health problems, as the water can create an inharmonious electro magnetic field. Hundreds of years ago, builders would watch carefully where sheep settled at night and would not build in places where sheep refused to sleep. Recent studies show rats also avoid areas of high electromagnetic fields.

Every time you turn on a light switch or any electrical equipment – your brain's rhythms change immediately. Spending too much time under fluorescent lighting or in front of a computer screen can suppress the brain chemical melatonin. This can have negative effects as diverse as infertility, depression, insomnia and increase the risk of cancer.

Foods to Avoid

■ Junk foods have a dull energy field frequency – which will eventually trigger negative symptoms if you eat junk foods to excess. But it is important to note that as all foods emit their own frequency and if you eat certain foods, whether considered healthy or not, which emit a frequency that is incompatible with your own frequency – this too can trigger symptoms in sensitive individuals.

Friendly Foods

■ Foods in as near a natural state as possible. For instance, if you look at the energy field of a raw cabbage it has a really bright energy field – but once cooked the energy field is greatly reduced. See *General Health Hints*.

Useful Remedies

■ A new device that took 20 years to develop for treating astronauts in space, called a *Scenar* is now available worldwide. It looks like a small hand-held TV remote device but don't let its size fool you. It marries state of the art Western technology with Eastern medicine. The machine is passed over the body by a trained therapist and higher disharmonic readings tell the therapist where any physical problems are situated. These disharmonic frequencies are then altered within the machine and a harmonic frequency is pulsed back into the problem area, which encourages the body to heal itself. The Russian scientists have presented a huge body of evidence stating the *Scenar* has proven, on average 80% successful in treating a huge range of conditions from back pain to eczema, psoriasis to prostate problems and has also proven effective in greatly reducing bruising from injury sites and healing scar tissue and wounds after surgery. For details of your nearest therapist in the UK call 01722 340221. www.life-energies.com

■ The *Bicom* machine developed in Germany picks up the electromagnetic frequencies within the body – it is able to separate the healthy frequencies from the unhealthy frequencies and the healthy frequencies are then amplified back into the body again to encourage self healing. Cells carry a memory of certain diseases that you thought long ago had left your body. For instance when I was tested with the *Bicom* (at the **Hale Clinic** in London 020 7631 0156) my cells showed a positive reading for the memory of glandular fever which I suffered in my teens – so the therapist inverted the frequency of the Epstein Barr virus (from a tiny phial containing Epstein Barr) back into my body which neutralises any remaining memory. The *Bicom* is brilliant for helping people eliminate allergies, chronic fatigue, endometriosis, treating intestinal parasites and eczema. As of going to press, I have been unable to trace Bicom practitioners in the UK, but you could ask Peter Smith at the Hale Clinic on 0207 6310156 as his secretary may be able to help you.

■ Electro crystal healing works on similar principles except that the therapist pulses the calming or stimulating frequencies through crystals that are held in a saline solution. I have interviewed dozens of people who have been crippled with arthritis and other conditions who have been greatly helped by this type of therapy. I personally see Mark Lester in London. Tel: 0208 349 4730. www.thefinchleyclinic.co.uk or to find your nearest electro crystal therapist in the UK send a large SAE to *The School of Electro Crystal Therapy*, 117, Long Drive, South Ruislip, Middlesex. HA4 OHL.

Helpful Hints

■ The subject of energy medicine is now becoming a mainstream subject and for those who want to know more, I recommend you read *Virtual Medicine* by Dr Keith Scott-Mumby, Thorsons or *The Complete Book of Energy Medicine* by Dr Helen Dziemidko. Gaia Books.

■ The basic rule is that moving electric fields are harmful ie mobile phones or power lines, and static magnetic fields, like the earth on which we all evolved are beneficial to health.

■ Avoid using a mobile phone inside a car, building or any enclosed space, because the phone is forced to increase its output power, which can affect health more quickly. Never use a mobile for more than 20 minutes at a time.

- Tecno AO aluminium antennas can be attached to mobile phones – this helps the body resist the affects of the negative electromagnetic frequencies emitted by the phones. (£29-00 inc VAT) For details call 01793 741080 www:tecnoaouk.com

- **Microshield** makes a leather case incorporating shielding materials used in the radiation industry that have been proven to reduce the amount of radiation entering the head. For details call 0208 363 3333. www: microshield.co.uk

- Keep electrical appliances in the bedroom to a minimum. Turn off all mains switches in the bedroom at night. If you live near an electrical power station, put large copper jugs or ornaments in the windows.

- Avoid sleeping with an electric blanket on, warm the bed thoroughly before you get into bed and then switch it off for the night. However, if you are over 60 and have poor circulation and have been specifically told to sleep with it on, for goodness sake don't get too cold!

- Studies show that microwave ovens alter the chemistry of food. Irradiating (X-raying) food could, in the long run, prove very dangerous. If any foods like strawberries are still healthy looking after being in your fridge for a few days, then they have most likely been irradiated.

- The **Coghill Research Laboratories** have invented a small, easy to use, instrument called *The Coghill Fieldmouse* (£100 plus VAT), which tells you if you are in a high electrical energy atmosphere. For details, send a large SAE to Coghill Research, Lower Race, Pontypool, Gwent, NP4 5UF. Tel 01495 752122. Or read Roger's fascinating book *Healing Energies of Light*, Gaia Books. For more information on how electricity can harm or heal log onto Roger's website: www.cogreslab.co.uk

- For the latest updates on electrical pollution, log onto www.em-hazard-therapy.com or call **Electro Magnetic Hazard and Therapy Helpline** on premium-rate line 0906 4010237.

- Have your home dowsed by an expert if you are worried about suffering from over-exposure from electricity. Send an SAE to **The British Society of Dowsers**, Sycamore Barn, Hastingleigh, Ashford, Kent, TN25 5HW. Tel: 01233 750253. Office is open from 9.00am–1.00pm and 2.00pm–5.00pm. Website: www.dowsers.demon.co.uk Email: bsd@dowsers.co.uk

Energy flows where your attention goes.

Stephen Langley

EMPHYSEMA

Emphysema is a condition that usually occurs in middle and old age, which affects the lungs reducing their capacity to absorb oxygen and difficulty in expelling air. Normally, sufferers complain about increasing breathlessness, which is exacerbated by exercise. It is nearly always caused by smoking or exposure to other atmospheric pollutants and chemicals. Having an ioniser in the home may be useful for lowering levels of dust in the house.

Foods to Avoid

- Any foods to which you have an intolerance – the most common being wheat and dairy from cows.

- If you find you are making too much phlegm, this is almost always linked to high-fat foods including full-fat cheese, chocolate, milk, white bread and croissants etc.

- Generally cut down your intake of red meat and if you choose to eat meat always cut off the fat first.

- Eggs are hard to digest for some people and it's well worth being tested to see if they are a problem.

- Sugary foods and drinks suppress immune function which leaves you more susceptible to infections. Also, most foods high in sugar are also high in fat and many low-fat foods are high in sugar which is converted to a hard fat within the body.

Friendly Foods

- People who eat fruit and vegetables on a regular basis seem less likely to develop emphysema, particularly foods rich in natural source carotenes such as apricots, mangos, green vegetables, watercress, parsley, red peppers, spinach, sweet potatoes, watercress and cantaloupe melon.

- Use low-fat soya or organic rice milk as non-dairy alternatives.

- Choose low-fat dishes including cottage cheese and replace too much butter with healthier spreads such as *Biona* and *Vitaquell*.

- Use olive oil for salad dressings and eat plenty of brown rice, lentils, barley, oat-based dishes, wheat-free breakfast cereals – **Nature's Path** make a great range. There are also plenty of wheat-free pastas available such as lentil, rice, corn and potato pasta and flour.

- See *General Health Hints*.

Useful Remedies

- *N-Acetyl Cysteine* (NAC) 500mg 1–2 times a day. This amino acid is one of the best researched nutrients for emphysema, as it helps protect lung tissue and improve breathing.

- Vitamin C. Take 1–2 grams daily with food in an ascorbate form to help clear mucous and improve respiratory ailments.

- L-carnitine, 2grams daily, if breathing is made worse by exercise.

- *Mullein* formula, 2–3ml a day, contains a blend of herbs including mullein which are antiviral and expectorant that help to ease breathing and congestion. HC

- *Microcell Nutri Guard Plus* contains high potency lycopene, selenium, zinc, alpha lipoic acid vitamins A, C, E which all help to support lung tissue. **BC**

- Include a high potency multi-vitamin and mineral in your regimen.

Helpful Hints

- Stabilised liquid oxygen helps to re-alkalise the body and gets more oxygen into the system. Available from all good health stores or call 0208 886 6555

- Try using an *Ultrabreathe* – a small inexpensive device that helps to exercise the lungs. For details call 0870 608 9019. Details can be found on their Website: www.ultrabreathe.com

- Gentle exercise can help relieve the symptoms of this condition, especially regular walking, swimming or cycling. Start slowly and build up gradually. Reflexology has proved successful with some sufferers. Yoga can also be beneficial as this therapy will teach you relaxation techniques and how to breathe properly (see *Useful Information*).

- Aromatherapy has also been of benefit to some sufferers. Fill a basin with boiling water and add three drops of eucalyptus essential oil. Put your head over the basin with a towel over you to trap the steam and inhale deeply for two to five minutes, keeping your eyes closed.

Adaptable, positive people tend to live longer.

ENDOMETRIOSIS

Endometriosis is a condition where tissue, which normally lines the womb, is found outside the womb, in places such as the ovaries, fallopian tubes or pelvis. It is not certain what causes this condition but some doctors theorise that during menstruation womb tissue flows not only down to the vagina but up through the fallopian tubes eventually sticking to other structures. It can cause a lot of pain particularly during ovulation and sexual intercourse. It is one of the more common causes of infertility. As excessive bleeding and pain are associated with endometriosis, internal examinations are often necessary which in most cases aggravates the condition. Unfortunately it is necessary to eliminate anything more serious. Most nutritional practitioners believe there is a strong link between endometriosis and candida overgrowth which when treated greatly alleviates symptoms. Many of the women suffering this condition, note that symptoms are definitely worse when they are stressed or really tired. The chemical dioxin and numerous other toxic chemicals have been linked to this condition – always use pure cotton towels that are guaranteed free from dioxin. Tampons can exacerbate symptoms.

Foods to Avoid

- Avoid alcohol and animal fats which can elevate oestrogen levels and place a strain on the liver, which in turn can increase the pain and inflammation.

- Caffeine reduces the body's ability to cope with pain.

- If you suspect candida – symptoms include bloating, constipation and/or diarrhoea, thrush, food cravings and chronic fatigue – avoid sugar, refined carbohydrates, cheese, mushrooms, concentrated fruit juice and yeasted breads for a couple of weeks to see if this helps. See also *Candida*.

- As with so many other conditions, if there is a food intolerance it will almost certainly aggravate the problem.
- Also avoid eggs for at least two weeks. Keep a food diary to see when symptoms are worse.

Friendly Foods

- Soya-based foods have an ability to control excessive oestrogen levels; as do beans, lentils, chickpeas, cauliflower, Brussels sprouts and broccoli.
- Add sunflower, pumpkin, sesame and linseeds to your breakfast cereal which provide essential fatty acids and zinc that is vital for soft tissue healing. Nuts with the exception of peanuts, again a good source of fatty acids and zinc.
- Eat more oily fish for its anti-inflammatory properties.
- Pineapple is rich in bromelain, a highly anti-inflammatory enzyme.
- Ginger and turmeric are also anti-inflammatory and ginger is very soothing within the gut.
- Eat foods high in natural carotenes – spinach, carrots, apricots, parsley, mango, cantaloupe melons and sweet potatoes.
- Natural wheatgerm and avocados are rich in vitamin E.

Useful Remedies

- Take 3 grams of evening primrose, as the fatty acids help regulate hormones and reduce discomfort.
- Most sufferers are lacking in the mineral magnesium. Take 200–600mg daily.
- Zinc, 30mg, as most sufferers are deficient and zinc ensures proper absorption of fatty acids.
- A strong B complex helps absorption of fatty acids
- Soya isoflavones, 50–100mg, a day to help regulate hormone levels.
- Wild yam 1–3ml of tincture or 1–3 grams a day of tablets, has been shown to reduce the discomfort of endometriosis and help reduce excessive bleeding.
- 500mg of the amino acid L-methionine which helps de-toxify oestrogen in the liver.
- Include a high-strength multi-vitamin and mineral in your regimen. **HN**
- *Vitex* (also known as *Agnus Castus*) help to balance hormones naturally 5 mls daily.

Helpful Hints

- Natureopathy and Chinese Medicine have proven beneficial to many sufferers. If you decide to try Chinese Herbs make sure your doctor keeps an eye on your liver function. (see *Useful Information*).
- Contact the **Women's Nutritional Advisory Service** Mon–Fri 9am–5.30pm. Tel: 01273 487366.
- Further help is available from **The National Endometriosis Society**, 50 Westminster Palace Gardens, Artillery Row, London, SW1P 1RL or call their help line on 0207 222 2776 which is open every day, 365 days a year. Website: www.endo.org.uk

*Don't you find that when people give of their time and energy to you in a
loving way without asking what's in it for them, you feel more inclined to do the
same for them? What you give out is what you get back.*

EXHAUSTION

(see also *ME* and *Stress*)

Out of the 50,000 letters I have answered during my 9 years as a health journalist, the most common without doubt have been from people, particularly women who feel tired all the time.

A huge majority of people are working longer hours, having shorter breaks and eating the wrong foods, which are all taking a cumulative toll on our bodies. One of the most common problems is simply lack of sleep. When you are under pressure you have more difficulty getting to sleep and then you have to get up for work feeling almost as tired as you did the night before. There is no right or wrong amount of sleep, we are all unique, Margaret Thatcher could manage on four hours, but I need eight. Everyone knows how much sleep they need to be fully functioning the next day.

Obviously there are varying levels of exhaustion, but if you find you suffer from palpitations regularly during the day, chronic headaches, have an urgency to keep going to the loo and experience a red flushing in your upper chest and throat area- this is most likely your adrenal glands telling you that your body is on limits. You need to listen and take note of the signals or worse is to come. Your immune system is lowered and you are more likely to pick up anything that's going. Rest is your best option at this point. Know when to walk away. It's not worth dying for ... literally.

Have your thyroid checked as chronic exhaustion is also linked to an underactive thyroid.

Foods to Avoid

■ Unfortunately, stimulants like coffee, tea, alcohol and sugar give a short-term energy boost but this soon wears off, leaving you craving more sugary, refined foods. Therefore greatly reduce your intake of colas and fizzy drinks, black tea, chocolates biscuits, cakes, snacks, croissants and mass-produced refined foods. Not only do they leave us feeling tired but they also deplete important nutrients like magnesium, chromium and the B vitamins, and we become even more exhausted.

■ Don't eat heavy protein meals late at night as they take a long time to digest.

Friendly Foods

■ Eat more high-energy foods such as alfalfa or aduki bean sprouts, wheat grass and fresh fruits and vegetables.

■ Include more whole-grains like brown rice, oat-based cereals and millet packed with B vitamins which help support your nerves.

- Magnesium and calcium are known as nature's tranquillisers so eat more green vegetables like kale, cabbage and broccoli plus almonds, Brazil nuts, soya flour, sesame seeds, pineapple, papaya, Parmesan cheese, fish, dried apricots, pilchards and skimmed milk. Chocolate is also high in calcium, but the benefits are offset by the caffeine content. Just eat in moderation.

- At night, eat wholewheat pastas and jacket potatoes which are more calming. Make thick vegetable soups which are easier on the digestion.

- Generally by controlling your blood sugar levels by eating small meals regularly instead of binging on junk foods will help to reduce the constant exhaustion. See *Low Blood Sugar*.

- Drink herbal teas throughout the day which are free from caffeine and choose a calming blend such as camomile and apple.

- As your digestive system is bound to be stressed eat a low-fat, live yoghurt with meals.

Useful Remedies

- Take a strong B complex to help calm your nerves and aid digestion plus 500mg of pantothenic acid (B5) which helps support adrenal function.

- As the digestive system begins malfunctioning when we are really tired take a digestive enzyme or betaine hydrochloride (stomach acid) with meals to improve the absorption of nutrients. Do not take the betaine if you have active stomach ulcers, instead take a digestive enzyme capsule with main meals.

- Co-enzyme Q 10 is a supplement well proven to improve energy levels. The body produces Co Q 10 naturally but as we age or when stressed we produce less. And as most people no longer eat organ meats, rich in Co-enzyme Q 10 it is best taken as a supplement of 100mg daily. **PN**

- Calcium and magnesium are often depleted – take 500mg of calcium with 200–300mg of magnesium an hour before going to bed. Most companies sell them in one formula.

- *Siberian Ginseng* is useful as a general tonic that helps to support adrenal function. There are plenty of liquid formulas and this can be taken for a month.

- A supplement originally devised to help Parkinson's patients reduce their chronic fatigue called *ENADA* – the co-enzyme form of vitamin B3 – has proven in numerous independent medical trials successful for raising energy levels, mental alertness, proper brain function and enhanced immunity. Two tablets can be taken daily on an empty stomach. Once energy levels return then one tablet daily is fine. This supplement should not be taken if you suffer regular palpitations due to stress. **NC FSC**

Helpful Hints

- If you are at rock bottom, a few vitamin pills and a couple of nights sleep will help but are not the long-term solution. You must try and address the root cause of your exhaustion.

- Generally try and take at least one day a week out for yourself and makes dates in your diary for exercise or time simply to call your own.

- Breathe deeply into your tummy every hour. Get up walk around, have a stretch.

■ If your exhaustion is linked to personal problems, ask your doctor to refer you to a counsellor. Talking problems through gives you a better perspective. See also *Depression*.

■ *Homeopathic Phos Ac 30c* twice daily for 3 days helps restore energy levels.

■ Never take work to bed and always finish work at least one hour before going to bed – otherwise your mind simply keeps churning your thoughts over and over.

■ Gentle exercise like yoga, t'ai chi (qigong) or walking at leisure in nature helps to make you feel more positive and re-build energy levels.

■ Find a practitioner who can really sort out your diet, such as a nutritionist or naturopath and make a determined effort to improve your food intake (see *Useful Information*).

■ If at all practical treat yourself to three days at a health spa to rejuvenate and rest.

If you wake regularly between 3–5 am, this can be linked to adrenal exhaustion.

EYE PROBLEMS

(see also *Cataracts*)

EYE PROBLEMS – Dark circles under the eyes.

Dark circles can be caused by a food intolerance, mainly to wheat or an underactive thyroid. The obvious cause is lack of sleep but if this problem continues then the adrenal glands become exhausted which can further darken the eyes.

Foods to Avoid

■ Cut down on alcohol and salt and drink plenty of water to flush toxins from the body.

■ If you are sleeping well but still have circles after 3 or 4 good night's sleep, then eliminate wheat for 4 days and see if this helps. Try eliminating cow's milk. These are the most common triggers.

Friendly Foods

■ Drink plenty of water to eliminate toxins and generally eat a clean diet avoiding too much refined food and sugar. See *General Health Hints*.

Useful Remedies

■ If you are totally exhausted see Useful Remedies under *Exhaustion*.

■ *Eyecare* contains bilberry extract, antioxidants (vitamins A E and C plus selenium) potassium, grapeseed extract, ginkgo biloba, lycopene and chromium. **BC**

■ Try *Calendula Under Eye Therapy*, a formula devised by Dr Peter Theiss in Germany containing marigold extract and hyaluronic acid (levels within the skin drop as skin ages) which helps to reduce dark circles and puffy eyes. To find your nearest stockist call 02890 662551.

EYE PROBLEMS – Itchy eyes

Itching of the eyes can be due to an infection like conjunctivitis, allergies or hayfever, or exposure to a smoky or polluted atmosphere. It can also be due to over-exposure to computer screens – as well I know as I sit typing this book!

If the problem is linked to your PC, then take regular breaks, get out in the sunshine and get some rest.

Foods to Avoid
- Avoid dehydrating beverages like caffeine and alcohol. Just like every other part of the body the eyes need plenty of fluid intake to keep them in good shape – drink more water.

Friendly Foods
- Eat plenty of dark purple fruits like bilberries, blueberries, blackberries and cherries as the bioflavonoids in these fruits not only protect and strengthen the eyes but they help reduce the risk of eye damage from other diseases.

- Eat more green vegetables, sweet potatoes and carrots as they are very rich in the carotenes which nourish the eyes.

- Eat more oily fish which are rich in vitamin A and essential fats which help prevent the eyes from drying out.

- Eat more unsalted nuts (not peanuts) and seeds which are high in zinc and selenium.

Useful Remedies

- Vitamin A, 25,000iu a day for 1 month. If you are pregnant limit, to 5000iu per day.
- Zinc, 30mg a day, is essential for enhancing vitamin A absorption.
- A strong B complex, B vitamins – in particular B2 – are necessary for the prevention of dry eyes.

Helpful Hints
- Eyebright herb or tincture can be made into a tea and when cooled, used as an eye lotion. It has anti-flammatory, astringent and anti-catarrhal properties.

- The homeopathic version of eyebright, *Euphrasia*, can be used for bathing the eyes and is very soothing. Use *Euphrasia Mother Tincture* about four times a day using a disposable eye bath. Most good health stores should stock this.

- Another way of relieving itchy eyes is to brew a pot of camomile tea and lay the tea bags, when they've cooled, on the eyelid. Ideally, leave on the eye for about 15 minutes.

- Don't use anyone else's face cloth or towel just in case the problem is infectious. If your eyes are inflamed, *Chloride Compound* is useful to reduce redness around the eyes. **BLK**

- *Traynore Pinhole Glasses* help to take the strain off the eyes and help your eyes to focus properly. Sold at all good health stores or call **The NutriCentre** (see page 15).

EYE PROBLEMS – Macular degeneration
Macular degeneration happens when the macula, an oval-shaped depression in the central area of the retina begins to deteriorate. Symptoms can include blurred vision.

and blind spots. It is linked to hardening of the arteries and poor circulation, excessive exposure to sunlight and smoking. Sitting too long at computer screens, household chemicals and low levels of antioxidant nutrients are also a factor. Copper is vital for healthy eyes but women who take the Pill or HRT can have too much copper in their system which can deplete zinc levels.

Foods to Avoid
■ Avoid sodium-based salt and high-saturated-fat foods.
■ See *Diet* under *Circulation*.

Friendly Foods
■ Eat more oily fish, carrots, pumpkins, tomatoes, cantaloupe melon, apricots, green leafy vegetables – especially cabbage, spring greens, kale, pak choi and spinach.
■ Bilberries, blueberries and blackberries are all great eye foods.
■ Generally eat more organic fruits and vegetables which are rich in antioxidant nutrients.
■ Wheat germ and avocados are rich in vitamin E.
■ Sunflower, pumpkin and sesame seeds, and linseeds and their unrefined oils are rich in essential fats, zinc and selenium, needed for healthy eyes.
■ Use a sea salt that is magnesium and potassium based.

Useful remedies
■ 2 grams of vitamin C with bioflavonoids daily with food.
■ A high potency antioxidant formula that contains 30mg of zinc plus 200mcg of selenium NL
■ A multi-vitamin and mineral formula made especially for your sex and age. S
■ The amino acid taurine helps to keep the retina healthy. 500mg daily.
■ A natural source carotene complex, one daily. BC
■ Formulas such as *Eyecare* containing vitamin A, ginkgo and bilberry are usful to nourish the eyes. BC

Helpful Hints
■ If you spend a lot of time outside wear a hat to cover your eyes and wear UVA/UVB protective sunglasses.
■ Have your copper levels checked.
■ Reduce your exposure to electromagnetic fields from computers and mobile phones.

EYE PROBLEMS – Optic neuritis
This is an inflammation of the optic nerve which carries the inflammation from the seeing part of the eye, the retina, to the brain. It can cause partial or complete loss of vision which comes on over a few hours or days and may be accompanied by a pain

in the eye. Optic neuritis can be one of the symptoms of multiple sclerosis.

Foods to Avoid

■ Foods which would aggravate inflammation including animal fats, meat, butter, cheese.

■ Try to avoid alcohol and caffeine which can interfere with blood circulation to the eyes.

Friendly Foods

■ Pineapple is a rich source of bromelain, an anti-inflammatory enzyme.

■ Oily fish is rich in vitamin A which nourishes the eye and the fatty acids can reduce inflammation.

■ Spices like ginger, turmeric and cayenne, all of which can reduce inflammation as well as improving circulation to the eye.

■ Bilberries, blueberries, blackberries, all blue and orange fruits will help to nourish the eyes.

Useful Remedies

■ Bromelain, 2,000–3,000 mcu a day, can reduce the inflammation and improve circulation.

■ The herb *Ginkgo Biloba* helps strengthen the capillaries in the eye and improve the circulation 120–240mg of standardised extract a day.

■ Vitamin A 10,000–25,000 units a day, for one month (only 5000iu if you are pregnant).

■ A good antioxidant formula to prevent further degeneration in the eye and reduce inflammation. NL

EYE PROBLEMS – Puffy eyes

Puffiness and bags under the eyes can denote kidney problems and a build up of toxins within the body. It also signifies that the sodium, potassium balance within the body is upset, in which case take 100mg of potassium for a week or so and reduce your intake of sodium-based salts. It can also be associated with food intolerances and conditions such as hayfever. Drink more water to flush the kidneys and for at least three days, avoid wheat and dairy products and note if your eyes go down. Puffy eyes can also indicate an underactive thyroid, therefore if the problem continues after making these changes, see a doctor.

Foods to Avoid

■ If underneath the eyes is both puffy and dark, it is very likely that you have food allergies or intolerances so it is important to identify these. The most common being dairy from cows, wheat, citrus fruits, eggs and nuts.

■ Salt is a major trigger which definitely exacerbates any water retention and increases swelling in all parts of the body if you suffer fluid retention.

■ Mass-produced breakfast cereals often contain more salt than the average bag of crisps.

■ Dairy products from cows, cheese and cottage cheese are high in sodium.

- Most pre-packaged, refined foods will have additional salt and a lot of foods which are naturally sweet have salt added partly as a preservative but also to take the edge off the sweeteners.

- Cut down on all foods and drinks containing caffeine and alcohol which further dehydrate the body.

- Reduce heavy red meat meals to reduce the burden on the kidneys.

Friendly Foods

- Water is really important, drink 6–8 glasses a day.

- Fruit and green vegetables – especially celery and dark green leafy vegetables, dried fruits, nuts, sunflower seeds and seafood which are all rich in potassium that can improve the balance of minerals in the body, particularly if your salt intake is high.

- Eat more artichokes, beetroot, celeriac, celery and fennel.

- If you are not a big fan of fruit and vegetables, at least try drinking a couple of glasses of fruit juice or freshly made vegetable juice daily. Don't use oranges for the juice as orange juice is a common allergen.

Useful Remedies

- Dandelion tea or tincture taken with every meal. Total 5mls daily.

- Take a digestive enzyme with all main meals.

- A strong multi-vitamin and mineral.

- Vitamin C, 1gram daily, as potassium ascorbate to encourage lymph drainage.

- *Celery Seed Extract.*, 500 mg twice daily to aid drainage **BC**

Helpful Hints

- Manual lymph drainage (MLD) can also aid this condition (see *Useful Information*). A herbal supplement like *Lympherba* is also useful for relieving congestion in the lymphatic system. **NC**

- Make an infusion with camomile tea bags and, when cool, apply to the eyes.

- **Bach** flower remedies have been found very useful for this condition, as has reflexology and facial acupuncture (see *Useful Information*).

- Lymph drainage done mechanically either through massage, reflexology or even bouncing up and down on a rebounder can be quite helpful.

- The puffy eyes may be related to an underactive thyroid so it is worth checking with your GP and getting a thyroid test.

EYE PROBLEMS – Red-rimmed eyes

- Consistently red-rimmed eyes can be a sign of malnutrition or lack of B vitamins. It can also be a sign of malabsorption of nutrients within the gut from your diet (see *Leaky Gut*).

Foods to Avoid
- Refined carbohydrates like biscuits, cakes, white bread, pizza and pasta, which all deplete the B vitamins you need for good eye health.
- Avoid caffeine in foods and drinks as these tend to over-stimulate the system and deplete B vitamins still further.

Friendly Foods
- Brown rice, wholemeal bread and pastas, lentils, barley, oat-based cereals, nuts and seeds, are rich in B vitamins which help maintain healthy eyes.
- See *Friendly Foods* under *Itchy Eyes*

Useful Remedies
- A strong B complex.
- *Dandelion and burdock tincture*, 1–3mls a day. **FSC** If the red-rimmed eyes are due to a build up of toxins, these herbs can help eliminate them from the body as well as improving liver function and digestion.
- As red-rimmed eyes can also indicate toxicity or allergies. Try Herbal Clear containing dandelion, burdock, milk thistle, vitamin C and niacin to detoxify the liver. **HN**

Helpful Hints
- Bathe the eyes in cooled camomile tea which is very soothing.
- Soak some pads in witch hazel and rose water and lay them on the eyes for 10 minutes. Use a soothing eye balm made from cucumber extract. **Body Shop** make some great natural creams.

General hints for eye problems
- If the whites of your eyes are dull or yellowish in colour – this indicates that your liver is struggling. Eat more green vegetables, fruits and wholegrains and take the herbs milk thistle and dandelion to help cleanse the liver. Eat less saturated fats, alcohol and coffee.
- *Trayner Pinhole Glasses* help strengthen weak eye muscles. Write to **Trayner Pinhole Glasses**, 12-14 Old Mill Road, Portishead, Bristol, BS20 7EG. Tel: 01749 850822.
- Try using some vibrating eye goggles, which can be placed over the eyes for a few minutes daily. They massage the area encouraging drainage of toxins and help the eyes not to feel so tired. For details call **Shakti Chakra Ltd**. 106 West Street, Erith, Kent. DA8 1AQ Tel 01322 447610. £34.50 inc p&p.
- For people like me who spend a lot of time reading and working in front of a computer screen, take breaks as often as you can, preferably in fresh air and natural sunlight.
- Get plenty of sleep.

Resolve that all situations shall turn into opportunities.

Barbara Marciniak

FATIGUE

(see *Exhaustion* and Stress)

FATS YOU NEED TO EAT

The majority of us understand that we shouldn't eat too much fat, but there is a mass of confusion about which fats we should eat and which to avoid. Most people in the West consume about 42% of their calories from fat. Unfortunately, the majority of these fats are saturated and/or animal fat which can, over time, cause hardening of the arteries. Having said this, many children especially girls are becoming obsessed with giving up all fat – this is really dangerous. If the body becomes too low in fat then chronic depression can result. The body needs the right kind of fats to encourage weight loss. Children need fat for many vital functions, to manufacture hormones in their teens and for energy production. Obviously, I do not encourage really overweight children who do little or no exercise and live on burgers, but I would never recommend that children give up all fats. Treats are fine so long as they are not living on treats.

It is very important that we ingest a good supply of essential fatty acids (EFAs) which we cannot manufacture within the body and therefore must take them in from external sources. According to Dr Udo Erasmus the world's leading authority on fats and oils 'If you have dry skin, water retention, increased thirst, physical and mental exhaustion, emotional imbalance plus inflammatory conditions such as eczema and arthritis, frequent infections, allergies, behavioural or cardiovascular disease, these are all signs of EFA deficiency'.

Various factors can interfere with the absorption of EFAs: they include ageing, saturated fats, hydrogenated oils, blood sugar problems and inadequate levels of various nutrients including magnesium, zinc, plus vitamins B and C.

There are three types of EFAs. The two biggest groups are omega 3 and omega 6. The Omega 3s are found primarily in oily fish and linseeds, also known as flax seeds. Omega 3 helps to transfer oxygen around the body, relax blood vessels, are vital for hormone production and a healthy heart. Omega 6 are found in evening primrose, starflower, blackcurrant, walnut and sesame oils. Walnuts, Brazil nuts, pecans, almonds, sunflower, pumpkin and sesame seeds are all rich in omega 6 oils which help to keep your hormones healthy. Omega 9 is the third EFA and is found in unrefined, extra virgin olive oil. Because we eat 80% less oily fish now than we did in the 1940s most people are deficient in omega 3 EFA's. A perfect ratio for good health is two parts omega 3 to one part omega 6.

Polyunsaturated oils also contain essential fatty acids, but what makes them unhealthy is if you expose them to heat or sunlight. All essential fats need to be kept cool and never heated. Mass-produced refined oils such as sunflower, safflower and vegetable oils are heated to high temperatures during the extraction process and any health benefits are long gone. Many people cook with polyunsaturated fats, margarines and oils believing this is healthier, but it is not so. Butter is actually better for cooking at low temperatures as it does not turn rancid like the essential fats. Olive oil is a monounsaturated fat which is far more stable for cooking, but never heat until it spits and produces smoke.

Foods to Avoid

■ Reduce the amount of fat in your diet from meats in general, and if you eat meat choose a lean cut, with chicken and duck always cut off the skin. If you eat bacon, grill it and cut off the fat.

■ Reduce your intake of full-fat milks, cheeses, sausages and meat pies and refined, mass-produced cakes and biscuits which are usually high in hydrogenated or trans fats, which are very bad for your health.

■ Avoid as much as possible all refined vegetable oils typically found in margarines, biscuits, cakes and shortening.

■ Eliminate or greatly reduce fried foods.

■ Remember that sugar, if not used up during exercise, turns to a hard fat inside the body.

Friendly Foods

■ If you need to shallow fry, use a little olive oil or butter – although butter is a saturated fat it does not turn rancid like vegetable oils when heated. I also use a little butter for baking cakes. For wonderful biscuits, I use olive oil.

■ Try stir frying. Use a little olive oil, heat through but not until 'spitting or smoking' then add vegetables etc and stir for a minute, I then add a little water and 'steam fry' for a couple more minutes. This helps to reduce the amounts of free radicals that are produced when you fry food.

■ Nuts like walnuts, pecans, almonds, but not peanuts are all rich in omega 6 fats.

■ Oily fish, like mackerel, salmon, sardines, tuna and herring are all rich in omega 3 fats.

■ Seeds like sunflower, pumpkin, linseeds (flax) can be eaten as a snack in their own right or just sprinkled on soups, salads and added to meals.

■ Hemp seed and hemp-seed oil are now readily available and contains both omega 3 and 6 fatty acids. They are available at all health stores or call **Viridian**. Tel: 01327 878050.

■ Eat more mono-unsaturated fats such as those found in avocados and olive oil.

■ Look for non-hydrogenated vegetable oil based spreads such as *Vitaquell* and *Biona*.

■ Only use cold pressed or extra virgin oils – as all others have been heat treated and need to be avoided. Buy high-quality sunflower, walnut, sesame and olive oils and only use them for salad dressings. Keep them in the fridge to protect the EFAs.

Useful Remedies

- *Udo's Choice Oil* is made from organic flax, sunflower and sesame seeds in the perfect ratio for good health. It is available either as an oil that can be used to mix with olive oil for salad dressings or a little can be drizzled over cooked dishes that are ready to serve. It is also available in capsules. These oils are highly unstable, they should never be heated and need to be kept in the fridge. *Udo's Choice* is available from health stores worldwide or to find your nearest stockist in the UK call 0845 0606070. **Savant Distribution Limited**, 15 Iveson Approach, Leeds, LS16 6LJ. Fax: 0113 230 1915. Website: www.savant-health.com Email: info@savant-health.com

- Other good blends of oils include *Efalex* from **Efamol** and *Essential Balance* from **Higher Nature**.

- For people who do not like the taste of these oils, you can now find butterscotch flavoured ones aimed at children and even chilli, garlic and linseed oil which are all ideal for adding to meals and dressings. **HN**

- When supplementing with fatty acids either in capsule or liquid form, it is very important to take extra vitamin E at least 100iu a day

Helpful Hints

- I use these oils for my salad dressings and they taste delicious if mixed with a drop of balsamic vinegar, extra virgin olive oil and a little honey, mustard or garlic.

- For anyone who has had their gall bladder removed, suffers Crohn's disease, colitis, has a sensitive gut, irritable bowel and cannot tolerate too much oil (as the liver has to metabolise all fats and oils) use *Dri-Celle Omega Plex* essential fatty acid powder. The EFAs have been micro-encapsulated into water-soluble fibre and then freeze-dried using no oxygen or heat. This powdered formula is therefore totally stable, which increases absorption dramatically. It bypasses the liver and is 100% absorbed in the intestines. **BC**

- For those who want to know more about this subject, Dr Udo Erasmus has written *Fats That Heal and Fats That Kill!*, Alive Books (£16-95). To order call 0845 0606070 or log onto www.savant-health.com

Every moment holds the potential for you to think of a new option.

Barbara Marciniak

FIBROIDS

A fibroid is a benign tumour made up of muscle and fibrous tissue which grows in the muscular wall of the womb. Fibroids often produce no symptoms at all but they are known to cause heavy menstrual bleeding and may contribute to infertility. The growth of fibroids seems to be related to a hormone imbalance, especially an excess of the hormone oestrogen. If you are on the combined pill or HRT, both of which contain oestrogen, you may wish to discuss coming off these drugs with your GP in order to prevent further growth. If you suffer heavy periods over several months please have this checked out. With any condition that is linked to hormones you really need to detoxify and support the liver.

Foods to Avoid

■ Any foods, which can cause elevated oestrogen levels or will recycle oestrogen into its aggressive form. These include alcohol, animal fats such as cheese, milk other than fully skimmed, most meats, cream, ice cream, butter and chocolates.

■ Don't eat and heat ready-made meals in plastic containers as the plastic residues leach into the food which, again has an oestrogen affect.

■ Avoid as much as possible non-organic foods that are often high in pesticides and herbicides – which migrate to fatty tissue and increase oestrogen activity in the body.

Friendly Foods

■ Soya-based foods such as tofu and soya beans have a regulating effect on oestrogen levels and are protective against aggressive oestrogens.

■ Chickpeas, broccoli, cabbage, Brussels sprouts and cauliflower are all beneficial foods.

■ Linseeds contain lignan which also helps to balance hormones naturally – I add a tablespoon of *Linusit Gold*, available from most supermarkets and health stores, to my breakfast cereals and vegetable juices.

■ Don't overcook your vegetables and make fresh vegetable juices every day, drink immediately after juicing.

■ Eat plenty of foods containing natural carotenes such as cantaloupe melons, apricots, sweet potatoes, parsley, carrots, spring greens, watercress and spinach. Eat more almonds, cod liver oil, avocados, wheat germ and hazelnuts which are all rich in vitamin E.

Useful Remedies

■ Soya isoflavones, 50–100mg, for regulation of hormone levels, and wild yam to help kerb excessive bleeding, 1–3ml of tincture or 1–3 grams of tablets.

■ *Agnus castus*, 1–3ml in tincture or 1–3 grams of tablets daily, a herb traditionally used to balance hormones.

■ A high-strength multi-vitamin and mineral for women. **BC HN S FSC**

■ Some women stop ovulating after 35 to 40 and therefore no longer make progesterone but continue to make oestrogen. Talk to your GP about using natural progesterone cream which can help reverse fibroids. This cream is freely available to buy outside Britain but you can order it for your own use (see under **PharmWest PW** page 15). Within the UK you need a prescription. For a list of doctors who work with natural progesterone send a SAE with a first class stamp to NPIS P.O. Box 24. Buxton. SK 17 9FB.

■ Silica and calcium fluoride tissue salts can help to break the fibroids down. 4 of each daily.

Helpful Hints

- Once you go through menopause the fibroids should shrink naturally.
- Homeopathic *Aur-mur-nat* 6x taken 3 times daily can help if there are no actual physical symptoms.

If you keep finding yourself in similar dramas – stand back and look at why you keep inviting these situations into your life.

FLATULENCE

(see also *Candida* and *Constipation*)

Flatulence, wind and bloating is to say the least unsociable and sometimes extremely uncomfortable. It can be due to partly digested foods being fermented in the gut and/or from an imbalance of the organisms that reside in the bowel. The yeast fungal overgrowth candida is often the root cause as unhealthy bacteria thrive on less healthy foods, particularly sugar, but also the bi-products of partial digestion.

It is very important that you chew your food properly as the digestive process begins in the mouth. Almost 60% of carbohydrate digestion is done in the mouth if foods are properly chewed. The majority of protein digestion is done in the stomach, so it is crucial that we have adequate levels of stomach acids and enzymes to break down the foods. Various factors can weaken our ability to digest foods properly, smoking is notorious, alcohol, sugary foods, high fat foods, caffeinated beverages and prolonged stress can all progressively weaken the digestion.

Foods to Avoid

- Beans such as cannellini, kidney, black eyed etc, plus lentils, artichokes, broccoli, Brussels sprouts, fizzy drinks and beer are all famous for causing wind. Others have problems with cabbage and onions.
- Also any food to which you have an allergy or intolerance, the most common being dairy products from cows.
- Try to note any foods which make you feel bloated or cause a lot of wind and see if there is a common denominator.
- If you have eaten a large meal, don't eat large amounts fruit directly after the meal as the fruit will ferment in the gut as it becomes stuck behind the other food, and fruit likes a fast passage through the gut. Eat fruit before or in-between meals.
- I often begin a meal with a few chunks of fresh pineapple or papaya which aid digestion.

Friendly Foods

- Certain foods help to improve digestion, noticeably fennel, celeriac, radiccio, young green celery and watercress help to stimulate gastric juices and aid digestion.

- Drinking peppermint, fennel or camomile teas or a combination after meals can often make digestion easier and make you feel more comfortable.
- Add a strip of dried *Kombu* seaweed when cooking any bean dishes, this helps to pre-digest the enzymes that cause the wind and bloating. Throw away after cooking.
- Include more fresh root ginger in your cooking which aids digestion.
- Eat more low-fat, live yoghurts.

Useful Remedies

- *Beano*, is a digestive enzyme based on alphagalactase which helps to digest plant carbohydrates, a common cause of fermentation and wind. **NC**
- Peppermint formula, a blend of herbs which help to stimulate digestion. Take 1–2mls before meals. This is also very useful if you have simply overeaten and feel uncomfortable 1–2mls generally alleviates the discomfort. **FSC**
- *Betain Hydrochloride* 1 capsule, taken prior to meals with a glass of water. This helps improve digestion which tends to weaken as we get older. If you have active stomach ulcers do not take this remedy – take the digestive enzyme instead. **FSC**
- *Acidophilus/bifidus* 1–2 capsules, taken at the end of a meal helps replace healthy gut flora which in turn helps manufacture gastric enzymes and helps to keep candida under control if this is the root cause of the problem. **BC**

Helpful Hints

- Try to eat smaller meals which place less strain on the digestive tract and liver.
- Many people have benefited from following the principle of food combining, separating carbohydrates and proteins.
- Chronic flatulence can also be a symptom of food intolerance, irritable bowel syndrome, candida or gut infections. If you are concerned, see a qualified nutritionist (see *Useful Information*).

FLU

(see *Colds*)

If you have had a heart attack, eating oily fish three times a week effectively halves your risk of having another.

Patrick Holford

FLUID RETENTION

(see *Water Retention*)

FLUORIDE

(see also *Bleeding Gums*)

Calcium fluoride occurs naturally in most drinking water and in small quantities is relatively harmless. However, artificial fluoride – hexaflurosilicilic acid is toxic. Added to drinking water in areas such as Birmingham and Newcastle it is literally a waste product scrubbed from the chimneys of phosphate fertiliser plants, brick works and aluminium smelters. Fluoride is used to make pesticides and rat poisons, it is also found in low concentrations in Californian table wines. Fluoride accumulates in bone and soft tissue and can have a devastating affect on the brain, bones and teeth. Dental fluorosis or mottling teeth is common in areas where the water is fluoridated. Since 1997 the FDA in America has required a poison label on all toothpastes containing fluoride, but in Britain there is currently no such requirement. Both the American and British Dental Associations make considerable amounts of money by endorsing fluoride toothpastes and mouth washes. The problem today is that so many products contain fluoride including toothpastes, mouthwashes, medicines (Prozac is fluoxetine), anaesthetics, pesticides and in our polluted air – and it is the accumulation of this toxin that is causing so many health problems. Currently no testing facilities to determine existing levels are available under the NHS.

In July 1997 the Union of 1500 government scientists working at the US Environmental Protection Agency issued a statement saying: 'Our review of eleven years evidence including animal and human studies indicates a causal link between fluoride/fluoridation and cancer, genetic damage and neurological impairment.' In 1994 the World Health Organisation warned 'Dental and public health administrators should be aware of the total fluoride exposure in the population before introducing any additional fluoride programmes.' Most European countries have now banned fluoride and I believe that Britain should do the same.

Foods To Avoid

■ Read labels carefully and note that tea, salmon and sardines are rich in fluorides. As much as possible avoid non-organic foods that have more than likely been sprayed with pesticides containing fluoride. If you live in a fluoridated area as much as possible drink bottled water.

Friendly Foods

■ Organic foods that are free of harmful pesticides and herbicides. Drink plenty of fluoride-free water in between meals.

■ See **General Health Hints**.

Helpful Hints

■ If you drink fluoridated tap water, do not use fluoridated toothpastes or mouthwashes.

■ Buy fluoride-free toothpastes – I found one in my local health store called *Aloe Dent* that contains aloe vera, co-enzyme Q10, tea tree Oil, silica etc which all promote healthy gums and teeth. They also make a brilliant mouthwash and for your nearest stockist log onto www.optimahealthcare.co.uk Otherwise ask at your local health store as there are several good natural brands available.

■ Young children tend to swallow toothpaste – therefore make sure it is fluoride free. To avoid fillings greatly limit your child's intake of sugary foods and drinks.

■ If you would like to test your fluoride levels there is a simple urine test. Contact **Good Health Keeping** on 01507 329100. Fax 01507 606655. Write to them at Fluoride Testing Service, Garrod House, Mamby Park, Mamby, Louth, Lincs LN11 8UT. www.good-healthkeeping.co.uk

■ For further information and the latest updates on the dangers of fluoride, log onto the **National Pure Water Association** Website on: www.npwa.freeserve.co.uk

FOOT PROBLEMS

All too many of us spend far too long on our feet. A typical person would walk 71,000 miles during their lifetime. Our feet contain 26 bones, 56 ligaments and 38 muscles so there is an awful lot that can go wrong with our often neglected feet.

Foods to Avoid

■ Refined carbohydrates and white foods like white rice, bread and pasta, sugar and refined grains. Reduce your intake of alcohol and sugary foods which also deplete vitamins and minerals that are vital for healthy bones.

■ Generally the more acid-forming the foods such as meat and dairy, the more problems you will have with your bones in later life.

■ See *General Health Hints* and *Osteoporosis*.

Friendly Foods

■ Seeds like sunflower, sesame, pumpkin and linseed are all good sources of fatty acids and calcium.

■ Nuts with the exception of peanuts are very rich sources of magnesium and fatty acids.

■ Whole grains particularly brown rice, brewer's yeast and leafy green vegetables as these are very good sources of magnesium and B vitamins.

■ Oily fish, bananas and pulses such as lentils and beans are all great bone foods.

FOOT PROBLEMS – Fallen arches

Find a good local health clinic that deals with sports injuries. If they have an in-house chiropodist or podiatrist you can be fitted for individual orthotics – inserts made specifically for your feet that give you all the support you need. Otherwise large chemists and foot specialists like **Scholl** offer a variety of inserts.

FOOT PROBLEMS – Hot burning feet

Poor circulation can cause this problem (see *Circulation*). People suffering from diabetes often have problems with circulation or nerves within the feet. Improving circulation to the feet often relieves symptoms. It can also be due to a lack of essential fatty acids found in seeds, nuts and oily fish and their unrefined oils. (see *Fats You Need To Eat*).

Useful Remedies

■ High-potency B complex daily.

Helpful Hints

■ Try using an *Energy Roller* (£23.50 inc p&p) a wooden spiked roller developed over ten years by a reflexologist. It hurts a little initially, but stimulates pressure points and many people, especially diabetics have said it has proven very helpful. For details, send a SAE to *Shakti Chakra*, 106 West Street, Erith, Kent DA8 1AQ. Tel: 01322 447610.

■ Acupuncture and reflexology are also very useful for alleviating this condition (see *Useful Information*).

FOOT PROBLEMS – Numb and tingling feet

■ If you have numb and tingling feet, take the vitamins suggested under *Circulation*, get plenty of exercise such as walking, skipping or rebounding which really help bring more blood to the feet.

■ Try reflexology and acupuncture to further improve circulation. If you have a pinched nerve you would need to see an osteopath or chiropracter. (see *Useful Information*)

■ It is very important if you have this problem for more than a few days that you see your GP to find out if there is anything more serious going on, as numb or tingling feet can be due to peripheral neuropathy which can denote late onset diabetes. A simple urine test is all that's needed. This problem could also be a calcium deficiency. Try taking 1000mg daily for a couple of weeks.

FOOT PROBLEMS – Swollen feet and ankles

(see also *Water Retention*)

This problem is common in middle-aged and older ladies.

Foods to Avoid

■ Avoid all foods high in salt such as preserved meats and fish, crisps etc. and greatly reduce the amount of salt you use in cooking. Red meat is high in sodium, so avoid meat for a few weeks. Eat chicken only once a week.

■ Don't eat any burger-type meals that are high in salt and fat also avoid sausages, mass-produced pies, cakes and biscuits.

■ Caffeine in any form, plus tea and alcohol will dehydrate the body.

■ See *General Health Hints*.

Friendly Foods.

■ Eat foods rich in potassium such as green vegetables, fresh fruit, dried fruits, nuts (not peanuts and any mass-produced nuts containing lots of salt) seafoods, and sunflower and pumpkin seeds.

■ Eat more oily fish and use unrefined walnut, olive and sunflower oils for your salad dressings.

■ Try a little magnesium-rich *Solo Salt*.

Useful Remedies

■ Celery seed extract acts like a diuretic. Take 2 capsules twice daily until symptoms ease.

■ Also take 1 gram of vitamin C as potassium ascorbate to improve lymph drainage. **BC**

■ Silica and sulphur compound for three months will help to improve tissue tone. **BLK**

■ On days when your ankles are very swollen, take *Herbal Fluid Balance* containing dandelion leaves – a potassium rich diuretic which also help to cleanse the liver. **BLK**

■ As lack of B vitamins are linked to this problem, also take a B complex plus an extra 50mg of vitamin B6 daily.

Helpful Hints

■ Sit with your feet at hip level for 15 minutes every day, moving your feet back and forth to improve circulation.

■ Rebounding (mini-trampolining) is especially good for boosting lymph drainage. Deep tissue lymphatic drainage can help if the problem is one of a stagnant lymph system.

■ If the symptoms persist after following the advice given here for more than six weeks, ask your GP for a thorough check-up as, occasionally, swollen feet and ankles may be a sign of heart, liver or kidney problems.

Taking mineral supplements at night with your evening meal increases absorption.

FROZEN SHOULDER

This condition is often characterised by pain and limited movement in one and very rarely both shoulders. It is due to the inflammation of the muscles, ligaments or tendons around the shoulders. Exercise is often very painful, however, gentle exercise which encourages blood flow and does not overstrain the joint or tendons is often helpful. It is common between the ages of 40 to 60 and affects between 2 and 5 % of the population.

Foods to Avoid

■ Avoid any foods and drinks containing caffeine which greatly reduces our body's ability to make painkilling endorphins.

■ Animal fats from meat, butter, cheese and milk will tend to increase inflammation in the body as they are acid forming.

Friendly Foods

■ Oily fish contain anti-inflammatory essential fatty acids.

■ Cherries are high in bioflavonoids which are mildly anti-inflammatory. Eat more pineapple for its bromelain content which is also anti-inflammatory.

■ Ginger, turmeric and cayenne pepper are all spices which can help decrease pain when used liberally.

Useful Remedies

■ Ginger, curcumin and boswelia, 4 or more tablets a day as needed should help reduce the inflammation. **FSC.**

■ Magnesium helps to relax the muscles – while symptoms are acute take 1000mg per day.

Helpful Hints

■ Creams made with cayenne pepper can bring rapid pain relief.

■ Bags of cherry stones or wheat can be either heated or frozen and then applied to the affected area for 10 minutes at a time to ease pain and inflammation.

■ Traditionally, frozen shoulder is treated with physiotherapy. Alternatives are chiropractice and osteopathy, which are available on the National Health in some areas

■ Magnets make powerful pain relievers – they encourage oxygenated blood to the painful area which speeds the healing process. **Homedics** make a great shoulder wrap that can easily be worn under clothes all day long (£19.99). For details call 0161 798 5876. www.homedics.co.uk

■ Use your local swimming pool, as gentle movement in warm water loosens the shoulder.

■ Acupuncture, Bowen Technique massage and aromatherapy massage with essential oil of eucalyptus, ginger and juniper are all helpful (see *Useful Information*).

Lecithin granules help to emulsify the bad fats (LDL) and improve memory.

GALL-BLADDER PROBLEMS

(see also *Gall Stones*)

The gall bladder is a small pear-shaped organ/sack, which sits underneath and is connected to the liver. The gall bladder's main function is to store bile, which is made in the liver. The gall bladder passes bile into the small bowel where it helps break down fat during digestion. If the liver is overloaded, toxins tend to get dumped in the gall bladder, a major cause of gall bladder disease. The gall bladder can be affected by gallstones, inflammation and infection. Each of the problems may produce pain on the right side encasing the centre of the abdomen. In some cases the pain can be so severe that the patient feels nauseous and faint.

Foods to Avoid
■ High-fat and fried foods put an extra load on the gall bladder and its ability to digest fats. See *General Health Hints*.

■ Alcohol and coffee place an extra strain on the liver which can make the problem worse. Many people who have gall bladder problems are overweight and tend to love creamy naughty foods – you know what I mean! Cut them out and generally eat less. Otherwise you end up having your gall bladder removed and then your body finds it difficult to metabolise fats and you will put on even more weight.

Friendly Foods
■ People who eat more beans and lentils are much less likely to end up with gall bladder or liver problems. Foods like celeriac, artichokes, beetroot and celery are all good for liver and gall bladder function.

■ Try making fresh vegetable juices daily with celery, artichoke, parsley, raw beetroot, apples, carrots, and any green vegetables you have in your fridge. Add this to half a cup of organic aloe vera and drink daily to help detoxify your liver and gall bladder.

■ Regular consumption of unrefined extra virgin olive, walnut or flax oil diminishes the risk of developing problems. Use for salad dressings.

■ Drink at least 6 glasses of water daily.

Useful Remedies
■ Milk thistle and dandelion are very effective for maintaining a healthy gall bladder. They both have the ability to enhance bile production, flow and activity. 1ml with each meal. **FSC**

■ Sprinkle one tablespoon of lecithin granules over breakfast cereals, fruit whips or yoghurts, which helps to emulsify the bad fats within the body.

■ Artichoke is a bitter tonic which aids the liver by enhancing the flow of bile. One tablet daily. **NC**

■ *Sodiphos* contains sodium sulphate and sodium phosphate which helps the flow of bile 3 tablets daily. **BLK**

■ See also *Useful Remedies* under *Gall Stones*.

Helpful Hints

■ Generally, to avoid gall bladder problems you need to control your LDL cholesterol levels and stress. See also *Cholesterol* and *Stress*.

GALLSTONES

Although up to 25% of the population have gallstones, only 15–20 % eventually develop symptoms. Gallstones are twice as common in women especially after forty. People who tend to eat high saturated fat and sugary diets that do not include sufficient fibre, are obese, constantly dieting but rapidly gain weight or suffer Crohn's Disease are at a higher risk. Multiple pregnancies, the Pill and HRT are other factors, as is a high stress level. The gall bladder gets rid of unwanted substances such as cholesterol and bilirubin into the bile duct, which in turn drains into the intestine. Most gallstones consist of a sediment made up primarily of cholesterol, bilirubin and bile salts, and occur in individuals with excess cholesterol in the bloodstream or as a result of stagnation in the gall bladder

Small gallstones produce often produce no symptoms, but if they become large enough to obstruct the bile duct they can cause jaundice, inflammation, intense pain and vomiting. Symptoms tend to be much worse after high fat meals or foods to which the individual has a sensitivity such as eggs. Constipation can be linked to the risk of gallstones so it is very important that adequate fibre is eaten to reduce the likelihood of constipation and thereby reduce the risk of developing gallstones.

Foods to Avoid

■ To avoid gall bladder attacks and gallstones you really do have to stick to a low-fat diet by greatly reducing your intake of animal fats from any source.

■ Low-fibre foods such as white bread, cakes, biscuits, ice cream, most puddings and pre-packaged meals should be avoided as much as possible.

■ Foods like eggs, pork, onions, pickles, spicy foods, peanuts, citrus fruits and sometimes coffee are likely triggers.

■ Ironically, regular coffee drinkers (that's real coffee, not decaffeinated) have a much lower risk of developing gallstones, but if you have a sensitivity to coffee then you do need to avoid it completely.

Friendly foods

■ Most important: drink plenty of water to prevent the bile from becoming too concentrated – at least 8 glasses daily.

- Small amounts of lamb plus brown rice, peas, pears and broccoli are usually no problem.
- Keep a food diary and eliminate any foods to which you have a reaction within an hour of eating them.
- Other foods which help the function of the gall bladder include beetroot, artichoke, dandelion, dried beans and legumes, linseeds, oat bran and psyllium husks, all of which are high-fibre foods ensuring you don't get constipation. Sprinkle a good tablespoonful of lecithin granules over a low-sugar oat-based muesli or cereal, as soya lecithin helps to break down the fat in foods.
- Drink dandelion tea three or four times a day. It's rather bitter so add a little honey or ginger to make it more palatable – but it helps to cleanse and stimulate the gall bladder.
- Use wholemeal bread and pasta made from corn, lentil, rice and potato flour. Include fresh fish, a little chicken without the skin, plenty of salads and fresh fruit in your diet.
- Replace full-fat milks with skimmed and try more herbal teas. Use organic rice milk.
- Enjoy one glass of white wine daily –but if you drink to excess especially on long flights – again you could be in trouble!
- Use organic extra virgin olive, sunflower and walnut oils for salad dressings – these are all rich in essential fats which help to dissolve stones.

Useful Remedies

- Milk thistle and dandelion in combination as tablets or capsules or dandelion formula. Take 1 or 2 tablets with every meal or a measure 10–20 drops of tincture with every meal. **FSC**
- People with gall stones tend to be deficient in vitamin C and E. Take 1 gram of C daily with food which is needed for the conversion of cholesterol to bile acids. 200–400iu of vitamin E.
- *Betaine Hydrochloride* (stomach acid), 1–2 capsules with meals as many people with gallstones have food intolerances and digestive problems. Many practitioners find that gall stone sufferers are deficient in stomach acid. Don't take this remedy if you have active stomach ulcers – instead take a digestive enzyme capsule with main meals. **BC**
- *Livatone Plus* is a formulation of milk thistle and other nutrients which are known to enhance the detoxification of the liver. If you take it in a powder form, try one teaspoonful twice a day or two capsules twice a day. **NC**
- Silica and calcium fluoride tissue salts can help to break down and expel the stones. 4 of each daily. **NC**

Helpful Hints

- As multiple food sensitivities are linked to gall bladder problems, it is well worth your while to consult a qualified nutritionist or naturopath who can sort out your diet. The initial few weeks may be hard but there are plenty of foods you can eat. See *Useful Information* for details.
- A reader sent the following gall bladder flush remedy to me after being advised by a top

American nutritionist. Only attempt this remedy after discussing it with your GP and it should not be tried by people who suffer Crohn's disease, colitis or irritable bowel.

1. For five days prior to the 'flush', drink 3½ pints (2 litres) of fresh, organic apple juice daily. Eat normally but avoid all saturated fats.

2. On the sixth day, have no evening meal. At 9pm take one or two tablespoons of *Epsom salts* (a laxative) dissolved in 1–2 tablespoons of warm water. At 10pm mix 115 grams unrefined olive oil with 50 grams lemon juice. Immediately upon finishing the olive oil and juice go to bed and lie on your right side with your right knee drawn up towards your chin. Remain in this position for 30 minutes before going to sleep. This encourages the olive oil to drain from your stomach, helping the contents of the gall bladder and/or liver to move into the small intestine.

3. Next morning the stones should pass. They should be green in colour and soft like putty.

Between 20,000 and 2000 BC, the average human consumed around 225 different foods annually. Today in the West up to 90% of our average calorie intake comes from just 18 different foods.

GENERAL HEALTH HINTS

■ Eat as great a variety of foods as possible, preferably locally grown and organic which contain higher levels of nutrients than foods flown thousands of miles. At last the price of organic foods is coming down and I believe that 100% organic food will help reduce many cancers and greatly alleviate the toxic load on the planet and its inhabitants.

■ In winter, eat heart-warming cooked foods and in summer choose lighter meals with plenty of raw foods and fresh fruit. In winter, I make fruit compotes and grill fruit which makes it easier to digest.

■ Make time for breakfast which is the most important meal of the day. You are literally breaking a fast and to keep your blood sugar on an even keel you need to eat, or you will end up craving sugary snacks by mid morning. Oat, spelt, quinoa, kamut and low-sugar based cereals or sugar-free muesli make an ideal breakfast for most people with skimmed milk or try organic oat, rice, soya, sheep's or goat's milk. Protein helps to wake up your brain, hence why eggs, grilled fish or lean meat also make great breakfasts. Otherwise wholemeal bread toasted with a non-hydrogenated spread such as *Vitaquell* or *Biona* and a little honey or low-sugar jam is fine. If you cannot face breakfast, at least take with you an apple or a couple of bananas and a yoghurt to eat later.

- Drink at least six glasses of filtered, bottled or distilled water daily. If you suffer from digestive problems, avoid drinking too much fluid with food because it dilutes the digestive juices, which can lead to poor digestion of food and reduced absorption of nutrients.

- Cut down on tea, coffee, alcohol and caffeinated soft drinks, which dehydrate the body. For every caffeinated or alcoholic drink – you need 8ozs (250ml) of water.

- The additives, artificial sweeteners (especially aspartame) and sugar in soft drinks and foods can cause hyperactivity and mood swings. Sugar depletes the body of vital minerals such as chromium and magnesium. Forget low-calorie drinks, they are a waste of time, they place a strain on your liver which slows weight loss. If you find yourself craving sweet foods take 200 mcg of chromium daily. After a few days it will kick in and you will crave sugar less.

- Remember it's the foods and drinks you crave the most that are often causing most of your health problems.

- Drink more herbal teas, dandelion coffee or barley drinks.

- Aim to eat at least three pieces of fresh, whole fruit and three portions of vegetables plus a salad daily. The darker green the leaves, the more nourishing they are. Three portions of cabbage a week can reduce the incidence of colon cancer by as much as 60%

- Steam vegetables when possible, as boiling destroys vitamins. Many pesticides, especially the organophosphates (OPs) seep right through the vegetables and fruit and cannot be washed off. They are now linked with many cancers and lowered sperm counts.

- Keep food simple – say 'no' to rich foods with rich sauces and to fried and barbecued and burnt foods which are carcinogenic.

- Avoid pre-packaged, takeaway and tinned foods whenever possible, as they are often packed with fat, salt, sugar and additives. Also a great majority of these foods are packed in aluminium containers, and aluminium has long been linked to Alzheimer's and senile dementia.

- Do not add sodium-based salt to your food as it can aggravate water retention and cause blood pressure to rise. Our typical diet contains 9 grams of salt a day and it has been estimated that if we can reduce salt consumption to 3 grams per person per day it would save 70,000 deaths in Britain each year. There are plenty of magnesium- and potassium-based sea salts freely available from supermarkets and health stores.

- Do not become fanatical about fad diets. Everything in moderation and keep a balance of foods at all times for good nutrition. I love cakes but try and bake them only once a week! I bake cakes with butter, which does not become rancid like some hard margarines when cooked. Use organic rice syrup, honey or fresh fruit instead of sugar. Or soak some dried fruits in warm water, drain, chop and add to the cake mix.

- Use extra virgin cold-pressed olive oil in cooking and try walnut or cold-pressed sunflower or sesame oils for salad dressings. These oils have many health benefits from lowering cholesterol to keeping your skin looking younger (see *Fat You Need to Eat*).

- Eat your meals sitting down – or at least standing still! Chew your food thoroughly, if you bolt your food your body will tell you. Aid digestion by eating fruit between meals and not as a dessert. Fruit can ferment when eaten after a large meal causing wind and bloating.

- Cow's milk is often a problem for many people. Skimmed milk is higher in sugar (lactose) and many people are intolerant to this. Try organic oat, soya, pea or rice milk which are non-dairy. Also use sheep's or goat's products and eat plenty of live, low-fat yoghurt, which contain beneficial gut bacteria and is a rich source of calcium.

- Avoid any foods and oils that contain hydrogenated or trans fats – these are the bad guys.

- Wheat-based cereals, especially wheat bran, seem to cause bowel problems for many people. Use oat-based cereals, oat and rice bran or wheat germ instead. Try lentil, rice, corn, spinach and potato based flours and pastas.

- Try to avoid red meat, which can putrefy in the gut and may contain antibiotic and chemical residues. If you adore meat gentlemen, please don't eat more than 100 grams at one meal and ladies keep it to 50–75 grams. Other great proteins are fish, free range eggs, low-fat cheese, chicken, turkey, tofu, beans and lentils.

- Avoid smoking and smoky atmospheres.

- Make time to relax. When we are stressed the body starts pumping the hormone adrenalin ready for the fight or flight response. Eventually this can cause us to blow a fuse. It can be a gastric fuse, leading to ulcers, or a heart fuse causing heart attacks, etc. The body and mind are one. If you are stressed, something has got to give in the end. Vitamins, minerals and diet alone will not keep you healthy. Stress is a major factor. Remember you are special, give yourself the odd treat and make space every day in your diary for yourself.

- Get plenty of fresh air and learn to breathe deeply; this aids relaxation. Deep breathing also helps to alkalise the body. Stress makes it too acid.

- Sunlight is great for your health and without it you can become very ill indeed. Moderate sunbathing is fine with sun screens; just stay out of the mid-day sun. As a general rule never let your skin go red.

- Learn to have a good laugh regularly and don't be afraid to laugh at yourself – lighten up.

- Take regular, sensible exercise which is one of the best favours you can do for your health. Brisk walking, cycling, light jogging, swimming, skipping, aerobics and aqua aerobics as these exercises have the most health-related benefits. You will be amazed at the difference regular exercise can make to your overall well-being. If you do nothing else, try to walk for 30 minutes daily, preferably away from main roads

- Gradual lifestyle changes are of much greater benefits than 2 –4 day fad diets.

- Over time your taste buds will come to love healthier foods.

- Generally eat smaller meals more regularly rather than eating huge meals which place an enormous strain on the liver and digestive system. Losing weight is easier if you practise this way of eating which also keeps blood sugar on an even keel thus preventing mood swings.

- Get into blending and juicing. This is a fantastic way to ingest huge amounts of nutrients quickly. Buy yourself a blender and twice a week make the following cocktail; 1 table-spoon of sunflower or flax seeds, 1 teaspoon of a green powder mix, 1 dessertspoon of organic GM-free lecithin granules, a teaspoon of raw wheat germ, 2 ready-

g

to-eat prunes or apricots, one box of blueberries, a fresh or dried fig, half a chopped apple, a kiwi, a banana, or any fruit you love. To this add half a cup of aloe vera juice and half a cup of organic rice or soya milk. Blend the lot for a minute and drink as a meal replacement. It's neat fibre and vitamins, minerals and essential fats.

- With a juicer, on alternate days make yourself fresh raw vegetable juices, again adding any extras such as the aloe, fresh root ginger, a few drops of any herbal tinctures you like especially dandelion and burdock to cleanse the liver and drink immediately after juicing whilst the beneficial enzymes are still alive.

No-one ever had engraved on their tomb stone 'I wish I had spent more time at the office' – get a balance in your life. Enjoy the journey.

GENERAL SUPPLEMENTS FOR BETTER HEALTH

Supplements that I take every day.

1. An organic dried green food supplement powder made up from ingredients such as alfalfa, wheat grass, chlorella, broccoli, seaweed, seeds and so on which are all packed with vitamins, minerals, essential fats and fibre in a highly digestible form. In the West the majority of us eat too many acid-forming foods such as bread, cakes and animal protein which triggers acid conditions such as arthritis. My current favourites are Dr Gillian McKeith's *Living Food Energy Powder*, available from any health store. Or *Alkalife* powder and *Alkaherb* tea both of which are available from most health stores or call 01342 410303 or www info@bestcare-uk.com for your nearest stockists. Most importantly these super-rich green foods are alkaline as well as helping to detoxify the system. They are also a rich source of protein, iron, calcium, vitamin C, natural carotenes and fibre.

2. Many people believe that low-fat or no-fat diets are healthy. In fact we all need essential fats to function. Take one tablespoon of organic sunflower, pumpkin, sesame or linseeds every day or take an essential fatty acid supplement like evening primrose oil, starflower oil, GLA or linseed oil. For details of all types of EFA's see under *Fats You Need to Eat*). These essential fats protect your heart, digestive system, keep your skin supple and improve hormone and brain function.

3. Give your immune system a boost by taking 1 gram of vitamin C in an ascorbate form, plus a multi-vitamin/mineral each day such as Kudos 24 nutrient powder – Tel: 0800 389 5476. Any multi you take should contain 200-400iu of natural source vitamin E, 10–30mg of natural beta-carotene and 100–200mcg of selenium. Co-enzyme Q

10 helps protect against cancer and heart disease and raises energy levels, 30–60mg daily. These levels are not available in a normal diet. Prevention is always better than cure!

4. Take one acidophilus/bifidus capsule daily. This replenishes the good bacteria in the gut and helps prevent many problems like candida, yeast overgrowth, constipation and an over-acid system, caused not only by our diet but the chemicals we inhale from the air. Acidophilus/bifidus capsules should always be kept in the fridge and taken with meals for four to six weeks, periodically.

The more fats healthy or otherwise you ingest the more natural vitamin E you need. Take 200iu a day.

GLANDULAR FEVER

Glandular fever is caused by the Epstein Barr virus. It usually affects people between the ages of 15 and 25 when the immune system is developing, hence the nickname of the 'kissing virus'. Symptoms include a severe sore throat, fever, swollen glands in the neck and a feeling of overwhelming exhaustion. Initially it can appear similar to a bad dose of flu but after a few days it becomes obvious that it is not flu and symptoms can continue for several months. The liver can be affected and some sufferers develop a mild hepatitis caused by the virus. Antibiotics are inappropriate because it is a viral infection, and certain strengths of antibiotics can actually make this illness much worse.

Bed rest and good nutrition are essential to help prevent a relapse, but unfortunately this often coincides with stressful academic studies making life rather difficult. It is one of those diseases where you can appear to make a recovery then a month later experience a relapse. For some individuals this can lead to chronic fatigue syndrome or ME (see under *ME*). The more you rest when the problem is first diagnosed the more likely you are to make a complete recovery. The yeast fungal overgrowth Candida often occurs with Glandular fever (see *Candida*).

Foods to Avoid
- I'm afraid it's a question of really cleaning up the diet.
- Avoid all pre-packaged ready-made meals unless they are freshly prepared.
- No more hamburgers and eating sugary snacks on the run.
- Colas and fizzy drinks often contain up to 10 teaspoons of sugar, and sugar in any form will greatly deplete immune function.
- White bread, croissants, Danish pastries, cakes, chocolate snacks, crisps, pork and sausage pies and all these instant type foods should be avoided for a few weeks.

149

- If you know you have a problem with certain foods, the most common being wheat and dairy from cow's milk, eliminate them for two weeks.
- Stimulants like caffeine, colas, alcohol and tea can overload the body giving brief bursts of energy but actually reducing it in the long-term.

Friendly Foods

- Try to eat plenty of fresh fruit and vegetables rich in magnesium and natural source carotenes such as spring greens, cabbage, sweet potatoes, dried apricots, parsley, broccoli, spinach, and all orange fruits.
- If you have a juicer, try a mixture of carrots, beetroot, tomatoes, green pepper, a little bit of garlic and onion. Cook with garlic and onions.
- Make rich soups and stews with added fresh ginger.
- If you prefer fruit juices try lemon, orange, kiwi, banana and pineapple to which you could add a teaspoon of dried wheat grass powder.
- Plenty of good quality high-protein foods such as fresh fish, chicken, tofu, beans and lentils, plus free range eggs all help to support the immune system.
- Eat more wholemeal breads and pastas, jacket potatoes plus brown rice, porridge made with rice milk and low-sugar cereals.
- Eat more low-fat, live yoghurts to help replenish healthy bacteria in the gut.
- Drink at least 6 glasses of water daily
- Coriander and parsley are packed with nutrients.

Useful Remedies

- Vitamin C is anti-viral and anti-bacterial. While symptoms are acute take 5–6 grams daily with food in an ascorbate form and after a couple of weeks reduce this to 1 gram daily for several months. If this causes loose bowels reduce dose to just below bowel tolerance. **BC**
- A high strength multi-mineral and vitamin, as when we're fighting an infection we are often depleted in minerals especially calcium, magnesium and zinc. **HN**
- Vitamin A 25,000iu can be taken daily for one month to help fight the infection. Only take 5,000iu if you are pregnant.
- Anti-viral herbs such echinacea, hypericum, astragalus, liquorice and Siberian ginseng are all anti-viral. 5mls daily of each.

Helpful Hints

- A gradual return to normal life is necessary because over-activity too soon can cause a relapse.
- Homeopathic Ailanthus glandulosa 6c three times daily for 10 days should help reduce symptoms dramatically.
- Check for possible iron deficiency with your doctor and take iron if necessary (see

Anaemia). If, after two months, your energy and appetite have not returned, contact a qualified nutritionist (see *Useful Information*).

GLUE EAR (OTITIS MEDIA)
(see also *Earache*)

The Eustachian tube is a pathway that allows the equalisation of air pressure between the middle ear and the back of the throat, through which bacteria can enter the middle ear. Ear infections are one of the most common childhood ailments. They are also likely to re-occur over a relatively short space of time. These infections can be very painful. It is understandable that parents would want to give the child immediate relief, the normal treatment being either antibiotics or the insertion of a grommet in the ear drum. Neither of these treatments is particularly effective. In fact almost 90% of children with glue ear have food allergies (see *Allergies*). Identifying allergies is often very difficult and it's also very important you don't suddenly eliminate a whole group of foods and leave the child malnourished. The most common culprits are wheat and dairy from cows. Children who are breast fed are less likely to develop ear infections.

One other odd thing that seems to increase the risk of inner ear infections is the use of dummies when children are very young.

Foods to Avoid
■ Sugar is top of the list, as it weakens the immune system leaving people more prone to infections. Other than sugar it is very important that the food intolerances or allergies are identified as these are likely to be the primary cause. Typically they would include dairy from cows, eggs, wheat and citrus fruits such as oranges, grapefruit, lemons and limes, but it could be any one of a number of other food groups.

■ Keep your child off mucous-forming foods such as full-fat cheeses, pizzas, Greek yoghurts, white breads and cakes, full-fat milk, chocolates and so on.

■ Remember that many canned drinks contain up to 10 spoonfuls of sugar, and artificial sweeteners are a nightmare for individuals with allergies.

■ Try to avoid preservative and additives.

■ Don't fry food.

Friendly Foods
■ Fresh fruit and vegetables are rich in vitamin C, which will boost the immune system.

■ Garlic helps to fight infections

■ Chewing gum made with xylitol seems beneficial as children who chew xylitol-sweetened chewing gum have a much lower rate of inner ear infections.

■ Introduce your child to lower saturated fat but highly nutritious foods such as brown rice, barley, lentils, pulses and as a treat give them rice or oat cakes.

- There are numerous health cookery books giving great recipes for cookies, biscuits and cakes that are low in fat and sugar.
- There are plenty of low-fat, live fruit yoghurts freely available that replenish healthy bacteria in the gut which helps fight infection.
- Use rice or oat milk and bake cakes with barley, rice, potato or spelt flours.
- Use non-hydrogenated spreads such as Vitaquell or Biona.

Useful Remedies

- Echinacea either as tincture or tablets. Tincture is often easier for children as it can be added to fruit juice or yoghurt. If the child is very small use one drop per 6kilos of body weight. It can be used several times a day but shouldn't be used for longer than 2–3 weeks without a break.
- Vitamin C 1–2 grams daily with food during an infection, half to 1 gram as a maintenance. Again, as a lot of children don't like tablets, vitamin C is often available as a powder, some of them fairly pleasant tasting or you can find ones that can be added to fruit juice and the flavour of the fruit juice is what the child will taste. Alternatively use a vitamin crusher. For details call **Health Plus** on 01323 737374.
- Zinc lozenges and zinc supplements can be given to a child. 1–2 lozenges a day while the child has an infection. Zinc boosts the immune function and helps to fight the infection. 25mg daily.
- A child's chewable multi-vitamin and mineral. **HN**
- *Potassium Chloride* helps to unblock the Eustachian tube – 100mg daily. **BLK**

Helpful Hints

- A humidifier placed in the main living room or the child's bedroom has been found to reduce the risk of inner ear infections.
- Many nutritionalist doctors advocate that your child should not be subjected to vaccinations until the cycle of ear infections is cleared, as vaccines place a strain on the child's immune system.
- Use *Mullein Flower oil* as ear drops – available from health stores.
- Use *Hopi Ear Candles* to remove excess wax. This is a pain-free way to reduce some of the pain and must be done by a responsible or qualified adult. **NC**
- Cranial osteopathy helps as it encourages lymph drainage. See *Useful Information*.
- Do not let the child be exposed to cigarette smoke – it increases the incidence of glue ear by 80%.

*If you sweat to excess when you are not exercising you may be low in
zinc – take 30mg daily.*

GOUT

Gout is a form of joint inflammation, which is caused by high levels of uric acid in the blood causing crystal deposits in the joints. It is very common in the big toe but can also affect other joints and the kidneys. The vast majority of gout sufferers are men but more and more women are beginning to suffer gout. An attack can be triggered by eating overly rich food, typically this would include shellfish, cheeses like Stilton, port, red meat and red wine. Most people who suffer gout tend to drink a lot anyway – especially champagne. Occasionally an accident or trauma to the body can precipitate an attack.

In the 18th century you were considered fortunate to develop gout as they thought this prevented you from contracting fatal diseases. It was seen as a rich person's disease because only those who could afford large amounts of meat, cheese and wine were likely to suffer.

Foods to Avoid

■ Any foods which are rich in purines, found in high protein foods such as offal, oily fish including anchovies, chicken, caffeine, shellfish including crab, lobster, scallops, roe and mussels, kidney, lima or navy beans, yeast based drinks like Marmite and Bovril, oatmeal porridge and lentils.

■ Avoid full-fat cheeses especially Stilton and goat's cheeses.

■ Most forms of arthritis usually benefit from taking cod liver oil or eating oily fish, however, with gout these foods would almost certainly make it worse.

■ Malted drinks such as *Horlicks* are a problem for some people.

Friendly Foods

■ Cherries and pineapple should be eaten on a daily basis, cherries in particular. They are one of the easiest ways of keeping gout under control and preventing it, as they increase excretion of uric acid from the body.

■ If you are not a fan of cherries, try eating blueberries or bilberries, both are very rich in bioflavonoids which help reduce uric acid levels in the body.

■ A macrobiotic diet, although hard to follow, would almost certainly eliminate the gout.

■ Eat plenty of fruit and vegetables especially celery, quinoa, millet, brown rice and pastas made from corn, rice potato and buckwheat flours.

■ Free range eggs, soya tofu and lamb should not cause any problems.

■ Make a healthy drink containing a small boxful of blueberries, pineapple, frozen or fresh pipped cherries, a pear, an apple and a banana. Add a teaspoon of a green food powder and a tiny piece of fresh root ginger. Put in a blender with half a cup of rice or light soya milk, whizz for one minute and drink immediately.

■ Drink at least 6 glasses of water every day to encourage excretion of the uric acid.

Useful Remedies

■ Vitamin C, 1–2 grams a day taken with food will gradually help lower uric acid levels.

■ Bromelain 2,000–4,000mcu a day, this is a very powerful anti-inflammatory.

■ Ginger, curcumin and boswelia 4 capsules, or more, a day. These herbs in combination provide relief from any type of inflammation discomfort. **HN**

■ Devils claw, 400mg 3 times a day for at least 3 months or more. This herb can gradually help lower uric acid levels as well as improving bowel function. Do not take this herb if you are pregnant. **FSC**

Helpful Hints

■ Lose weight as this is quite often part of the problem. Remember the gout is pretty much self-inflicted and almost entirely brought on by a poor diet. Be prepared to make some changes.

■ Nettle tea will also excretion of uric acid.

■ Massage the painful joint with essential oil of Roman camomile, juniper and ginger to help reduce the pain and inflammation.

■ Homeopathic *Ledum 30c* twice daily for 2–3 days will reduce symptoms.

■ Do not take aspirin if taking anti-gout drugs.

GUMS

(see *Bleeding Gums*)

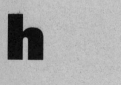

HAEMORRHOIDS

(see *Piles*)

Regular deep breathing helps to re-alkalise the body.

HAIR LOSS

The health of the hair depends on the circulation to the root of the hair and the amount of nutrients present in the blood. Hair is composed of protein and minerals and requires a healthy balanced diet for proper nourishment. It is thought that men lose hair on the top of their heads rather than the back and sides because the blood flow to the top of their scalp is reduced in comparison to lower down. When a person is very stressed the scalp becomes very tight resulting in restricted circulation and the hair follicle becomes malnourished resulting in further hair loss. Adrenal exhaustion is definitely a factor in hair loss.

Hair loss amongst middle aged female and male executives is becoming increasingly common, demonstrating that stress is definitely a trigger for hair loss. Another important factor is the male hormone testosterone. Although this is the hormone responsible for making men hairy during puberty, it also has a big part to play in hair loss from the scalp in later life. Hereditary factors are also important. The more hair loss there is/was in your father, uncles and grandfather, the more likely you are to lose your own hair, however, dietary supplements and regular daily firm scalp massage can help slow down hair loss. Hair loss in women often follows childbirth, the menopause; and protein deficiency can thin hair or cause it to fall out. Hair loss is also linked to heavy metal toxicity.

Foods to Avoid

- Greatly reduce the amount of caffeine from any source, which increases stress and weakens the adrenal glands.
- Avoid sugar and refined carbohydrates which all deplete the nutrients that we need for hair growth. See *General Health Hints*.

Friendly Foods

- Include plenty of high quality protein foods like lean meat, fish and proteins from vegetable sources like beans and pulses.
- Iron deficiency is sometimes linked with hair loss. Foods which are rich in iron include egg yolks, green leafy vegetables, whole-grain breads, cereals, meat and fish.
- Try adding some seaweeds like kombu, hiziki and arame to meals. Use them as you would a green vegetable, as they are a very rich source of minerals needed for healthy hair.
- Essential fats are vital for healthy hair therefore eat more oily fish, unsalted nuts and seeds.
- Use unrefined organic walnut, sunflower or linseed oils and olive oil for salad dressings.
- Coriander detoxifies the body of heavy metals and is full of nutrients especially B vitamins.
- Muesli, cereals and oats are all high in B vitamins.

Useful Remedies

- Zinc 30mg daily is essential for hair and nail growth.
- Vitamin B6, 50mg per day is helpful for women taking the contraceptive pill which can affect hair loss.
- Have a test and see if you are low in iron, in which case take a liquid easily absorbable formula such as *Spatone*. Available from health shops worldwide.

- *CT 241* plus *Colleginase* which contain vitamin C, rutin, hesperidin, cellulose, silica, vitamins A and D to strengthen hair and nails. **BC.**

- If you are stressed and with age, the body's ability to absorb nutrients is often impaired. *Betaine Hydrochloride* (stomach acid), 1 capsule with meals, helps enhance absorption of nutrients from a good diet. Do not take stomach acid if you have active stomach ulcers – use a digestive enzyme instead.

- A high strength B complex as a lack of B group vitamins such as biotin and folic acid are linked to hair loss **BLK**

Helpful Hints

- Take regular aerobic exercise, which will stimulate your heart and circulation increasing oxygen flow, reducing stress and promoting scalp and hair health.

- Jojoba oil mixed with a little essential oil of rosemary and massaged into the scalp removes old layers of cells and increases circulation.

- Uri Geller keeps his hair thick and healthy by practising daily yoga head or shoulder stands which increases circulation to the scalp.

- Some people suffering alopecia as a side effect of severe stress have found hypnotherapy really helpful (see *Useful Information*).

- For further information contact *Action Against Alopecia*, 7 West Terrace, Eastbourne, East Sussex, BN21 4QX. Tel: 0845 055 1402. Website: www.eucaderm.com Email: hair@mistral.co.uk

- To find your nearest qualified trichologist call 08706 070602 or visit the **Institute of Trichologists** at www.trichologists.org.uk. I highly recommend Mr Philip Kingsley in London on 0207 6294004.

- Contact Mr Chris Pick who is a naturopath and clinical nutritionist on 01798 343568. Website: www.life-force-clinical-nutrition.com

- Many people report that using *Romanda* lotion and shampoos, along with *Romanda* hair formula vitamins, improves hair growth. Call Jan Adams on the Romanda Advice Line on 020 8346 0784, or write to *Romanda Healthcare*, Romanda House, Ashley Walk, London, NW7 1DU. Jan really is incredibly helpful and formed the company after suffering hair loss. She really is a gem, www.romanda-healthcare.com

As lack of vitamin D is linked to SAD syndrome, take cod liver oil daily in the winter.

HALITOSIS (Bad Breath)

Bad breath is often caused by poor dental hygiene. A build up of plaque, infected gums, abscesses, and insufficient brushing and flossing are mostly to blame. Make sure you see a qualified dental hygienist at least twice a year. Use fluoride free floss and mouth wash daily, change your toothbrush regularly and clean your teeth at least twice a day, preferably after every meal.

Poor digestion, a sluggish bowel and liver can also cause bad breath. Foods such as meat take a long time to digest and can putrefy in the bowel. One of the simple things you can do is to chew properly as this enhances carbohydrate digestion and makes it easier for the rest of the digestive process. Try not to eat too much food at one sitting which overloads the stomach and bowel.

Some people find their digestion has improved if they avoid eating proteins and carbohydrates together in one meal. for example, If you are eating chicken or fish (protein) eat them only with vegetables – conversely if you eat rice or pasta eat them only with vegetables and not protein. Long-term bad breath can indicate problems with the liver, kidneys or diabetes in which case you must consult a doctor.

Foods to Avoid

- Avoid too much caffeine, sugar and low-fibre, high-fat foods which all weaken the digestion and cause sluggish bowel movements.
- Smoking not only causes bad breath directly it can also in the long term as it weakens digestion.
- Cut down on the amount of milk and dairy produce from cows which is mucous forming and slows bowel function.

Friendly Foods

- Leafy green vegetables such as pak choi, spring greens, kale, cabbage etc are rich in chlorophyll. Chlorophyll is useful in helping to clear the bowel and make breath smell fresher.
- Eat more artichokes and chicory.
- Eat plenty of fresh whole fruits. Pineapple or papaya eaten as a dessert at the end of a meal is a good idea as the enzymes in these fruits can help break down the proteins ensuring proper digestion.
- A 'bio' or live yoghurt either for breakfast or as a dessert containing acidophilus and bifidus improves the quality of the bacteria in the bowel enhancing digestion and making bad breath less likely.
- Add more coriander and fresh mint to foods and eat fennel or caraway seeds which help kill the bacteria that cause bad breath.
- Drink fenugreek tea.
- Drink plenty of water.

Useful Remedies

- *Betaine Hydrochloride* (stomach acid), 1 capsule taken with a meal improves protein digestion and ensures that foods completely digested don't arrive at the bowel causing fermentation. Not to be taken if you have active stomach ulcers.

- Take a *Digestaid*, containing enzymes that help break down foods, at the end of a meal to improve digestion. **BC**

- *Acidophilus and Bifidus* capsules with FOS (fructo-oligosaccharides) which increase healthy baceria. 1–2 capsules taken at the end of the meal can increase healthy bacteria in the bowel and enhance digestion. **BC**

- Take 5–6 drops of *Chlorophyll* daily to help eliminate bad breath.

- Sprinkle 1–3 dessert spoonfuls of linseeds or sunflower seeds over salads, breakfast cereals and so on to encourage toxins to move more quickly through the bowel.

Helpful Hints

- Make up your own healthy mouthwash using a few drops of essential oils of tea tree, peppermint, thyme and lemon. Mix with warm water and use regularly after meals and before bed. I make mine up with boiled water, allow it to cool and then I keep the blend in a dark bottle in my bathroom and it lasts for ages.

- Exercise regularly as this ensures healthy bowel function.

- If the bad breath is severe, with your doctor's permission, have a colonic irrigation, which gently washes out the bowel helping to reduce toxicity (see *Useful Information*).

- Contact the *Fresh Breath Centre*, Conan Doyle House, 2 Devonshire Place, London, W1N 1PA or call 020 7935 1666. Website: www.freshbreath.co.uk

HANGOVERS

(see *Alcohol*)

The herb *Kudzu* helps reduce cravings for alcohol and reduces hangovers.

HAYFEVER

(see also *Allergies and Allergic Rhinitis*)

Hayfever is caused by an allergic reaction to pollen produced by grasses and trees that mainly flower in the spring and summer. Symptoms vary from sore, puffy, itchy, watering eyes, to continual sneezing and a runny or congested nose. Hay fever is sometimes confused with a condition called allergic or perennial rhinitis, as the symptoms are similar to hayfever but occur all year round. Common causes of allergic rhinitis include dust, food allergies and atmospheric pollution. Many people with hayfever and allergic rhinitis are also likely to have a sensitivity to certain foods, the most common being wheat and dairy, but some sufferers have problems with anything from eggs to bananas. As this has been linked to digestive problems for some people, see also *Leaky Gut*.

Foods to Avoid

- Any foods to which you have an allergy or intolerance; typically these would include wheat, dairy products, eggs and citrus fruits – especially oranges.

- Dairy foods are mucous forming and without doubt can exacerbate the problem. While symptoms are acute avoid milk in any form for at least one week, plus cheeses, chocolate, foods high in saturated fats such as croissants, Danish pastries, meat pies and white-flour-based cakes and biscuits.

- Many foods high in sugar such as puddings and sweets are also high in dairy and fats. Too much sugar will greatly lower immune function.

- Reduce salt, additives, caffeine and alcohol.

Friendly Foods

- Garlic and onions are high in the flavonoid quercetin which can help reduce the severity of allergic reactions.

- Nettle tea helps to ease the symptoms of allergic rhinitis.

- Dairy-free alternatives to cow's milk are rice, oat and pea milk.

- Have a freshly squeezed vegetable juice in the morning, especially beetroot, artichoke, a little garlic, ginger, apple and carrot which boosts the immune system and help eliminate toxins.

- Bioflavonoids are important protectors of mucous membranes, therefore eat plenty of blueberries, blackberries, strawberries, kiwi fruit and include plenty of fresh vegetables, brown rice and whole grains in your diet.

Useful Remedies

- *Quercetin* 400mg 3 times a day, is a natural anti-histamine which can helps reduce puffy eyes and reduce irritation in the nose.

- While symptoms are acute, take up to 2–3 grams of vitamin C daily in an ascorbate form with food, which acts like a mild anti-histamine.

- Nettle tablets or tincture 3 times a day has proven to be effective for allergic rhinitis.

- Garlic, ginger and horseradish tincture as all of these herbs can ease congestion and reduce the symptoms of hay fever, take 1–2ml as needed. **FSC**

- *Oralmat* is an extract of the rye plant which has proven in medical trials to be hugely successful in reducing allergies of all kinds. It supports healthy respiratory function by strengthening defences against allergens. Dr Princetta, a specialist in the treatment of allergies in Atlanta, Georgia, reports: 'The South-eastern United States, and Atlanta, Georgia, in particular, is a well-known allergy area of the world. Even some of my worst allergy patients responded very well to the drops and suffered a minimum of 50 percent less this past spring.' Take 3 drops under the tongue (hold 30 seconds or longer) 3 times daily. Children can use one drop. **NC**

- *Histazyme* contains calcium, vitamin C, the amino acid lysine, zinc, vitamin B6, silica,

159

bromelain, vitamin A and manganese which all help if you suffer seasonal disorders. Take one capsule twice daily. This formula is not to be taken if you are pregnant. **BC**

■ If nothing else, take a high-strength multi-vitamin and mineral that contains plenty of the B group vitamins, at least 200iu of vitamin E, 7500 iu of vitamin A and 500mg of C. **HN S**

Helpful Hints

■ Buy a pot of honey from your local area, preferably with the honeycomb still in it, and take a dessertspoonful daily for about a month before the onset of the hayfever season. The pollen in the honey may protect you from developing full-blown hayfever. New research shows that the plant extract Butterbur helps relieve the cold-like symptoms associated with hayfever.

■ *Alka Life* is a green herbal food supplement rich in bee pollen. Sprinkle daily over breakfast cereal for at least one month prior to the hayfever season to help reduce the severity or onset of an attack. Available from all good health stores or call *Best Care Products* on 01342 410303. Fax 01342 410909. e mail: info@bestcare-uk.com

■ Homeopathy has been successful in treating hayfever with remedies like allium cepa, euphrasia and arundo. Ask for details at your local homeopathic pharmacy or to find a qualified practitioner in your area (see *Useful Information*).

■ Place a few drops of essential oil of basil and melissa on a handkerchief to help clear the sinuses. Massage these oils into the chest and throat once mixed with a base carrier oil such as almond or jojoba.

■ A company specialising in indoor air quality equipment is the **Air Improvement Centre Ltd**. They can be contacted at 23 Denbigh Street, Victoria, London, SW1V 2HF. Tel: 020 7834 2834. Fax: 020 7630 8485. Website: www.air-improvement.co.uk

■ It is always a good idea to check for food allergies when you suffer severe hayfever as many foods 'cross-react' with pollen. See a kinesiologist who can help you to find specific allergens (see *Useful Information*) or call **Noma** on 023 8077 0513 for details of the nearest Vega test (allergy test) practitioner in your area (8.30 am–4.30 pm, Monday to Friday and 8.30am–1.00pm on Fridays).

Imagination is more Important than knowledge.
Albert Einstein

HEADLICE

(see *Scalp Problems*)

Deadlines kill people. Don't accept unreasonable deadlines.

HEALING AND HEALERS

Research from the University of Maryland's School of Medicine in 2000 has confirmed what healers have known intuitively for over 2000 years, that hands on healing and the power of prayer are not figments of our imagination. Many people still believe that healing cannot work unless one has a specific religious belief or strong faith that the healing will work. Yet there are hundreds of documented cases where young babies, children and animals have benefitted from healing. To understand how healing works, it is imperative for us all to understand that we are all electrical beings in a physical shell. If you take a photograph using Kirlian cameras you can clearly see the energy or auric field surrounding a person, animal, plant, vegetable – in fact any object, even a stone will have an auric field. Roger Coghill, a bio-electromagnetics research scientist based in Gwent in the UK, says 'The entire universe is filled with tiny charged particles called electrons and when one single electron moves, it affects every single electron in the universe. Human beings are filled with electrons, and an individual's electronic energy field or aura, is as unique to them as their DNA. When we become ill, our field's characteristics change, this was proven by the American neurologist Albert Abrams in 1916.'

After my near-death experience in 1998, which is well documented in my book *Divine Intervention, Cima Books*, I truly began to comprehend how healing works. In my heightened spiritual state, which lasted for several months, I knew that there is an invisible part of every one of us that is always in a state of perfection. And this perfection is a frequency. When we become sick, cells begin emitting a disharmonic frequency which can clearly be seen in our energy field. I was able to see auric fields and when I saw a large blob of red, for instance near someone's liver area, I knew this was where their health problem lay. Also if I scanned my hands over a person, I could feel painful emissions from injury sites.

A healer simply pulses a correcting frequency into the patient's energy field, which encourages the body to heal itself. There are now electronic devices such as the *Bicom* (available at the *Hale Clinic* in London on 0207 631 0156) and electro crystal healing, that mimic this process and undoubtedly 21st-century medicine will be electromagnetic in nature. See also *Electrical Pollution and Healing*.

This is how dolphins heal. They have been on the planet for 30 million years longer than humans and their brains are highly developed. They can 'scan' someone, much the same as a good healer can and they then pulse harmonic, healing frequencies into the patient, which encourages the body to heal itself.

Of course healing does not work for everyone and some healers are better than others, just as there are better pianists, computer experts, or surgeons.

Recalling that we all emit our own unique frequency – you need to find a healer who is on a compatible frequency with your own, then you generally receive a more beneficial effect. You will soon know after three or four sessions whether their healing is making any difference, and if you are no better, simply find another healer. Also it greatly depends on how much harmonic frequency the healer is able to hold and channel through their body and out through their hands.

As we all emit a unique frequency and our brains act as both a receiver and a transmitter, by tuning into a person it appears we can also facilitate a transfer of healing energies over distances. Remember, energy can neither be created nor destroyed – it can only change into other forms of energy. Your thoughts are energy – they go somewhere – and when the intention is done with the whole heart and is for the receiver's greater good, your prayers will reach their destination. And the more people who pray at the same time with the same intention, the more powerful the prayer becomes. According to well-known healers such as Matthew Manning and Uri Geller, it is imperative we only transmit positive thoughts and visualise the person as looking 100% well in our mind's eye or imagination.

Helpful Hints

- To further understand healing read Roger Coghill's books: *The book of Magnet Healing*, Gaia Books (£10-99), or his fascinating book *Healing Energies of Light*, Gaia Books, available from all major bookshops or call 01495 752122

- The human mind is far more powerful than most people can even begin to imagine, therefore if you also truly believe the healing will work this really helps. Remember there is a huge difference between wanting something to work and believing it will.

- I find healing a great additional therapy used in conjunction with eating the right diet and so on. It literally recharges your internal batteries, which gives your body more energy to heal itself. Most healers find that the great majority are looking for a single magic bullet to heal their ills. But if they continue eating junk foods, which emit a disharmonic frequency, take no exercise and so on, obviously it's like trying to put a fire out while you remain standing in the flames.

- Then again, I have witnessed many miracles. Cancers have disappeared, crippled people walked again. How can this happen? I firmly believe this a combination of the power of the sick person's mind believing they are well and the ability of the healer to transmit a strong healing signal. But I also know that if a person believes 100% with their mind and heart they are truly healed, in that instant they are. You can hypnotise someone and tell them you are putting lighted cigarettes on their skin which will cause blisters. When the therapy is over their skin can be covered in blisters, but no such torture was ever applied. The blisters emanate from the power of the mind. We all have the ability to heal others and ourselves. All we need is an honourable intention and to keep an open mind.

- To find your nearest registered, insured healer call the **National Federation of Spiritual Healers** on 0845 123777. For general information, call 01932 783164. They have a world wide network of healers – check their website on www.nfsh.org.uk

- Reiki healing is also becoming very popular. To find your nearest qualified therapist call the **Reiki Association** on 01584 891197.

- Although there are hundreds of really amazing healers in the UK alone, there are two I have interviewed and seen for myself who are exceptional. The first is Seka Nikolic who practises at the **Kailash Clinic** in London. For details, call 020 7722 3939 or 020 8632 9466. The second is Kelvin Heard who specialises in chronic fatigue or ME. His number is 07710 794627.

HEARTBURN

(see *Acid Stomach, Indigestion* and *Low Stomach Acid*)

Taking 400iu of natural source vitamin E daily has been shown to reduce the incidence of heart attacks by 40% when taken for 2 years or more.

HEART DISEASE

(see also *Angina, Cholesterol, Circulation* and *High Blood Pressure*)

Heart disease is one of the biggest killers in Britain, killing 140,000 people every year, and the saddest part is that 90% of these deaths are totally preventable through diet and exercise. The majority of younger people who die with heart disease are male. Once women go through menopause their risk of dying from heart disease increases three fold. For some people there is a genetic predisposition of developing heart disease, others simply repeat the awful dietary habits of their parents. The majority of people with heart disease have high **LDL** cholesterol levels. High cholesterol levels and hardening of the arteries tend to go hand in hand, particularly if people are over 50 because cholesterol levels can vary dramatically over a short period of time and it can take many years for the arteries to harden. Having said this, there are a few lucky people who can eat high cholesterol foods and still maintain low cholesterol levels. Once people are over 85,, a higher cholesterol level has been associated with longevity. There are many factors to consider, and cholesterol is only part of the story.

Another factor now known to trigger heart disease and strokes is high levels of homocysteine, a toxic amino acid formed as a by-product of the metabolism of proteins. Levels are higher in people who have a genetic pre-disposition and those who eat a lot of animal protein including eggs. There are also links to heart disease via inflammatory conditions caused by the parasite *Chlamydia pneumonia*, and the organism *Helibacter pylori* – known to cause stomach ulcers.

Also if you have high-blood pressure or diabetes, you are much more susceptible to heart disease. The heart, like any other muscle, needs its own blood supply and receives this via three main vessels called the coronary arteries which we see on the surface of the heart. Over time, one of more of the arteries can become blocked. If an artery is blocked completely, some of the heart muscle may die during a heart attack. Typically symptoms of a heart attack include a severe pressing band of pain across the chest which can spread up the neck and into the jaw or across the shoulders and down into the left arm. Pain can be associated with sweating, breathlessness and a feeling of nausea. Immediate medical attention must be sought.

The heart, like any other muscle in the body, needs regular exercise which is one of the simplest ways of preventing a heart attack. It does not need to be intense, walking for 30 – 40 minutes a day is a good start. Recent research has shown that even moderate exercise after having a heart attack is one very effective way of preventing a second one. If you have had any heart problems only undertake an exercise programme under professional supervision. Being overweight greatly increases the risk for heart disease – a general rule (unless you are over 1.95m tall) is for men not to let their waistline go above 99cm and for women 90cm.

Foods to Avoid

- Saturated fats either animal or vegetable which includes butter, cheese, cream, hard margarines and red meats.
- Especially avoid any foods and refined oils containing hydrogenated or trans fats.
- Don't add salt to food. Use a low-salt alternative or a little magnesium rich sea salt.
- Stop smoking and avoid places where you will be exposed to second hand smoke as both increase the risk for heart disease.
- Greatly reduce your intake of mass-produced burgers, pies, sausages, pastries, cakes and desserts.
- Avoid excessive alcohol consumption, even though a moderate intake i.e. one glass a day is slightly protective, large amounts of alcohol frequently leads to heart disease.
- If you are going to cook in oil use unrefined olive or walnut oil.
- Avoid all fried foods.
- See *Fats You Need to Eat* and *General Health Hints*.

Friendly Foods

- Eat more fish of any description but try to have at least two portions of oily fish a week as they are rich in omega 3 essential fats.
- Eat plenty of fruits and vegetables containing carotenes: carrots, asparagus, French beans, broccoli, Brussels sprouts, watercress, spinach, cress, sweet potato, spring greens, dried apricots, mangos, tomato puree etc. which lower your risk of heart disease.
- Include brown rice and pastas, beans, wholemeal bread and other grains such as quinoa, amaranth, barley, oats and spelt in your diet.
- Fibre derived from fruits and vegetables is very protective and additional fibre from linseeds, oat or rice bran or psyllium husks all help lower the risk.
- Eating pistachios, walnuts, Brazil nuts, or macadamia nuts on a regular basis have been shown to help lower cholesterol.
- Wheat germ is rich in natural vitamin E which has been shown to reduce the risk of heart disease.
- Eat soya-based foods at least once a week.

- Use unrefined organic linseed (flax) oil for salad dressings as people who consume more linseed oil, which contains alpha-linolenic acid, have a lower risk of developing heart disease.

- Use healthier non-hydrogenated spreads such as *Biona* and *Vitaquell*.

- Use skimmed milk or organic rice milk and low-fat dairy produce.

- A vegetarian diet having no dairy or eggs but using a lot of beans, vegetables and grains, dramatically lowers your risk of developing heart disease.

- Sprinkle lecithin granules which emulsifies bad fats over breakfast cereals and desserts.

- Drink more water and try hawthorn tea which gently improves circulation.

Useful Remedies

- *Cardioflow* contains garlic, vitamin E, co-enzyme Q10, lipoic acid, magnesium and hawthorn. This formula can help to lower cholesterol, reduce angina and help lower the risk of heart disease. 2 daily. **NL**.

- Take a high-strength B complex as B6, B12 and folic acid reduce homocysteine levels in the blood. **BLK**

- Vitamin C and the amino acid lysine can help to reverse arterial blockages. You would need approximately 3 grams of each per day. **HN**

- Dimethylglycine (DMG) supplementation has been found very beneficial for circulation and cardiovascular problems. DMG enhances oxygen delivery to the heart. Clinical studies have reported major improvements in the areas of artherosclerosis, angina pectoris and high blood pressure upon administration of DMG. Take 50–90mg daily. **NC**

- Include a good quality multi-vitamin/mineral that contains at least 400iu of vitamin E, 150mcg of selenium, 30mg of zinc, 100mcg of chromium, 400mg of magnesium. **BLK**

Helpful Hints

- After the age of 50, do not take any supplements containing iron unless you have a medical condition that requires iron. Iron is stored in the body and excess is now linked to heart disease.

- Stop smoking.

- Reduce your exposure to toxic metals such as lead, cadmium and mercury.

- Homeopathic *Arnica 6x*, twice daily for up to 3 months helps to strengthen the heart.

- For a healthy heart, don't become overweight. Take regular exercise, which not only aids the heart, but also reduces stress which is a major cause of heart problems. Stress thickens the blood, so you could be playing squash, running etc and feel really fit but if you are also under excessive stress and eating the wrong diet you could still be at risk.

- People who are angry and argumentative have more heart problems.

- T'ai chi and yoga are great forms of exercise for reducing stress.

- See a doctor who is also a nutritionist to re-balance your diet and check for parasites or other organisms. (see *Useful Information*).

■ Contact the *British Heart Foundation*, 14 Fitzhardinge Street, London, W1H 4DH or call the Heart Health Line on 0870 600 6566. Website: www.bhf.org.uk

HERPES
(see also *Cold Sores*)

There are two types of herpes simplex virus: Type 1 causes cold sores, Type 2 is sexually transmitted and is the most common. It can cause extreme pain and swelling of the genital area and is sometimes accompanied by fever. You never eradicate the virus once you have it but you can keep attacks under control using supplements and eating a healthier diet.

Foods to Avoid
(See under *Cold Sores*)

Friendly Foods
(See under *Cold Sores*)

Useful Remedies
■ Vitamin C, take 1gram as a preventative and between 2–3 grams daily during an attack.

■ The amino acid lysine inhibits multiplication of the virus. Take 500mg as a preventative and up to 3 grams daily while suffering an attack.

■ Lemon balm applied topically and taken internally is very useful. Normally available in tincture form. If you use it externally, dilute it in warmish water first or douch in lemon balm tea. If you are unable to find lemon balm, liquorice is a good alternative as it is a strong anti-viral.

■ Vitamin E, either as a pure oil or a broken capsule applied 3–4 times a day, can rapidly alleviate the pain from the cold sores.

■ *Olive Leaf Extract* acts like a natural antibiotic and boosts immune function. Take 2–3 capsules daily. **NC**

■ *Larreastat*, an extract of the larrea bush has had a 97.5% success rate in treating herpes simplex 1,2 and herpes zoster, Available in capsules or as a lotion. Take one capsule up to three times a day and the lotion can be applied up to 5 times daily on to the lesions. **NC**

■ A multi-vitamin and mineral that contains 30 mg of zinc.

Helpful Hints
■ Avoidance of sexual intercourse when you have an attack is very important as it is extremely contagious. If you must have sex then use a condom, but you may well find it is too painful and need to wait until the sores have either healed or completely gone away. Remember that oral sex is one way of transferring a cold sore and turning it into genital herpes.

■ For further help, write to the **Herpes Viruses Association**, 41 North Road, London, N7 9DP, enclosing an SAE, or call their helpline on 020 7609 9061. Website: www.herpes.org.uk

Eat more celery which neutralises acid conditions such as arthritis and helps to lower blood pressure.

HIATUS HERNIA

The gullet or oesophagus takes food from the mouth to the stomach and passes through a sheet of muscle called the diaphragm. A hiatus hernia occurs when the part of the stomach pushes up through the diaphragm and allows acid to escape into the gullet causing heartburn, reflux of food and indigestion, especially when lying down. It can also cause a fair amount of chest pain which obviously needs looking at quickly. Most hiatus hernias can easily be seen on an X-ray.

Foods to Avoid

- Generally avoid large meals, especially ones containing red meat and fried foods such as chips and creamy type sauces.

- Alcohol, strong tea, coffee, fizzy drinks, tea, sugar, chocolate, dairy products and all high-fat foods can cause an 'acid' rebound reaction as they are all acid-forming foods within the body.

- Chew food thoroughly and don't drink too much fluid with food.

- If you are really stressed, don't eat or, at most, eat only lightly cooked small meals.

- Avoid artificial sweeteners like aspartame and artificial additives which can aggravate symptoms.

Friendly Foods

- Slippery elm and liquorice both soothe the oesophagus as well as providing a gentle fibre which can reduce discomfort.

- Try decaffeinated beverages and drink more herbal teas such as camomile and peppermint.

- Food combining has proved very useful to people who have this condition. There are numerous books on food combining the best being **The Complete Book of Food Combining** by Kathryn Marsden (Piatkus), www.piatkus.co.uk. The basic rule is to avoid eating proteins such as meat or fish with potatoes, pasta or bread. And when eating rice, pasta or bread do not eat proteins but eat vegetables and salads.

- A macrobiotic diet using a lot of brown rice, vegetables and beans although quite a difficult diet to follow, may be one way of avoiding symptoms.

- Eat more live, low-fat yoghurt after meals to soothe the digestive tract.

- Generally eat a low-fat diet but see under *Fats You Need to Eat* and *General Health Hints*.

- Steam, boil, poach, roast or grill your food.

- Eat more wheat germ, soya beans, alfalfa, dark green vegetables (especially cabbage which is rich in glutamine) plus a little avocado which are all rich in vitamin E.

- Sprinkle lecithin granules over your low-sugar breakfast cereal daily which helps to emulsify fats.

- Eat more garlic and fresh root ginger.

Useful Remedies

■ Deglycyrrhized liquorice, chew 1–2 tablets 20 minutes before a meal. The liquorice protects the mucous membranes, helps with digestion and can rapidly ease the discomfort of hiatus hernia. **FSC**

■ Slippery elm 2 tablets taken at the end of each meal can reduce any discomfort.

■ L-glutamine, found in cabbage, helps to heal any ulceration in the gut. Take 1–2 grams daily for 6 weeks.

■ Take a good quality multi-vitamin and mineral. **S**

■ Drink half a cup of aloe vera juice daily.

■ Calcium fluoride tissue salts, 4 a day to help strengthen the diaphragm.

Helpful Hints

■ Try to relax as much as possible and avoid lying down after eating.

■ Do not smoke near meal times.

■ Go for a gentle walk after meals but do not get involved in heavy exercise.

■ Many people report relief from symptoms after seeing a chiropractor.

Cabbage contains nutrients that help to heal stomach ulcers and improve varicose veins.

HIGH BLOOD PRESSURE

High blood pressure, otherwise known as hypertension, makes you more susceptible to coronary heart disease, arterial swelling which can eventually lead to eye damage, strokes and kidney disease. Blood pressure of 150 over 100 or more is classified as raised. A normal reading is 120/80, but 140/90 or less is deemed as acceptable. People who are overweight and don't get much exercise are at a much higher risk of having high blood pressure. 85% of all cases of high blood pressure can be treated without drugs if the person is willing to change their lifestyle and diet. In societies where salt is limited hypertension is rare. Too much caffeine, alcohol and smoking when combined with high blood pressure greatly increases your chances of suffering heart disease or stroke. Stress is a major factor in high blood pressure. Chemicals such as adrenaline and noradrenaline are released into the blood stream which increases heart beat, breathing and blood pressure. Blood cholesterol levels also rise and blood clots more easily. In stone age days all these symptoms were called 'fight or flight' when the hunter risked danger and had to run quickly, the adrenaline gave him the energy to do this. His ability to clot blood more quickly would help with any injuries he might incur. High blood pressure is also associated with pregnancy, which needs medical attention.

Foods to Avoid

- Avoid sodium-based salt as there is a clear link between the use of salt and high blood pressure. Unfortunately, it does need to be pretty much complete avoidance of salt to have any effect. You may cut it out at home and then be caught out by the fact that it's in every biscuit, pie, meal you eat out and any processed food you might consume out of the house.

- There are plenty of magnesium and potassium based salts such as Solo Salt available from health shops.

- Blood pressure has been shown to drop as much as 20 points when all caffeine was eliminated.

- Some de-caffinated drinks contains formaldehyde, so ask for de-caff drinks and coffee that has been de-caffinated using a more natural water method.

- Sugar is also a problem as sugar turns to a hard fat in the body if not used up during exercise.

- If you have eliminated all of the above and you still have a tendency towards high blood pressure, you might want to look towards the possibility of having an allergy or food intolerance test particularly if you are a migraine sufferer.

- People who are exposed to toxic metals like lead often have raised blood pressure.

Friendly Foods

- Potassium is needed to help lower blood pressure. If your GP has put you on a potassium diuretic then it is important you consult with them before consuming more fruit than normal.

- Two bananas a day have been shown to help lower blood pressure.

- Try *Solo* instead of table salt, which is potassium- and not sodium-based.

- Green vegetables, fresh fruit, unsalted nuts, seafood, soya flour, roast potatoes, butterbeans, currants, dried figs, ready-to-eat apricots, almonds, Brazil nuts, black treacle and sunflower seeds are all rich in potassium.

- If you are not a fan of eating fresh fruit and vegetables, at least drink a couple of glasses of freshly made fruit juice which contains potassium.

- Try switching to a more vegetarian-based diet as the more fruit, vegetables, beans and lentils you eat, the greater your potassium intake and, generally speaking, the lower your sodium intake. Long-term vegetarians tend to have much lower blood pressure.

- Eat more garlic, onions, broccoli and celery.

- Use unrefined organic virgin olive, walnut and sunflower oils for your salad dressings and eat oily fish. See *Fats You Need to Eat*.

- As high levels of toxic metals such as lead can lead to high blood pressure, buy a good quality water filter.

- Coriander helps to detoxify metals from the body.

- Natural source vitamin E helps to thin blood naturally, therefore eat more soya beans, wheat germ, alfalfa sprouts, dark green vegetables, hazelnuts, almonds and avocados.

Useful Remedies

■ Calcium, 1 gram daily with 500mg of magnesium, both of these minerals have been shown to lower blood pressure.

■ Co-enzyme Q10 is found in organ meats and as we age levels fall. Take 90–120mg. **PN**

■ EPA and DHA in a fish oil supplement. Unfortunately, at least 10 capsules a day, to provide the 3 grams of omega oil are needed to be effective.

■ Garlic, 900mg a day, when used long term, garlic can help gently lower blood pressure.

■ Hawthorn either as tincture or as tablets is a gentle way of bringing blood pressure back down to normal. 1–3mls of tincture or 1–2 grams of the tablets. **FSC**

■ If you are taking blood pressure medication you must have regular medical check ups as these supplements help to lower blood pressure naturally and you don't want the blood pressure to go too low!

■ If you have a craving for sweet foods such as cakes, biscuits etc then take 200mcg of chromium daily to help reduce the cravings.

■ Begin taking 100iu of natural source vitamin E and gradually increase to 500iu a day.

■ Jiaogulan is a herb that helps to modulate blood pressure, lowering it when it is too high and raising it when it is too low. In one study, 223 patients were divided into three groups. One group took ginseng, the next took jiaogulan and the last took blood pressure medication, *Indapamide*. The effectiveness was rated at 46% for ginseng, 82% for jiaogulan and 93% for *Indapamide*. Up to 4 tablets of jiagulan can be taken daily. **NC**

■ Include a high-strength multi-vitamin and mineral in your programme as the B vitamins help to support your nerves.

Helpful Hints

■ Liver congestion and constipation can aggravate high blood pressure.

■ Try to find a method of relaxation that you enjoy whether it's meditation, tai chi, yoga, exercising, walking or swimming.

■ Have a regular aromatherapy massage using rosewood, ylang ylang, clary, sage and majoram.

■ Cayenne pepper is anti-hypertensive. Use one teaspoon in daily cooking. (Do not use if you suffer from stomach ulcers.)

■ Exercise is vital in controlling this condition. With your doctor's permission start walking briskly for 30 minutes daily.

■ Rosemary and nettle tea sipped regularly can help to lower blood pressure.

HIRSUTISM

(see *Body Hair*)

Eating an organic apple daily can help reduce constipation and lower cholesterol.

HYPERACTIVITY

Hyperactivity, also known as attention deficit disorder is a condition that occurs predominantly in children but sometimes symptoms can continue into adulthood. There is no hard and fast definition of this disorder, consequently children who are merely rebellious or find it difficult to pay attention for great lengths of time may be labelled as hyperactive. Typical symptoms include an inability to concentrate or sit still for any length of time, rapid and severe mood swings, difficulty in keeping still or quietening down and will often need very little sleep. Stereotype hyperactivity is associated with an excessive intake of sugar, artificial sweeteners and ingestion of colourings and preservatives found in prescription medicines and foods. Sensitivities or allergic reactions to various foods and substances such as bubble bath, air fresheners, spray deodorants, perfumes and toothpastes can also trigger this problem. Many children are now given so many junk foods, they have become malnourished and deficient in many vital nutrients such as zinc, chromium and essential fats, a lack of which can have a dramatic effect on their behaviour. Exposure to neurotoxins such as lead from water pipes and car fumes, plus cadmium from cigarettes can make the problem worse.

The normal drug therapy is *Ritalin*, from the amphetamine family. Understandably many parents don't feel comfortable giving this to their child, however, others feel that this is their only weapon in making the child controllable or teachable. I believe there is a gross overuse of this drug which is leaving some children like zombies. It would be far healthier for all concerned if the parents could correct their child's diet with the help of a nutritionist and eliminate all triggers from the child. I realise this may take longer but I believe we are sitting on a time bomb with Ritalin.

Foods to Avoid

- Any foods containing large numbers of additives, particularly the strong colourings like tartrazine. Many sweets are bright rainbow colours such as red, green, purple, yellow and so on. The brighter the sweets the more they should be avoided.

- Greatly reduce or eliminate cola-type drinks and any foods or drinks containing the artificial sweetener aspartame.

- Generally cut out most foods containing sugar such as cakes, biscuits, chocolates, snack bars and so on. One specialist once compared giving sugar to hyperactive children as ' like putting rocket fuel in a Mini'. The odd treat is OK but try and buy organic, low-sugar snack bars that have been sweetened with apple juice or honey. Most of the mass-produced refined foods should go.

- Citrus fruits and juices are often a problem.

- If your child has a favourite food, be it cheese, eggs, wheat based foods, milk or orange juice, try cutting these out for 1–2 weeks and see if behaviour improves as it's usually the foods they eat and crave the most that are doing the greatest harm.

- Buy a book that gives you all E numbers and note which foods have the highest amounts and avoid them like the plague.

Friendly Foods

■ As much as possible feed your child on organic foods free from pesticides and herbicides.

■ Try buying corn, lentil, rice and spinach based pastas.

■ Introduce more whole foods and grains such as brown rice, millet and barley into your child's diet.

■ **Nature's Path** make great breakfast cereals that are sweetened with apple juice. Chop an apple or banana into the cereal for fibre and added nutrients.

■ Try organic rice, soya, oat, pea or goat's milk which are less likely to cause a problem.

■ Use diluted sugar-free pear, apple or even grape juice which are less likely than the citrus fruits to cause a problem.

■ Encourage the child to drink water in preference to fizzy drinks and try to encourage a taste for fresh fruit rather than sugary sweets.

■ Add low-sugar fruit yoghurts to fruit to make desserts more attractive. I make jellies with low-sugar cranberry juice and chop fresh fruit into the jelly.

■ Top desserts with chopped nuts which are a rich source of minerals. Avoid peanuts. I use organic hazelnuts, almonds, chopped coconut, sunflower seeds, walnuts and whizz them all in a blender. Keep in an air tight jar in the fridge and sprinkle over breakfast cereals and desserts.

■ Give your child quality protein such as chicken, fresh fish, tofu or lentils and beans.

■ Essential fats found in oily fish, seeds and nuts are really important in controlling this type of behaviour.

■ Use unrefined olive, sunflower, walnut and sesame oils for salad dressings or drizzle over cooked foods.

Useful Remedies

■ Magnesium is known as nature's tranquilliser and many children are low in this vital mineral. 200mg daily.

■ Essential fatty acids are vital. Either use **Essential Balance Junior** butterscotch-flavoured oil **(HN)** or *Efalex* 1–2 spoons a day over cooked food or add to salad dressings.

■ Give your child a good quality chewable multi-vitamin and mineral that is free from artificial additives **HN**

■ Siberian ginseng has worked well for some children. 10–60 drops of tincture or 1–3 grams in tablets, use for 60 days and then rest for 30 days. If you use too much ginseng the worst that seems to happen is that the child feels sleepy.

Helpful Hints

■ Try to avoid smoking and drinking during pregnancy as both of these have been linked with an increased likelihood of the child having hyperactivity.

■ If the child has allergies or food intolerances, explain to the child how they affect their behaviour and tell everyone in the school or relatives who might be giving the child food or drinks, which they think perfectly harmless.

- Homoeopathy has a great track record of dealing with ADD and hyperactivity so, if you can, get your child along to a good homoeopath. Be prepared to be patient as it may not be an overnight success. See *Useful Information*.

- Avoid air fresheners of all types, spray deodorants, pot-pourri, perfumed fabric conditioners, washing powders and liquids. Try **Ecover** products which contain far fewer chemicals, now available in all major supermarkets and health stores.

- For further information, contact the **Hyperactive Children's Support Group**, 71 Whyke Lane, Chichester, West Sussex, PO19 2LD. Tel: 01243 551313 between 10.00am – 1.00pm, Monday to Friday. Website: www.hacsg.org.uk Email: web@hacsg.org.uk

- If you cannot afford an allergy blood test, take your child to see a kinesiologist, who uses muscle testing to detect food and environmental allergens (see *Useful Information*).

- Serena Smith makes up flower remedies called *Little Miracles*, which have proven very helpful for reducing hyperactivity. For further information write to **Serena Smith at Little Miracles**, PO Box 3896, London, NW3 7DS. Tel/fax: 020 7431 6153. Website: www.littlemiracles.co.uk Email: info@littlemiracles.co.uk

HYPOGLYCAEMIA
(see Low Blood Sugar)

IMMUNE FUNCTION
(see also *Stress*)

Almost 25% of our body's cells are dedicated to the immune system, which protects us from invading bacteria, viruses and fungi. The single most important thing we can do to stay healthy is to look after our immune system. Prolonged stress, junk foods or lack of sleep are the immune system's biggest enemy. Stress alone can suppress immune function by up to 60% (see also *Stress*).

Foods to Avoid
- Avoid foods high in saturated fats which cause free radical damage to our cells.
- Sugar in any form lowers immune functioning.
- Alcohol and caffeine stress the immune system if taken to excess.

■ Avoid foods high in preservatives, artificial colourings, artificial sweeteners especially aspartame.

■ Reduce your intake of hydrogenated or trans fats and all mass-produced refined oils.

■ Avoid all smoked foods such as smoked meats and cheeses.

Friendly Foods

■ All fresh fruits, vegetables, whole grains, sprouts such as alfalfa, brown rice and algae such as spirulina and chlorella.

■ Eat more purple, red and orange foods – blueberries, bilberries and blackberries are a powerhouse of nutrients – plus sweet potatoes, apricots, papaya and red peppers.

■ Nuts (not processed peanuts and heavily salted nuts) and seeds are packed with essential fats and minerals like zinc and selenium.

■ Include more vitamin C rich foods, broccoli, peas, cabbage, lychees, lemons, kiwis, oranges and blueberries.

Useful remedies

■ An antioxidant formula containing at least 7,000 iu of vitamin A (only 5,000iu if pregnant), 400iu of vitamin E, 15mg zinc, 1gram of vitamin C and 200mcg of selenium.

■ 50mg daily of *Alpha Lipoic Acid* to help remove free radicals and reduces oxidative stress.

■ Take a good quality multi vitamin and mineral.

■ *Immunalive No 1 & No 3* is a formula containing IP6 (inositol hexaphosphate, extracted from brown rice), plus plant sterols and sterolins – plant fats (usually sold as *Moducare*) which dramatically enhance immune function. Take 4 of the No 1 formula and 3 of the No 3 formula for optimum benefits. Take at least 40 minutes before breakfast on an empty stomach. **PW**

■ Echinacea, astragalus and Siberian ginseng all support immune function. 5mls of each of the tincture when you are feeling low but only for a month at a time.

Helpful Hints

■ Make sure you get sufficient sleep.

■ If possible take 2 holidays a year in the sunshine, which really helps to boost your immune system.

■ Take regular exercise but not to excess. Don't over exercise if you are truly exhausted.

■ Learn to meditate or chant to calm your mind. Make time for yourself.

■ Breathe deeply every 20 minutes – it's hard for the body to stay stressed if you breathe properly.

■ Walk out in sunlight as much as possible at least 15 minutes a day – this helps boost brain melatonin levels, a hormone which helps boost the immune system.

■ See *General Health Hints* for more help.

IMPOTENCE

(see *Aphrodisiacs*)

Regular use of antiperspirants and deodorants containing aluminium can treble the risk of contracting Alzheimer's.

INCONTINENCE

(see also *Bladder Problems* and *Prostate Problems*)

Incontinence can lead to urine leaking out when the bladder is put under pressure when you laugh, cough, sneeze or exert yourself. It can also occur when you have eaten to excess and the bowel puts pressure on the bladder. This type of problem is referred to as stress incontinence and is usually associated with a weakness in the muscle in the pelvic floor. Exercise can help keep the pelvic floor strong and childbirth tends to weaken it, hence why it is a good idea to do plenty of pelvic exercises after giving birth. I suffered this problem during my twenties after giving birth to my daughter and it became so embarrassing that in my early thirties I found a gynaecologist who specialised in bladder repair and had surgery. It has really made a huge difference and I can now exercise without the embarrassment.

Urinary incontinence is also associated with candida (see also *Candida* and *Cystitis*).

Foods to Avoid

- Any food to which you have an allergy or intolerance can aggravate incontinence.
- Avoid fluoridated water, toothpastes and mouthwashes. I have received many letters from people who say that when fluoride is eliminated, the problem stops. It also seems to help with children who wet the bed.
- The biggest culprits are usually yeast, wheat, dairy, alcohol and sugar.

Friendly Foods

- Add a little cayenne pepper to your foods. It may initially aggravate the problem but in the long term usually helps.
- See *General Health Hints*.

Useful Remedies

- A high-strength multi-vitamin and mineral for women. **BC, S, HN, BLK**
- 500mg of calcium with 250mg of Magnesium to help muscle control. After 6 weeks you should see benefits.
- *Inurin* is a formula containing horsetail and sweet sumach which have proven very helpful for ladies who need to get up several times in the night. **NC**

■ The mineral silica 75mg and the herb aquisetum (horsetail) – take 5mls of each tincture a day to help strengthen the bladder.

Helpful Hints

■ Strengthening the pelvic floor muscles can reduce or eliminate stress incontinence. These muscles contract when you try to stop your urine flow. Squeeze this area and hold for at least 4 seconds, repeat as many times as you like throughout the day – even when you are sitting at a desk or use a pelvic toner developed by Dr. Steven Harvey, an incontinence specialist. For details call 0117 9687744 www.natural-woman.com (£29.99).

■ Try using a set of vaginal cones containing weights to help strengthen the muscles. For information on the *Aquaflex* system, call the order line on 0800 614 086. There is also a help line available on 0800 526177. One set costs £19-95 inc. P&P in the UK or log onto www.ssl-international.com

■ An osteopath or chiropractor can check the alignment of bones in the pubic area. This can help as if the bones are out of balance urine flow in both men and women can be affected. Acupuncture has proven helpful to some people. See *Useful Information*.

■ Contact the **Continence Foundation**, 307 Hatton Square, 16 Baldwins Gardens, London, EC1N 7RJ, enclosing a SAE. Tel: 020 7831 9831 (9.30am–4.30pm weekdays). Website: www.continence-foundation.org.uk Email: continence-foundation@dial.pipex.com

If you suffer cracked skin fissures in your heels, add a dessert spoonful of organic linseed oil to cooked foods daily.

INDIGESTION

(see also *Acid Stomach, Flatulence, Hiatus Hernia* and *Low Stomach Acid*)

Indigestion covers various symptoms from cramping in the stomach, heartburn, wind, belching and even pain in the bowel. It is usually a sign that the digestive system is having difficulty coping with food, and this is frequently due to a lack of stomach acid and digestive enzymes in the small intestine. The problem can be made worse if you eat too quickly and don't chew food thoroughly. Overeating, drinking to excess, eating poor food combinations or eating when stressed all exacerbate indigestion.

Foods to Avoid

■ Generally reduce your intake of sugar and sugary foods such as cakes, biscuits and rich puddings.

■ Red meat and fatty cuts of meat are hard to digest.

■ Coffee, tea, chocolates caffeine in any form, alcohol, peppers, citrus fruits onions and sometimes garlic can be difficult to digest.

■ Salt hinders digestion and assimilation of proteins, so cut down on sodium-based salts.

- Don't drink too much liquid with meals as this dilutes the stomach acid, which you need to digest your meal.
- Avoid fruit immediately after a large meal, unless it's a small chunk of pineapple or papaya.
- Avoid as much as possible rich, creamy foods and heavy desserts such as Christmas pudding.
- Avoid antacids which neutralise stomach acid – the very substance you need to digest your meals.
- Many people with indigestion have problems digesting wheat. Try try *Ryvita* low-salt crispbreads, rice cakes and amaranth crackers, available from health shops.

Friendly Foods

- Drink some ginger or dandelion root tea with or before meals to stimulate digestion.
- Small meals made from whole foods and small quantities of meat or fish are much easier on the digestion.
- Try eating small amounts of pineapple or papaya before a meal. They contain enzymes which can enhance digestion.
- Add more fresh root ginger to foods as it is very calming.
- If you like beans and pulses but they give you wind, then cook them with a strip of kombu seaweed which helps to pre-digest the beans.
- Eat more live, low-fat yoghurts.

Useful Remedies

- Take *Betaine Hydrochloride* (stomach acid) 1 capsule with main meals. If you have active stomach ulcers or the HCl causes a burning sensation then take a digestive enzyme instead.
- Chew 1–2 tablets of deglychyrrized liquorice before a meal. This soothes any symptoms of heartburn or indigestion. **FSC**
- Acidophilus and bifidus are healthy bacteria which encourage better digestion and elimination. Take 1–2 capsules at the end of a meal. **BC**
- Sip peppermint tea after meals.

Helpful Hints

- Sit down and eat food in a relaxed setting.
- Go for a walk after eating which really aids digestion.
- Eat fruit between meals but avoid fruits you know are a problem such as oranges and grapefruit.
- Don't eat if you are stressed or really upset.
- Sometimes when people suffer indigestion, it is because they are unable to digest some information or something going on in their lives. If this is the case it would be worth seeing a homoeopath who may be able to resolve the underlying issues. See also *Stress*. Meanwhile the homeopathic remedy *Nux Vomica 30c* helps reduce the incidence of indigestion.
- Consult a nutritionist who will help re-balance your system (see *Useful Information*).

Drinking more than 5 cups of coffee daily can reduce fertility in women by a third – but don't use this as an alternative contraceptive!

INFERTILITY

Sperm counts have dropped dramatically in the last fifty years. A quarter of all couples planning a baby have trouble conceiving. In four out of every ten cases the problems are on the male side. If the male sperm count is low this can sometimes be due to infection such as mumps. A low sperm count can be due to a poor diet and/or environmental toxins such as lead, mercury and cadmium. Food additives, smoking, alcohol, food intolerances, urinary tract infections plus stress can all affect fertility. Common organisms such as *Mycoplasma hominis* and *Ureaplasma* can infect the urinary tracts of men and women. They don't always cause infertility but there seems to be a higher number of these organisms in the secretions of couples who have unexplained fertility problems. Smoking and alcohol can also reduce sperm count. Many scientists now believe that sperm counts in the Western world are dropping because of overuse of herbicides and pesticides which have an oestrogen-boosting effect within the body that counteracts male testosterone.

Female infertility can be due to blockages in the fallopian tubes. This can be triggered by an infection such as thrush or cystitis, but whatever the cause it would need a medical examination. Sometimes there is a problem with ovulation, usually due to a hormone imbalance. Other conditions such as endometriosis, low thyroid function, a diet deficient in nutrients especially zinc and magnesium and/or environmental toxins are also a common cause of infertility in women. Candida, a yeast fungal overgrowth is also linked to infertility. When women are under a lot of stress and the body releases adrenalin, their endocrine system eventually becomes exhausted which can prevent conception.

Foods to Avoid
- Tea, coffee, chocolate and cola, which all contain caffeine, have been shown to reduce the chance of conception.
- Alcohol alone can reduce your chances of fertility and it's worse when combined with caffeine.
- Smokers are less likely to conceive particularly if their parents are also smokers.
- Avoid foods high in saturated fats, junk foods, pre-packaged meals, sugar and salt which deplete the body of the nutrients needed for conception.

Friendly Foods
- As the mineral zinc is vital for both partners eat plenty of fresh fish and eat oily fish such as mackerel, salmon, sardines or herrings at least once a week as they are rich in omega 3 essential fats.

- Add some sunflower seeds, pumpkin seeds and linseeds to any low-sugar breakfast cereal as they are high in minerals and essential fats.

- Use organic olive, sunflower, walnut and flax oils for your salad dressings.

- If you have any iron deficiency, eat more lean meats especially calf's liver, turkey and chicken plus eggs and dried apricots.

- Leafy green vegetables, cereals, honey, beans and nuts are all good sources of magnesium which may well be deficient.

- Try caffeine-free alternatives like dandelion tea or root coffee as these can have beneficial effects on the liver and consequently enhance hormone production.

- Ladies need to eat more organic tofu (soya), fennel and alfalfa which help balance hormones.

Useful Remedies

- A multi-vitamin and mineral – many companies now make special formulas for women who are trying to conceive. *The Pregnancy Pack* is available from **Health Plus** on 01323 737374. Web site www.healthplus.co.uk

- Any multi for men needs to contain at least 30mg of zinc, 200mcg of selenium and 250mg of magnesium.

- Both partners should take a B complex plus 5000iu of vitamin A which are needed for egg and sperm production.

- Vitamin E, 200iu a day has been shown to help reduce both male and female infertility.

- For women take 40 drops in the morning of *Agnus Castus*, or 1000mg in tablet form. This herb helps regulate the hormonal cycle. **FSC**

- Both partners should take 1 gram of vitamin C daily.

- The mineral potassium chloride 150mg can help clear the fallopian tubes. **BLK**

- For men there is a well-researched form of these minerals called ZMA (EAS) containing zinc and magnesium which research has shown to elevate testosterone levels. **NC**

- L- arginine and carnitine are two amino acids that are needed for sperm production and to prevent sperm becoming too 'sticky' which can interfere with conception. You could take 1.5–3 grams of each daily. Do not take the arginine if you have herpes or Shingles.

Helpful Hints

- For more help read *Natural Solutions to Infertility* by Dr Marilyn Glenville (Piatkus). For a postal consultation with Dr Glenville log onto www.marilynglenville.com.

- Stop smoking and reduce alcohol intake.

- Eat organic food free from pesticides and herbicides.

- Ask to be screened for any urinary infections.

- Limit the amount of chemicals in your home and garden such as wood preservatives, perfumes, insect sprays etc. Use eco-friendly products.

- Avoid too much exposure to mobile phones, computers, and electrical equipment.

- If the woman is overweight or extremely underweight it needs to be corrected as either extreme can lead to problems with fertility.

- If either partner is taking prescription drugs or regular over-the-counter remedies, check for their known side effects.

- Remember to try not to get too stressed as stress in either partner can lower the chances of conception. I have received letters from many couples who, when they gave up trying so hard to conceive, bought a pet or adopted a child – the next thing they knew a baby was on its way!

- Sitting for long periods raises the temperature in the testicles, which may reduce male fertility. If you are deskbound, for example a long-distance driver, wear loose fitting underwear and trousers and get plenty of exercise.

- As most tap water is contaminated with chemicals and antibiotic residues invest in a reverse osmosis water filter system. Contact *The Pure H2O Company* on 01784 221188 email: info@purewater.co.uk website: www.purewater.co.uk

- Contact **Foresight**, who specialise in giving couples information about how to plan for a healthy pregnancy and increase fertility naturally. The service includes nutritional status analysis, though this is usually done in consultation with a recognised Foresight practitioner. **Foresight** can be contacted by writing to 28 The Paddock, Godalming, Surrey, GU7 1XD. Tel: 01483 419468. Website: www.surreyweb.org.uk/foresight/home.html

Get plenty of exercise, as relaxed muscles mean relaxed nerves.

Dr Melvyn Werbach

INSECT BITES

Apart from the obvious discomfort that they cause, insect bites can occasionally transmit serious disease and cause severe allergic reactions like anaphylactic shock. If you know that you or a family member has a particular allergy to stings and bites it is important to discuss this with your GP to make sure you take the appropriate medication away with you. For people who suffer anaphylactic shock, you need to carry adrenalin injections with you at all times. For anyone travelling to tropical countries where malarial mosquitoes exist, take precautions seriously. In Africa a child dies every 30 seconds from malaria.

In the Caribbean both my husband and myself have suffered Dengue fever from mosquito bites and I would never want to feel that ill again as long as I live. The key, as always, lies in prevention.

If you are unfortunate enough to be attacked by a swarm of bees, immediately close your eyes and mouth and wait for help. If you happen to be near water and can swim jump in.

Foods to Avoid

■ Sugar makes your blood taste sweeter, especially to mosquitoes. If you are visiting the tropics, stop eating sugar at least a week before you travel.

Friendly Foods

■ Garlic eaten on a regular basis may well make you smell less appetizing to stinging insects.

■ Malaria-carrying beasties are attracted to the smell of human feet. Limburger cheese or other strong cheeses smell just like your feet, so by putting a bit of the cheese in your room at least five feet away from you the mosquitoes are distracted.

Useful Remedies

■ Thiamine (B1), 300mg per day and 50mg of zinc. Order from **GNC** on 01483 410611. When these are excreted they give off an odour that repels insects. As all the B vitamins work together, also take a B complex.

■ Brewer's yeast, either as tablets or powder is a rich source of vitamin B1 which changes the smell of your sweat, making you less attractive to insects.

■ Some people have found that taking feverfew, the herb which contains pyrethin – an effective insecticide, really helps. Also, the herb catnip repels mosquitoes.

■ Use *Bug Ban* by **Herbcraft** – spray liberally over the body as often as is needed.

■ *Quantum Buzz Away* is Deet Free and made from a combination of essential oils such as cedarwood, eucalyptus, lemongrass and peppermint. **NC**

Helpful Hints

■ Use lemongrass or citronella candles at dusk to repel insects.

■ Try an essential oil preparation for repelling insects. Mix 10 drops of lavender oil, 10 drops of orange oil, 5 drops of eucalyptus, 5 drops of citronella, 10 drops of neem oil into a base of 50ml apricot almond oil. Apply sparingly on exposed areas of skin, especially ankles and wrists. Most good health food stores will carry these oils.

■ Try *Alfresco* body lotion, containing melissa, geranium, lavender and other essential oils which has been proven to help repel insects. For details call 0208 348 6704.

■ Avoid wearing any perfumed toiletries at night and use cotton nightclothes that cover the arms and wrists.

■ Use a mosquito net. In Africa, trials on children showed incidence of malaria was cut by 80% when nets were used at night. These are easy to buy at travel shops.

■ **Ainsworth Homeopathic Pharmacy** can supply a general travel kit, which includes items for bites, traveller's tummy, sunstroke etc. They can also provide individual homeopathic remedies for tropical diseases such as homeopathic *Malaria*, and *Caladium* which changes the smell of your sweat making you less attractive to insects. Tel: 020 7935 5330 or write to 36 New Cavendish Street, London, W1M 7LH. Website: www.ainsworths.com E-mail: ainshom@msn.com

If you can expend just 1000 calories a week in exercise, this reduces the risk of heart disease by a fifth.

Patrick Holford

INSOMNIA

(see also *Sleeping Pills*)

If there is truly one subject I could fill a book on it's this one. I have suffered chronic insomnia for almost thirty years and I really do know what it's like not to be able to get to sleep because your mind is racing, and then when you do drop off to be wide awake again at 3 or 4 am. Thanks to our modern way of life – open all hours, stress and anxiety etc – one in every four people now say they experience regular sleep problems. To get to sleep, you need to switch your brain from its normal busy or beta brainwave state to a more relaxed alpha state. The best way to achieve this is by meditation, self hypnosis (see NLP under Helpful Hints) or relaxation tapes.

No-one functions well when they are short of sleep as it not only compromises your immune system but can severely affect your day-to-day performance. Recent studies have shown that lack of sleep can have almost as a drastic effect as drinking alcohol when it comes to driving.

Many people, including myself, when absolutely desperate, resort to prescription sleeping pills. The problem can then become chronic and addictive. Hence it's best only to use sleeping pills on the odd or occasional night – as when the body and brain become overtired it often becomes harder to get to sleep. Even though loath to take them, the need for sleep is more important. In the long term prescription pills can affect your memory and upset delicate brain chemistry.

It's worth noting that if you tend to wake regularly between 3 and 5am you are likely to be suffering adrenal exhaustion from stress. It can also mean that your liver is struggling in which case you need to cut down on fats, coffee and alcohol and eat really lightly for a few days.

Foods to Avoid

■ Caffeine is one of the most important substances to avoid after around 5 pm in the afternoon. Having said that, I have friends who can drink expresso and sleep like a log. I'm not one of them, if I drink filter coffee after early evening I can literally be awake until 3 or 4 am. Remember that caffeine is not just found in tea and coffee, it's also in cola, chocolate, cocoa and some over-the-counter cold remedies.

■ If you drink a fair amount of alcohol you tend to feel sleepy, but unfortunately because of the way it is metabolised in the body you might sleep for 2–3 hours and then wake up again and find it very difficult to get back to sleep.

■ Food intolerances can make the problem worse. In one study, cow's milk appeared to be the problem but it can be any food to which you have a sensitivity. Keep a food diary.

■ Don't eat big meals late at night.

■ Avoid red meat and too much protein, which tend to wake up the brain. Eat **protein for breakfast or lunch.**

Friendly Foods

■ Try to make the last meal of the day a carbohydrate-based one like pasta, potatoes or brown rice. These starchy foods can have a slight soporific effect. Eating carbohydrate rich foods before sleep also encourages the body to produce a brain chemical called serotonin which can help reduce anxiety and improve the quality of sleep.

■ Serotonin is made from a constituent of protein called tryptophan, so include more foods such as fish, turkey, chicken, cottage cheese, beans, avocados, bananas and wheat germ in your diet.

■ Sprinkle wheat germ over breakfast cereal; my favourite is **Nature's Path** who make great cereals from amaranth, quinoa and kamut that are sweetened with a little apple juice.

■ Some people find that a banana an hour before they go to sleep helps them sleep longer.

■ Many people have porridge for breakfast but often having it as a supper or late-night snack made with organic rice milk and a chopped banana encourages sound sleep.

■ If you are a regular tea or coffee drinker, gradually switch over to the decaffeinated varieties. Don't do this too quickly as caffeine withdrawal headaches can be quite unpleasant.

■ Drink camomile tea before going to bed or try one of the many night-time formulas freely available.

■ If you suffer low blood sugar problems then eat a banana or a *Ryvita*-type cracker with a little honey just before going to bed.

■ Eat more lettuce at night – it contains the natural sedative lactucarium which encourages deeper sleep. You can also heat crisp lettuce in stir fries etc, it's delicious.

Useful Remedies

■ Valerian and passiflora are two herbs which help enhance sleep patterns, and have been compared successfully with the prescription drug benzodiazepines. Benzodiazepines help people to get to sleep faster, enhance the quality of their sleep and leaves them less cloudy headed when they wake up. Try *Valerian Formula*. **FSC**

■ The herb *Kava Kava* has been proven to reduce stress but due to certain negative reports from Europe, it is no longer on sale in the UK. A new extract from greentea, L-theanine, helps promote relaxation. Take 50–200 mg daily. **NC**

■ Calcium and magnesium are nature's tranquillisers, take a two-in-one formula with your evening meal that includes 600mg of calcium and 300–400mg of magnesium .

■ Hops are a good alternative for people who don't get on with valerian. They are available generally in tincture form: take 1–2mls about an hour before you want to go to sleep.

■ Take 100mg of a plant extract 5 hydroxytryptphan (5HTP) derived from the plant griffonia twice daily to help boost serotonin levels naturally. The second pill should be taken at bedtime. **HN**

- Take a B complex every morning to support your nerves and keep you calmer.

- Melatonin is a hormone secreted by the pineal gland which regulates our sleep/wake cycle. It has been used successfully for years for jet lag and is freely available in health shops outside the UK but in Britain you would need a prescription. To fulfil your prescription call **The Nutricentre** Tel: 0207 436 5122. It can be ordered for your own use by calling **Pharm West** (see page 15). I take 3mg before bed as needed. Melatonin has been medically proven to aid restful sleep. Melatonin production is suppressed if we are not exposed to sufficient natural daylight. **PW**

- If you are one of those people who has tried all the above and not found them successful, try taking some ginseng in the morning. Although most people take ginseng for energy, because it is an adaptogenic herb and helps balance the body, taking it in the morning can actually help balance the body's sleep patterns by the end of the day. Take about 1000mg with breakfast for a month and see if this helps. Avoid Korean ginseng if you suffer from high blood pressure.

Helpful Hints

- One of the simplest things to do is to get into a regular routine, go to sleep at a similar time every night.

- Exercise on a regular basis can often improve sleep patterns but don't exercise too late in the day as the endorphins released by the brain can be quite stimulating.

- Find a way of reducing stress levels, as stressed individuals definitely have poorer sleep patterns.

- Try reading a novel before bed or watch television (but nothing too violent or stimulating). If you can't sleep, don't panic. Get up and do something relaxing like reading a few more pages of a novel until you start to relax and let go; then go back to bed. Don't try to go to sleep, allow yourself to fall asleep naturally.

- Meditation is particularly useful as it helps you clear the mind and get rid of all those extraneous thoughts. People who meditate on a regular basis enjoy better quality sleep.

- Smoking can also cause insomnia so if you want another reason for giving up, poor sleep patterns might be the last push you need.

- Massage your chest with a mixture of essential oils of lavender, clary sage, marjoram and basil, or add them to a relaxing bath. You can buy a burner and let the aroma fill your room.

- **Potter's** *Nodoff Mixture* is a traditional herbal remedy to promote natural sleep. It tastes awful but helps a lot of people. Available from all good health stores. For your nearest stockist contact **Potter's (Herbal Supplies) Ltd**. Tel: 01942 405100. Website: www.pottersherbal.co.uk

- Don't read any work papers close to bedtime – it stimulates your mind.

- Turn the bedside clock to the wall, so you will not panic about the time.

- Try *Flower Essences (Insomnia Blend)* containing crowea, boronia and black-eyed Susan. A few drops on the tongue before bed aid sleep by slowing an over-active mind. Contact

Serena Smith. Tel: 020 7431 6153. Serena also makes a blend for children called *Little Miracles* that contains no alcohol.

■ Reflexology, homeopathy, acupuncture and hypnotherapy have all proved useful in restoring natural sleep patterns (see *Useful Information*).

■ I find homeopathic *Lycopodium 30c* really great for shutting down my overactive mind. *Passiflora 6x* before bed helps to induce restful sleep.

■ I have found Neuro-linguistic programming (NLP) absolutely fantastic for helping to re-train my mind to aid restful sleep. It is so easy and there are many practitioners worldwide. To find your nearest practitioner send a large SAE to **The Association Neuro-Linguistic Programming** (**ANLP**), PO Box 10, Porthmadog, LL48 6ZB. Free information booklet is available. Public information line: 0870 870 4970.

■ Paul McKenna the world renowned hypnotherapist has made some great sleep CDs and tapes. Tel: 01455 852233. Website: www.mckenna-breen.com

■ Persistent insomnia can also be caused by food allergies in which case it would be wise to consult a doctor who is also a qualified nutritionist (see *Useful Information*).

■ Many people have found a herbal remedy called *Valerian Hops Complex* containing hops, oats and valerian very helpful. Take 20–30 drops in a little juice half an hour before bed. Contact **BioForce**. Tel: 01294 277344.

Homeopathic Arnica 6x taken twice daily for three months helps to strengthen the heart.

INTERMITTENT CLAUDICATION

(see also *Angina* and *Heart Disease*)

This condition is characterised by a pain in the legs, usually in the calves when walking. It is caused by blockages in the arteries supplying blood to the legs and is due to the hardening of the arteries in the lower body. To deal successfully with intermittent claudication you need to resolve the hardening of the arteries. Diets and therapies that help lower cholesterol levels and reduce the build up of deposits on the arteries are the most important treatment. See also *Cholesterol*.

Foods to Avoid

■ Greatly reduce your intake of animal fats and saturated fats including hard margarines and highly refined mass-produced cooking oils. Avoid red meat, chicken skin, too much butter, full-fat milk and most mass-produced pies, sausages, cakes and so on.

■ All fried foods should be avoided.

■ Cut down alcohol to only 2 units a day.

■ Percolated coffee or microwaved coffee elevate cholesterol which in turn can lead to intermittent claudication.

Friendly Foods

- Oily fish is rich in the omega 3 fats that help to thin the blood naturally.
- Garlic and onion should be used liberally in food as they help to lower LDL cholesterol levels.
- A diet rich in soluble and insoluble fibres from fruits and vegetables, nuts and seeds, linseeds, oat bran and psyllium husks.
- Eggs are fine as long as they are boiled and not fried.
- Look for non-hydrogenated spreads in the supermarket such as Biona and Vitaquell.
- Drink at least 6 glasses of water daily.
- See *Friendly Foods* under *Cholesterol*.

Useful Remedies

- Take natural source vitamin E, 400–600 units a day which has been shown to improve walking distance and decrease the discomfort of intermittent claudication. It probably needs to be taken for a minimum of six months to be effective. Check with your GP if you are on blood-thinning drugs as vitamin E will thin your blood naturally and reduce the risk for heart disease.
- Vitamin B3 in the form of *Inositol Hexaniacinate* 2 grams a day for at least three months. This form of B3 can help lower cholesterol and studies have shown it to be very effective for intermittent claudication. Order from **Country Life**. Tel: 0800 146 215. From outside the UK call 020 8614 1411. **Be sure to ask for no-flush B3**.
- *Gingko Biloba* 120mg of a standardised extract daily, has been shown to decrease pain and increase walking distance in sufferers.
- *Padma 28*, originally developed by Tibetan monks centuries ago, is an increasingly popular supplement with good research to show its beneficial effct on this condition. Initially 2 tablets can be taken three times daily and then after a month reduce to one tablet twice daily. **NC**
- Take the amino acid L-carnitine – 1 gram twice a day. L-carnitine is fairly expensive so try some of the other supplements first.
- Taken together *Lysine* 1500mg daily, and 2 grams of vitamin C help to clear the arteries.

Helpful Hints

- Don't smoke as there is a strong link between smoking and the development of intermittent claudication.
- Gentle exercise is definitely beneficial even though it may be uncomfortable. Do see your GP before starting on an exercise programme. People who exercise regularly are much less likely to develop intermittent claudication.

If you tend to feel light headed when you stand up –

you may have low blood pressure.

IRRITABLE BOWEL SYNDROME (IBS)
(see also *Diverticular Disease*)

Sometimes called a spastic colon, IBS is a disorder characterised by abdominal digestive problems which often cannot be explained by the conventional medical establishment. Symptoms vary greatly but include bloating, wind, abdominal pain, constipation and/or diarrhoea which are all exacerbated greatly by short- and long-term stress. IBS is most commonly due to food intolerance or allergy. Sometimes IBS can be due to poor gut bacteria, quite frequently this can happen after antibiotics or surgery and can sometimes be a result of candida (see *Candida*). Occasionally the symptoms of IBS can reflect a more serious underlying condition so it is very important to see your doctor in case you have Crohn's disease, ulcerative colitis or Diverticulitis which are often mistaken for IBS. People with IBS need to support their liver by watching their intake of fats, caffeine and alcohol.

Foods to Avoid
- Refined wheat is usually the biggest problem and cow's milk comes next. Cut these two foods from your diet for two weeks and see if there is any improvement.
- Other problem foods are eggs and citrus fruits, especially oranges.
- Foods with a high tyramine content such as cheese, port, red wine and sherry, beef, liver, herring, sauerkraut and yeast extracts.
- Flour from any source gunks up the bowel in sensitive individuals – hence why for the first seven days its a good idea to avoid any foods containing flour.
- If you suspect Candida see *Foods to Avoid* under *Candida*.

Friendly Foods
- There are plenty of alternatives to wheat. Ask at your health shop for wheat-free breads and use amaranth, oat and rye crisp breads and rice cakes which are delicious.
- If symptoms are severe, you might also need to drop oats, barley and rye – try a small amount and see what happens.
- You can now buy lentil, corn, rice and potato based pastas.
- Try organic rice, soya, pea or oat milk,
- Eat more brown rice, potatoes, fish, lean poultry, fruits and vegetables.
- Peppermint, fennel, camomile and rosemary teas can all enhance digestion and ease discomfort.
- Try to eat more foods that you wouldn't normally eat. Exotic grains like quinoa and amaranth are good protein sources and rarely cause problems.
- Instead of orange juice, try apple, pear or even pineapple juice.
- Add more ginger to your food which soothes your gut (see also *Leaky Gut*).
- Many sufferers report that eating a banana helps ease symptoms.

Useful Remedies

■ As absorption of nutrients is often a problem in IBS and you may be low in stomach acid, try taking one *Betaine hydrochloride* (stomach acid) capsule with meals, or if you don't like swallowing capsules then try *Peppermint Formula* 20 drops, prior to a meal. **FSC**

■ If you have active stomach ulcers do not take the *Betaine*, instead take a digestive enzyme formula. **BC**

■ Take 1–2 *Acidophilus* capsules at the end of meals to replace healthy bacteria in the gut and also improve digestion.

■ Take a high-strength B complex to make sure you have all the nutrients necessary to digest carbohydrates, proteins and fats. **BLK**

■ *Aloe Vera* juice, 20mls taken before meals, has helped a lot of people as it helps increase stool bulk, enhances digestion and eases the discomfort of IBS.

■ Take 1–3 dessert spoonfuls of Linseed in the form of *Linusit Gold* daily, providing 10–20 grams of linseeds. The mixture of soluble and insoluble fibres help stimulate the bowel gently while providing stool bulk enabling the bowel to function normally and comfortably. Linseed has been successful both in alleviating constipation and diarrhoea but it must be taken with plenty of water.

■ See other remedies under *Constipation* and *Diarrhoea* if either is your main problem.

■ *Seacure* is hydrolyzed protein from lean white fish which helps relieve the pain of multiple digestive dysfunctions by helping to repair the gut wall. Adults should take 6 capsules daily. Children may also take it. Break open capsules and mix with food. **NC**

Helpful Hints

■ *Oil of Peppermint* is anti-spasmodic – massage it on your abdomen and drink peppermint tea after meals.

■ Gentle exercise on a regular basis enhances bowel function. Yoga, swimming or walking are all good forms of exercise which do not overtax the system and enhance relaxation.

■ Remember to eat in a relaxed fashion; being stressed while you eat makes it very difficult for normal digestion. Try to avoid eating food on the run.

■ Remember, if you have an intolerance to one food, its likely to be more than one. Very few of us react to just one food and in most cases we react to 4 or 5. Try to identify them with the aid of a nutritionist or kinesiologist. See *Useful Information* for details.

■ Call the *Woman's Nutritional Advisory Service*, who offer help to IBS sufferers, on 01273 487366. 9–5pm Monday to Friday. www.wnas.org.uk

j

JET LAG

When we move time zones our internal body clock and production of the hormone melatonin can be disrupted. Long haul flights are very dehydrating and cramped. Lack of sleep and the change in times can cause extreme fatigue and poor concentration. The sooner you adjust to the local time the better.

Foods to Avoid
- On long flights eat small meals and reduce your intake of tea, coffee, alcohol and cola-type fizzy drinks which all dehydrate the body. Caffeine can contribute to poor sleep patterns, so ask for decaffeinated varieties. Sugar depletes minerals and lowers immune function which can be a real problem in the airless cabins where bacteria and viruses spread so quickly.

Friendly Foods
- I realise that airline food often leaves a lot to be desired – but eat light and healthy food the day prior to travel and drink plenty of water
- Foods that help you to calm you down and aid restful sleep are turkey, cottage cheese, avocados, pasta, bananas and skimmed milk
- Camomile tea is great if you can get it or take a few tea bags with you.
- Ask the cabin crew to give you a bottle of mineral water and drink it throughout the flight.

Useful Remedies
- Take one gram of vitamin C with bioflavonoids every 2–3 hours with a full glass of water.
- Take a high-strength multi-vitamin and mineral
- Try *Emergen C*, a powdered vitamin C and electrolyte formula that helps replenish depleted minerals.
- The amino acid L-glutamine helps improve concentration on long flights if you are on business – take 1–3 grams during the flight.
- *Melatonin* produced in the pineal gland, has proven highly effective for reducing jet lag. Take 3mg one hour before sleep. In the UK this is only available on prescription but can be bought at virtually any American airport or health store. And you can order from **PharmWest** for your own use by post in the UK. **PW**
- If you are worried about being cramped in a seat, take some *Ginkgo Biloba* and *Gotu Kola* a few days before and during your flight as they increase circulation.

■ Natural source vitamin E thins the blood and reduces the risk of clotting on long flights. Take 400iu at least a week prior to travel and during the journey.

Helpful Hints

■ To help reset your body clock attach a super magnet to the top of your head for 15 minutes before landing. One of the reasons you get jet lag is because your body clock is trying to adjust to the new magnetic field. By using the magnet you can reset your body clock to the local magnetic field. To order a *Super Magnet* call **Coghill Research** on 01495 752122.

■ Try and stay up until the local time to go to bed. When I travel west I usually manage to stay up until the local bedtime but if I'm going east I find this harder and often take a nap. Basically, the sooner you get onto local time the better. Get as much sunlight as you can as soon as you arrive which helps to re-set your body clock.

■ Homeopathic *Arnica 200c* can be taken one dose before the flight and every few hours during flight and then 4 doses during the 24 hours after landing to reduce jet lag.

■ Think positive.

■ **Australian Bush Flower Essences** make a formula called *Travel Essence* – available from health stores.

■ Have a small meal when you arrive to help you to sleep.

■ While you are on the plane, get up and walk around as much as your can, touch your toes and have a good stretch.

Eating too much animal protein depletes calcium from the bones

KIDNEY STONES

Kidney stones are usually made of insoluble crystals and minerals which are found in the urine. Most stones are made from calcium where lime salts form around small mucous masses or other tissue fragments, but stones can be also be made from other substances such as uric acid. Stones form in the kidney, the bladder or the urethra (the tubes which connect the kidneys to the bladder). They can cause almost no pain when they are tiny but if they begin to pass through the urinary tract the pain can be excruciating. Having kidney stones in the body makes bladder infections much more likely. If you ever pass blood in your urine or have persistent back pain, then it's very important that you see your GP. People who live in soft water areas are more likely to suffer kidney stones. Hard water areas have less incidence of this problem. The calcium content of both types of water are usually similar but the hard water may simply have low levels of other minerals which causes more calcium to be dumped into the kidneys.

Foods to Avoid

■ As kidney stones are linked to a high-acid diet it is best to reduce acid forming foods such as animal protein, dairy from cows, sugar, alcohol, tea and refined white foods should be kept to a minimum.

■ Foods high in oxalates should be avoided as much as possible. These include rhubarb, beetroot, spinach, parsley, instant coffee, beans, chocolate, celery, dried figs, grapefruit, oranges, gooseberries, raspberries, lemon peel, peanuts, peppers, sweet potato, tea, strawberries and bran.

■ Avoid sodium-based table salts, try *Solo Salt* which is based on magnesium and potassium.

■ Try to avoid all caffeinated and fizzy drinks as they increase calcium loss through the urine.

Friendly Foods

■ Replace animal protein with more vegetarian-type foods, such as tofu (soya bean curd) and quorn.

■ Eat more calcium- and magnesium-rich foods such as fresh fish, pilchards, curried vegetables, black strap molasses, honey, watercress, soya flour, yoghurt, muesli and sesame seeds.

■ Raw wheat germ is rich in magnesium and vitamin E.

■ Include more leafy green vegetables, brown rice and pastas made from corn and rice in your diet.

■ Wholemeal bread is fine: Use non-hydrogenated spreads such as *Biona* or *Vitaquell*.

■ Ask at your health shop for quinoa, millet, amaranth, spelt and other grain breads, cakes and crackers.

- As dairy from cows is one of your biggest problems try soya light milk or organic rice milk. Try the rice milk on cereal for a couple of days and you will never want ordinary milk again! Soya light is great with tea and for desserts.

- Use unrefined extra virgin olive oil for salad dressings.

- Add lecithin granules to your breakfast cereals or yoghurt as they help to emulsify the bad fats.

- Drink at least 8 glasses of water every day.

- Use *Alka* herb tea and *Alka Life* granules to help re-alkalise your system. For details call **Best Care Products** Tel: 01342 410 303 Website: www.bestcare-uk.com

- Eat more barley- and lentil-based dishes.

Useful Remedies

- Most people with kidney stones are low in magnesium and vitamin B6 which helps prevent calcium depositing in the joints and kidneys. Take a 100mg of magnesium three times a day and 50mg of B6 daily. **FSC**

- Take calcium citrate, 500mg, with each meal as the calcium binds to the oxalate and reduces the likelihood of kidney stones being formed. However, calcium taken on an empty stomach can increase the risk of kidney stones so it is very important it is taken with a meal.

- An extract of brown rice called IP6 has been shown to reduce the risk of developing kidney stones. Take 800mg daily. **NC**

- Take a high-strength multi-vitamin which includes plenty of B vitamins.

- A good liquid multi-mineral is vital for controlling kidney stones. I use mineral drops called *ConcenTrace* available from 01342 824684 or call **Higher Nature** (see page 15).

- Horsetail, either as tincture or as tablets historically has been used to help reduce kidney stones.

- The amino acid lysine helps decrease urinary calcium. Take 1500mg daily.

- The tissue salts silica and calcium fluoride help to break down kidney stones. Take 4 of each a day.

Helpful Hints

- Exercise on a regular basis. Inactivity is more likely to lead to a calcium build up, leaving you more prone to developing kidney stones.

Essential oil of Indian sandalwood blended with a little grapeseed oil helps dry skin retain more moisture. It is effective for dry skin conditions such as eczema.

LEAKY GUT

Over time, we have a tendency to build up various toxins in our body, especially in the small intestine and large bowel. The build up tends to be a combination of undigested food, impacted faeces, bacteria, fungi, parasites and dead cells. As the toxins accumulate, the gut wall can become irritated and damaged which enables partly digested food molecules to cross the gut (small intestine) wall into the bloodstream. These undigested food molecules are treated as foreign invaders and provoke an immune response. In other words our body now reacts to foods as though it were an infection entering our system and sends out antibodies to fight it. This is one of the possible mechanisms that trigger rheumatoid arthritis and is now recognised as a major trigger for most food intolerances, see under (*Allergies* and *Candida*).

Leaky gut syndrome has now reached epidemic proportions, thanks mostly to stress, eating too many of the wrong foods, eating in a hurry and so on. People with irritable bowel tend to have a leaky gut. Generally, if you suffer bloating, constipation and/or diarrhoea, crave sugary, refined foods, feel tired all the time and notice that your food comes out the other end looking fairly much the same as it went it in you may well have a leaky gut.

Foods to Avoid

- I'm afraid it's the same old song! You need to cut down on low-fibre foods such as jellies, ice cream, burgers, biscuits, cakes, pies and pastries.
- Sugar encourages fermentation and growth of unfriendly bacteria in the bowel, so keep sugary foods and drinks to a minimum.
- If you tend to bloat a lot after meals, don't eat large amounts of fruit directly after a large meal as fruit likes a quick passage through the gut. If it gets stuck behind proteins such as meat, the fruit will ferment which adds to the problem.
- Alcohol increases fermentation.
- Any foods to which you have an allergy or intolerance will only aggravate the problem, the most common being wheat, citrus fruits and sometimes cow's milk.
- Particularly bad is melon, this should only ever be eaten on its own.
- Avoid heavy large meals which place too much strain on the digestive system.

Friendly Foods

- Eat more natural low-fat, live yoghurt containing the friendly bacteria acidophilus/bifidus.
- Pineapple and papaya are rich in enzymes which improve protein digestion making it less likely that undigested proteins end up in the bowel.

193

- Beetroots, artichokes, radishes and celeriac are all very good liver cleansers which also improve digestion. They contain inulin, which helps encourage the growth of bifidus within the large bowel. This helps to reduce the load on the liver in the long term.

- Sunflower, pumpkin, sesame and linseeds and nuts (always buy the unsalted ones, preferably organic) are all rich sources of fibre, both soluble and insoluble helping the bowel move regularly and easily. I toast the sunflower and pumpkin seeds and throw them over salads and snacks. Also add them raw to breakfast cereals and fruit whips.

- Drink plenty of fluids, not tea, coffee and fizzy canned drinks which dehydrate the bowel, but water, at least 6–8 glasses a day.

- Garlic helps fight infections and encourages growth of friendly bacteria in the bowel.

- Seaweed, spirulina and chlorella sprinkled on meals is another good way of detoxifying the system. You do need to use liberal amounts and it is better in powder form than taking tablets.

- Use more fresh root ginger in your cooking which soothes and heals the gut.

- Green cabbage is rich in the amino acid L-glutamine which helps heal a leaky gut. Eat more raw and steamed cabbage and use the liquid from the cooking to make gravy.

- Eat plenty of fresh vegetables, grains and fruits between meals.

- Figs, apricots, apples and bananas all help reduce constipation.

Useful Remedies

- Sprinkle Alkalife greenfood, rich in wheat germ and green foods that re-alkalise your system, over cereals and desserts. To order call **Best Care Products**. Tel: 01342 410303. Website: www.bestcare-uk.com

- Add 1–3 dessert spoonfuls of raw linseeds to your cereals or yoghurts every day.

- Take 2 acidophilus/bifidus capsules after main meals to replenish healthy bacteria aids digestion and elimination.

- Take 1 *Betaine Hydrochloride* (stomach acid) capsule with meals to enable the body to break down proteins adequately. If you have stomach ulcers or the Betaine causes a slight burning sensation then use a digestive enzyme capsule instead.

- L-glutamine, the amino acid, really helps to heal a leaky gut. Take between 1–4 grams a day for the first month and then reduce to 1 gram daily.

- Vitamin E 200–500 units a day, zinc 30–60mg a day and 1–3 grams of vitamin C daily with food.

- After taking these supplements for 3 months your gut should be in better shape and you could then reduce this regimen to a good multi-vitamin/mineral plus a digestive enzyme.

Helpful Hints

- Make sure you get plenty of regular exercise and always walk for 15 minutes after a meal to aid digestion.

- Reflexology and acupuncturecan help improve bowel function (see *Useful Information*).

- Remember not to eat on the move, enjoy meals in a relaxed comfortable situation.

- If you are anxious or upset just eat light soups. Never eat a heavy meal when stressed.

- I find colonic irrigation really helps this problem. To find your nearest practitioner see *Useful Information*.

Respect yourself, respect others and take responsibility for all your actions.
The Dalai Lama

LEG ULCERS

(see also *Circulation* and *Cholesterol*)

This common problem in the over sixties is caused by a restricted circulation and lack of oxygen and nutrients reaching the skin. Leg and foot ulcers are more common in diabetics due to changes in circulation and the nerve endings near the skin.

Foods to Avoid

- Foods which impede circulation including animal fats, especially red meats, sausages, meat pies, burgers, full-fat cheeses and dairy produce as well as hard margarines made from refined vegetable oils.

- Avoid all fried foods and don't use mass-produced vegetable oils.

- Cut down on alcohol and low-fibre foods such as jelly and ice cream, white breads, mass-produced pies and cakes.

- See diet under *Circulation* and *Cholesterol*.

Friendly Foods

- Eat more leafy greens especially cabbage, kale, celery, pak choi, spinach and broccoli which contain high levels of carotenes and minerals.

- Eat more salads and sprinkle sunflower, pumpkin and sesame seeds over them as these seeds are high in essential fatty acids, minerals and fibre.

- Oily fish are rich in omega 3 fats that thin the blood naturally and aid healing.

- Sprinkle wheat germ and lecithin over your breakfast cereals to lower bad cholesterol and emulsify the bad fats.

- Add almonds, Brazil nuts, hazelnuts and walnuts to fruit dips as they are all high in zinc which aids skin healing.

- High protein foods like whey protein are a very rich source of glutamine which speeds the healing process. You can buy powdered whey at all health shops.

Useful Remedies

- Take zinc 30mg 1–2 times a day with meals. This is absolutely essential if you are suffering slow wound healing.

■ *Gotu Kola* 500mg, 3 times a day, this herb has been used historically for wound healing and when combined with zinc can be very successful.

■ Vitamin C, taken 1 gram daily with food, is essential for healing connective tissue.

■ If the ulcers are superficial and not too deep, aloe-vera gel applied topically can speed healing, ease the discomfort and protect from infection.

■ Many elderly people cannot be bothered to cook proper meals, so if this is the case make sure you take a multi-vitamin and mineral.

■ A varied diet is always best but when needs must, the pills will make a difference.

■ *Ginkgo Biloba* helps to increase circulation. Take 120mg of standardised extract daily until symptoms ease.

■ *Oralmat* is a wound-healing spray, based on rye grass, it contains powerful wound healing, analgesic, anti-inflammatory, immune, anti-bacterial, anti-fungal and anti-viral properties. Apply up to 4 times daily. **NC**

Helpful Hints

■ Try *Bach Rescue Remedy* cream once the skin starts to heal – available from good health stores.

■ Place raw honey on the site of the ulcer, which will speed the healing process.

■ Raise legs above hip level when resting and move feet backwards and forwards slowly to increase circulation in lower legs. Try and walk for at least 15 minutes twice a day.

■ Many readers have found that acupuncture and reflexology improve circulation (see *Useful Information*).

■ Wearing magnets in your shoes greatly aids circulation. Tel: 0161 798 5876 Helpline: 0161 798 5885. Website: www.homedicsuk.com

If you stop supporting your body, it will stop supporting you.

LICHEN PLANUS

Lichen planus is a chronic condition of the skin and mucous membranes, typically the lining of the mouth. This is thought to be caused by a virus and has some features in common with other skin problems like eczema and psoriasis. Sores on the skin are often localised on the wrist and ankles but it can be widespread.

Foods to Avoid

■ Anything which weakens the immune system like concentrated sugars, refined carbohydrates, even concentrated fruit juices and any food to which you have an intolerance.

■ Foods which are a problem for many sufferers are tomatoes, pineapples, mushrooms, coffee, red meat, chocolate and ice cream. Keep a food diary and note when symptoms are worse, so you can identify and remove them from your diet.

- Alcohol, vinegars and oily, spicy foods can make the problem worse.
- Avoid dairy produce from cows as much as possible.

Friendly Foods

- Eat more fresh fish of any kind, but try and make it oily fish like salmon, tuna or mackerel twice a week; oily fish are rich in omega 3 essential fats and vitamin A.
- Beta carotene converts to vitamin A in the body and aids the healing process. Therefore eat plenty of carrots, green vegetables, a little butter, French beans, cress, spinach, spring greens, watercress, sweet potatoes, apricots (fresh and dried), parsley and mangos.
- Seeds and nuts are zinc-rich foods which can speed up healing.

Useful Remedies

- Vitamin A 20,000iu a day for up to 2 months as it has been speculated that lichen planus is due to vitamin A deficiency. If you are pregnant or planning a pregnancy only take 5000 iu daily.
- Take a good quality multi-vitamin and mineral.
- Take an additional 30mg of zinc in addition to the multi once a day. Zinc and vitamin A are complementary in their action. Zinc is essential for wound healing and a healthy immune system.
- Organic aloe vera juice taken as 20mls taken before every meal speeds healing, and reduces discomfort as well as boosting the immune system. **HN**
- Anti-viral herbs are echinacea, liquorice and St John's wort. They can all be used internally and applied topically to the skin.

Helpful Hints

- Try to rest as much as possible. Don't overwork and don't over stress your system as it is much harder for the body to heal.
- Use washing powders and detergents suitable for sensitive skin.
- Ultraviolet light often brings relief, but only try this under proper supervision.
- Moderate amounts of sunshine can help too, but avoid sunbathing between 11am and 3pm.
- Chickweed ointment has been useful to some people. **NC**
- Homeopathy has helped many sufferers (see *Useful Information*).

As liver toxicity is associated with virtually every health problem in this book, I suggest you read The Liver Cleansing Diet *by Dr Sandra Cabot. Tel: 0117 983 8851.*

LOW BLOOD PRESSURE (HYPOTENSION)
(see also *Low Blood Sugar*)

The most classic symptom of low blood pressure is a feeling of light-headedness on standing, especially from the ground up. It is more common in women. Low blood pressure is not thought of as a problem in Britain by orthodox doctors, however, in certain European countries it is often treated. Because the blood is responsible for carrying oxygen and nutrients to the body's tissues and organs, low blood pressure can often trigger problems with energy levels and mental function.

Low blood pressure is frequently a sign of weakness in the adrenal glands. These glands sit on top of your kidneys and have an important role to play in our hormonal system. Adrenal weakness is often due to overworking and excessive stresses compounded by dietary deficiencies. Far too many of us have a lifestyle which over stresses our adrenal glands. We work too many hours, don't get sufficient sleep and tend to rely on coffee and sugar to get us through the day or when our energy levels drop. In the long term all these factors weaken adrenal function.

One of the most common complaints received by staff in health food shops these days is that of feeling tired all the time. The first question you need to ask yourself is, do you start the day with a good breakfast or find that you can't face breakfast and the only thing that gets you going is two or three cups of tea or coffee. What you are doing is putting a stimulant into your body that puts even more stress on your adrenal glands.

Foods to Avoid
- Caffeine and sugar in any form will particularly deplete the adrenal glands. Remember that tea, coffee, chocolate and cola all contain caffeine. You might remember not to put sugar in your tea or coffee but are you having a biscuit with it? This will have a similar deleterious effect.
- Refined foods like bread, biscuits, cakes, pizza, burgers and pies all deplete the body of B vitamins necessary to keep the adrenal glands in good shape.

Friendly Foods
- Liquorice is one of the quickest and simplest ways of restoring adrenal glands to normal function.
- Eat more quality protein such as fresh fish, chicken, lentils, beans pulses and tofu – as protein helps to normalise blood pressure.
- Whole grains which include brown rice, quinoa, millet and amaranth are highly nutritious.
- Eat plenty of fresh fruit and vegetables particularly fresh juices – if you are feeling low in energy rather than reaching for coffee, try a glass of carrot, beetroot, apple and ginger juice.
- Eat more avocados and wheat germ which are rich in vitamin E.
- Use potassium and magnesium salt in your diet such as *Solo Salt*.

Useful Remedies

- *Liquorice Formula*, taken 1-3mls a day for up to three months, is a blend of herbs to nourish the adrenal glands. Over time it will help increase energy and can also help to normalise blood pressure. **FSC**

- Take high-potency B complex 1 twice daily with meals. Take B vitamins with breakfast and lunch, not supper as they keep you more alert.

- As the mineral magnesium is often lacking take 250–500mg daily with food.

- Siberian ginseng taken 1–3 grams a day for 60 days helps to balance the body. If the blood pressure is low it can help to bring it back up and ginseng has the added benefit of being an excellent adrenal restorative.

- The herb *Jiaogulan* is known as an adaptogen and antioxidant which modulates blood pressure, lowering it when it is too high and raising it when it is too low. Take up to 4 tablets daily. **NC**

- Vitamin E, 200iu per day, can help to normalise blood pressure.

Helpful Hints.

- Take sensible amounts of exercise but also make sure you are getting sufficient rest.
- See *General Health Hints*.

Don't let a small argument ruin a good friendship. Life is so short – make up.

LOW BLOOD SUGAR (HYPOGLYCAEMIA)

Low blood sugar, also known as hypoglycaemia, is something that 95% of us experience at some time if we go without food for too long – the most common cause is skipping breakfast. I have met a number of young women who suffer regular blackouts, fainting spells and dizziness which their doctor cannot explain. But when they relate their diet of missed meals, sugary drinks and snacks I know almost immediately what the problem is.

The level of sugar in the blood is critical to how you feel. If it is too low, you may well feel very tired, find concentration difficult, become shaky, feel very hungry, drowsy, possibly have headaches and feel anxious. These myriad symptoms can simply result from skipping breakfast.

If you are one of those people who won't eat breakfast for the sake of an extra 15 to 20 minutes in bed or simply can't face it in the mornings and then rush off to work, by mid-morning you are going to feel even hungrier than you did when you left the house. Most people then reach for coffee and a doughnut, tea and biscuits, something that will quickly raise blood-sugar levels. Unfortunately not long after consuming this type of food our blood sugar drops even lower than it was before, this is due to the body producing an excess of insulin to compensate for the sugar load. One of the problems with skipping breakfast is that even if your first meal of the day (lunch) is a good wholesome one, your blood-sugar levels are still likely to be very erratic, bouncing up and down all day long. This can lead your becoming irritable with your colleagues or extremely emotional in response to even small problems.

Other people with low blood sugar will find it crucial to have their meals at regular times. If their lunch hour is normally 12 o'clock and someone asks them to leave it until 2pm, they may feel weak, suffer memory problems or simply find it hard to concentrate. If they are dealing with the public, they are much more likely to be short-tempered and less approachable. If they are trying to complete a task, the work is likely to be of lower quality than it would have been if they had eaten at the regular time.

The brain's only food source is pure glucose and if you have not eaten for a while the hypothalamus area within the brain will just demand more sugar. Basically if your hypothalamus is not happy no amount of willpower will stop you craving something sweet. Nutritionists have known for years that the easiest way to control blood sugar is to eat small healthy meals more regularly but most people don't do this. The average person in the West eats 27lbs of snacks a year which cause weight gain and a very unstable blood sugar. The result is a huge increase in diabetes and as symptoms of low blood sugar are similar to high blood sugar diabetes – have a check up with your doctor. However, a single blood test is unlikely to show any problem with low blood sugar because unless you are actually suffering a dip in blood sugar at the time of the test, results could be normal.

Foods to Avoid

■ Most people with low blood sugar rush from one sugar fix to the next. In extreme cases they might eat 6 to 8 chocolate type snacks daily. Cravings for caffeine, sugar, refined carbohydrates such as croissants, biscuits, pastries and pizzas are all common. Not only do all these foods have a negative affect on blood sugar they are also low in fibre, vitamins and minerals.

Friendly Foods

■ Fibre helps to slow down the release of sugars, and if absent, the sugars in any foods get into the bloodstream too quickly.

■ Begin the day with a good breakfast such as low-sugar muesli or cereal, porridge, eggs or beans on toast.

■ If you only have time for a small meal, try to make sure it is high in protein rather than a carbohydrate-based meal which will keep you more satisfied in the long term.

■ At the very least eat a banana and a low-fat fruit yoghurt.

■ Eat more brown rice, barley, oats, lentils, amaranth, spelt, whole meal bread and pastas, also try corn, spinach and rice pastas.

■ Make sure you eat some good quality protein such as fish, chicken or tofu preferably in the middle of the day.

- Eat smaller meals more regularly.
- Snack on fresh fruit and low-sugar snack bars available from health shops.
- Drink freshly made or organic fruit and vegetable juices.
- Snack on low-fat yoghurts with added sunflower seeds and raisins to reduce sugar cravings.
- Have a piece of whole meal toast or an amaranth cracker with a little low-fat spread and low-sugar jam or honey.
- Drink more herbal teas and dandelion coffee.
- Drink more water.
- Make salad dressings with a combination of any unrefined organic oils such as sesame, walnut, olive or sunflower.

Useful Remedies

- In America studies have shown that when people who eat a refined Western diet, are given 200 mcg of the mineral chromium daily, the incidence of late onset diabetes was halved. Chromium is greatly depleted in the body by sugar and junk foods.
- During the first few days you are really going to be craving sweet foods and if you begin taking 400 mcg daily, it takes a few days to kick in but really does help reduce cravings.
- Take Magnesium 200–500mg once a day with food. Magnesium and chromium both help to regulate blood-sugar levels.
- A strong B complex with 30mg of niacinamide B3. (Make sure it's a no-flush type niacin). B3 is essential for the control of blood-sugar levels.
- Take vitamin E 500–600 units a day as vitamin E has been shown to help improve insulin response in the body.
- **Bio Care** make *Sucro Guard*, developed by Dr John Briffa. Taken between meals it contains all the above nutrients in one capsule. **BC**

Helpful Hints

- If you have acute symptoms such as fainting fits, blackouts, extreme weakness and trembling, it is important to restore blood-sugar levels as quickly as possible. In an emergency you need to get glucose into your body. While I would generally not recommend high-sugar foods and drinks this is one occasion when they can be used. Drink *Lucozade* or similar, or eat a sugary biscuit. This is not a long-term solution!
- Your own GP can refer you to the nearest doctor who is also a qualified nutritionist (see *Useful Information*).

If you have longitudinal ridges in your nails – you are likely to have low stomach acid.

LOW STOMACH ACID

(see also *Acid Stomach* and *Indigestion*)

When we eat food, particularly protein-based foods, our stomachs should produce a lot of gastric juice in response. This juice is a mixture of mucous which protects the stomach lining and a very strong acid, hydrochloric acid. High levels of hydrochloric acid are needed for proper digestion before the food goes on to the small intestine and the nutrients start to be absorbed. Due to various aspects of our diet, lifestyle and age, the amount of acid we produce over time tends to decline. Low levels of stomach acid are associated with poor digestion and more importantly absorption of nutrients we need for good health.

Three conditions strongly linked with low stomach acid levels are asthma, allergies and gall stones. Many people feel they make too much stomach acid whereas in reality they produce too little. A lot of people will take an antacid, which neutralises what little acid was available, making digestion even harder.

Undigested foods can end up leaking into the bloodstream causing food allergies. Undigested food can rot in the bowel causing wind, bloating, and overgrowth of unhealthy organisms such as candida.

Foods to Avoid

- Cut down on alcohol, sugar, caffeinated foods and drinks and cow's dairy products which can all cause an acid reflux.
- Don't eat in a rush and keep heavy, rich meals containing red meat and creamy sauces to a minimum.
- Avoid all fried foods which are hard to digest.
- Avoid eating proteins like fish or meat with potatoes or pasta.
- Avoid drinking too much liquids with meals.
- Stop chewing gum – this makes the stomach think that food is about to arrive which triggers stomach acid production.
- Don't eat a large amount of fruit directly after a large meal.

Friendly Foods

- Chew your food thoroughly and take your time eating.
- Eat fruit generally between meals or include a little papaya and pineapple with meals which are packed with digestive enzymes.
- Bitter-tasting vegetables are great for stimulating digestion, eat more *Rucola*, radiccio and celeriac plus ginger. These foods encourage gastric juice production.

Useful Remedies

■ As levels of stomach acid tend to drop as we age or when we are under stress, take one *Betaine Hydrochloride* (Stomach acid) capsule with main meals. Take with a glass of water just before the meal. If you have active stomach ulcers use a good quality digestive enzyme supplement instead.

■ *Peppermint Formula*, 10–20 drops before a meal. If you suffer with symptoms of overeating, feeling bloated and uncomfortable take 10–20 drops after a meal. **FSC**

■ Acidophilus/bifidus are the healthy bacteria which help to regulate digestion. 1–2 capsules taken at the end of the meal, if the gut flora is in good shape the body's ability to manufacture hydrochloric acid is improved.

Helpful Hints

■ Chewing food thoroughly really helps to improve the digestive process.

■ Some people have found separating proteins and carbohydrates at one meal has improved their digestion no end.

■ Eat small meals regularly, try 4 snack type meals daily. Avoid eating when stressed.

■ Dr John Briffa suggests this home test for low stomach acid in his book *Body Wise* (Cima Books). Take a level teaspoon of bicarbonate of soda and dissolve in some water. Drink this mixture on an empty stomach. If sufficient quantities of acid are present in the stomach, the bicarb mixture is converted into gas, producing significant bloating and belching within five to ten minutes of drinking the mix. Little or no belching denotes low stomach acid.

■ If you have pronounced longitudinal ridges in your nails, this is a common sign of low stomach acid.

■ Drink mint or peppermint herbal teas to aid digestion.

Walking for 30 minutes each day aids digestion.

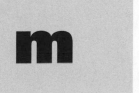

MACULAR DEGENERATION

(see *Eye Problems*)

Fresh cabbage contains the amino acid L-glutamine which helps to heal gut problems and can be applied externally to heal leg ulcers.

ME (MYALGIA ENCEPHALOMYELITIS) OR CHRONIC FATIGUE

Around 230,000 people in Britain are recognised as having chronic fatigue or ME, but I believe that hundreds of thousands more go undiagnosed. Many people feel tired all the time and just struggle on, but only when the crushing exhaustion becomes incapacitating do people seek medical help. Orthodox medicine basically offers anti-depressants which will not help in the long term and certainly do not address the root cause of the problem.

Symptoms range from chronic, debilitating tiredness to depression, muscle pain, headaches and decreased concentration to name but a few.

This condition appears multi-factorial in origin. If you are stressed, have suffered a viral illness such as flu, are exposed to a lot of electrical equipment or have running water under your home, any or all these factors can play a part. ME is also linked to the polio vaccine, low blood sugar, heavy metal toxicity, liver congestion, food intolerances, candida, adrenal exhaustion and deficiencies in minerals such as magnesium. If you have long-term low blood pressure this denotes your adrenal glands are struggling.

It is possible that some individuals could have all of these conditions which eventually result in chronic fatigue, and while it is true to say that there is no single answer for ME, there are a number of things that seem to help the majority. But as we are all unique, what helps one person may not work for another, but without doubt eating the right diet and taking the right supplements will make a difference. If you contract a viral infection – you must give your body a chance to rest and recover which gives you more chance of avoiding long-term illness.

Foods to Avoid

- Any foods and drinks containing caffeine, sugar and alcohol, all of which lower immune function, weaken the adrenal system and play havoc with blood-sugar levels. Also most pre-packaged foods high in sugar are also high in saturated fats, salt, additives and preservatives.

- Most mass-produced, tinned foods and takeaways (unless they are freshly made) are lacking in magnesium. 40% of ME patients have low levels of this vital mineral.

- Some people mistakenly use guarana as an energy source when they are very low in energy. Unfortunately, the primary reason it gives you energy is the caffeine content which will only serve to weaken you in the long term.

- If you find yourself constantly craving foods such as wheat, sugar and snacks, are bloated, have an urgency to urinate, suffer mood swings and are always tired, you may well have candida (see *Foods to Avoid* under *Candida*).

- Almost everyone with chronic fatigue will have multiple food intolerances. The most common being wheat and dairy from cow's milk.

- See *Useful Information*.

Friendly Foods

■ It is vital that you eat good quality protein such as organic meat, chicken or fresh fish, beans, and tofu at least twice a day. Protein helps to balance blood sugar for longer periods.

■ Include plenty of vegetables and fruits in the diet but don't eat too much fruit if you have candida.

■ Replace wheat with amaranth, oat and rice crackers and ask for wheat and yeast-free breads at your health shops. If you are too ill to leave home call *The Village Bakery* in Cumbria and order by mail. Tel: 01768 881515.

■ Try experimenting with other grains such as millet, quinoa, kamut, spelt and so on. **Nature's Path** make a great range of cereals from these grains which you can enjoy with organic rice or soya light milk.

■ Remember to include plenty of cereals, leafy greens such as cabbage, kale, spring greens, pak choi, broccoli, celery, wheat germ, soya-based biscuits and pastas, Brazil nuts, walnuts, almonds, curries, black strap molasses, honey and beans as they are rich in magnesium.

■ If you find you are intolerant to dairy there are now plenty of alternatives. Oat, rice, pea or light soya milk are all nutritious and can be used instead of cow's milk. Drink plenty of water even if you are not thirsty to help detoxify your system.

■ Eat sunflower, pumpkin and sesame seeds, packed with essential fats and fibre and use extra-virgin unrefined olive or sunflower oils for salad dressings.

■ Add coriander to your foods which really helps to detoxify heavy metals from the body.

Useful Remedies

■ Take Siberian ginseng 1–3 grams a day helps the body adapt to stressful circumstances. Take for 60 days and then stop for 30 days before starting again. Don't take ginseng if you are pregnant.

■ *Liquorice Formula* is a blend of herbs for the adrenal system, it is anti-viral, helps to alleviate pain and strengthens the adrenal glands. If your blood pressure is low, take for 3–6 months until the blood pressure is normal then take a rest. **FSC**

■ *Enada* is a stabilised form of vitamin B3 which was originally formulated at the Parkinson's Institute in Vienna to help alleviate the terrible fatigue that accompanies Parkinson's. In independent medical trials globally it has been found to raise energy levels and greatly reduce or eliminate the 'brain fog' often associated with ME for 70% of patients. Initially take 10mg every morning one hour before food and then after 2 months reduce to 5mg daily. **Springfield** *Enada* is available from health stores worldwide. **NC, FSC**

■ Take magnesium malate, 500–1000mg per day, helps to reduce muscle soreness.

■ Milk thistle and dandelion are two herbs which support and detoxify the liver which is often overloaded. Take 1ml 3 times daily.

■ Take a high-strength multi-vitamin and mineral twice daily **S**

■ Echinacea, either as a tincture or a tablet taken either Monday through Friday or three weeks on, one week off to boost the immune system and help fight off any other infections.

Helpful Hints

- Take some gentle exercise. One study found that people were able to walk for three minutes, rest for three minutes until they had done a total of 30 minutes walking without any negative effect on chronic fatigue.

- Try a gentle stretching programme, to gradually tone the muscles and help drain the lymph system which is often overloaded.

- Learn to relax. Meditation is a great way to give the body and brain a complete rest (see *Meditation*).

- Homeopathic *Sarco Lactic Acid 6x* taken twice daily for 7–10 days helps reduce symptoms.

- Stabilised liquid oxygen helps to re-alkalise the body, encourages healthy bacteria in the gut and has been shown to kill bacteria such as E coli, some viruses, parasites and fungi. Above all it helps to raise energy levels. Available from all good health stores or call 0208 886 6555.

- Have a friend massage your aching muscles with a mix of the essential oils of thyme and lemongrass, and to help lift depression try a mix of neroli and rose in a good base oil.

- For a free information pack, write to **Action for ME**, PO Box 1302, Wells, BA5 1YE or telephone 01749 670799. Website: www.afme.org.uk Email: info@afme.org.uk

- Many readers have been cured of ME by energy healers. One is Seka Nikolic. I know Seka personally and have interviewed many people (and their doctors), who are now free from ME thanks to Seka. Seka works from **The Kailash Clinic**, 7 Newcourt Street, London NW8 7AA. Tel: 020 7722 3939. The other is Kelvin Heard who suffered from ME for 3 years. After visiting a healer, he was cured and is now a qualified, registered healer who specialises in ME. Again, I have interviewed a number of his patients who are now living normal lives. Tel: 07710 794627.

- For more information on healing which is helpful for ME patients see *Healing*.

- If your symptoms persist, try having your house dowsed for electrical or geopathic stress. To find a dowser, call *The British Dowsing Society* Tel: 01233 750253. www.britishdowsers.org

- Cranial osteopathy has helped many people with ME, as it releases nerve endings which releases energy in the body. See under *Useful Information*.

- With ME, it is best to consult a doctor, who is also a qualified nutritionist, as you may need injections or magnesium and B12 (see *Useful Information*).

Persistent low blood pressure indicates that your adrenal glands are exhausted – get some rest.

MEDITATION

As stress is a contributing factor for practically every major disease, any way that we can find to reduce stress has got to be good news. Meditation costs nothing, you can practise it daily on your own or with friends and it has proven health benefits.

People who meditate regularly often look younger, enjoy more peace of mind, feel more contented with their lives, have a slower heart rate and lower blood pressure, they breathe more easily and if they become ill tend to recover more quickly. Under pressure they remain calm and are generally less anxious.

Researchers have also found that people who meditate regularly produce more of the hormone melatonin which lower levels of stress hormones.

The single biggest reason people don't meditate is because they do not have the time. Well, it seems if we could make time, the benefits would far outweigh the loss of 15–20minutes per day.

The basis of the benefits of meditation is that brain waves switch from their normal busy 'beta' state to a more relaxed 'alpha' state. This allows your right, intuitive, psychic brain to click in. Many spiritual masters are almost permanently in a theta state, which most doctors say would require you to be comatose!

In some areas meditation lessons are available on the NHS. Chronic insomniacs soon learn to shut off their 'brain chatter' which allows deeper more refreshing sleep

Foods to Avoid
■ Meditation is best done in the morning before you begin the rush of the day, even if you try for 10 minutes daily on an empty stomach, this will help.

■ Generally, don't meditate on a full stomach.

Friendly Foods
■ If you like to meditate before going to bed – make sure you eat a light meal early, go for a walk and then settle for your meditation.

Useful Remedies
■ *Isopogan* is an **Australian Bush Flower Essence** that helps integrate left and right brain activity. **NC**

■ *Bach Flower Remedies* – White Chestnut and Walnut will help still the mind.

Helpful Hints
■ There are now hundreds of books teaching you how to practice this age-old art. One of my favourites is *The Meditation Plan* by Dr Richard Lawrence (Piatkus).

■ Meanwhile, find a straight-backed comfortable chair. Sit with your back straight and your feet firmly on the ground. Take a few deep breaths – breathe in – close your eyes and RELAX, say the word to yourself and as you see the word in your mind allow the feeling of calm to flood from the top of your head right down to your toes. Then imagine a golden light flowing in through the top of your head down your body and out through your feet. Many people have a mantra such as 'Om' or 'I am', which they repeat over and over in their mind to keep their mind chatter at bay. It takes a while but with practice you will soon reap the benefits. There are thousands of meditations – it's just a question of finding which one really suits you.

If you hate swallowing pills, use a pill crusher. Call **Health Plus** *on 01323 737374*

MEMORY

(see also *Alzheimer's Disease*)

At the age of 51, I often forget people's names and why I started a sentence, so don't panic, help is at hand. The brain can be regenerated, and like any other muscle in the body, if you don't use it, you lose it. The secret to improving your memory is to keep your brain active and it will then become more efficient. There really is no need for your memory or brain function to decline with age – my mother in law is 86 and her brain is as sharp as a razor as she has spent 30 years regularly completing crosswords.

Temporary memory loss is not uncommon after drinking alcohol, if your blood sugar is low, after a high fever, surgery, an epileptic fit, or a diabetic coma. Depression and acute anxiety can also cause temporary memory loss.

More serious memory loss can occur after an accident, brain injury or stroke. Senile dementia involves progressive loss of short-term memory until the individual is unable to remember what they did or saw only a few moments before. Many prescription drugs affect memory.

Most memory loss is caused by years of eating the wrong foods, especially saturated fats, which clog the arteries until the small capillaries are affected, and if no fresh blood is reaching the brain it means the brain is being deprived of oxygen. Also most of us forget to breathe deeply on a regular basis. Lead is well-known to affect memory, hence why lead-free petrol was introduced. Mercury fillings are also linked to memory loss (see *Mercury Fillings*).

Foods to Avoid
- Stimulants like tea, excessive coffee plus alcohol all deplete the body of vital nutrients.
- Avoid excess sodium-based table salt and don't add salt to food once cooked.
- Greatly reduce your intake of refined pies, cakes, biscuits, red meat, full-fat dairy produce, white bread, pizzas, burgers etc which not only deplete nutrients but also contribute to clogging arteries, as most of these foods are usually high in fat, sugar and salt.

Friendly Foods
- To keep your blood sugar on an even keel eat a low-sugar cereal, such as muesli or porridge for breakfast. Cereals are rich in B vitamins, often lacking in dementia patients, especially B12.
- Omega 3 essential fats are rich in EPA and DHA, vital brain nutrients found in oily fish, so

eat tuna, salmon, herrings, mackerel or any oily fish twice a week.

■ In countries where olive oil is widely used people seem to maintain efficient memories for longer. Therefore use unrefined, preferably organic olive, sunflower, walnut and sesame oils for salad dressings and drizzle over cooked foods.

■ Caffeine is often criticised for its various problems but in terms of memory function it seems to help it, particularly in the elderly. Two cups of coffee a day is fine.

■ Foods rich in antioxidants like green leafy vegetables, particularly spinach, cabbage, pak choi, celery, broccoli, spring greens and red and purple fruits like strawberries, blueberries, blackberries, cherries and water melon help to slow age related memory decline.

■ Wholegrain foods such as brown pasta and rice, wholemeal bread and flour, barley and buckwheat, as the whole grains contain all the nutrients in their natural state.

■ If you find yourself craving sugar, use a little honey or brown rice syrup. Refined sugar is preferable to artificial sweeteners which contain aspartame.

■ Phosphatidyl choline is a really important brain nutrient found in lecithin granules that has the added benefit of emulsifying unhealthy fats. Sprinkle a tablespoon over your breakfast cereal, into salads or yoghurts. Make sure the brand you buy is a GM-free product with a high (at least 30%) phosphatidyl choline content such as *Cytoplan*. **NC**

■ Eat more ginger and live, low-fat yoghurt to aid digestion.

Useful Remedies

■ If you are on blood-thinning drugs have regular check-ups with your doctor once you begin this programme.

■ The herb *Ginkgo Biloba* is proven to increase memory. Take 1–3 times a day either as tincture or tablets, around 60–300mg of standardised extract.

■ *Phosphatidyl Serine*, 100mg up to 3 times a day, has been shown to improve mental function. Take early in the day, as at night this can increase dreaming and delay your getting to sleep.

■ The amino acid acetyl-L-carnitine, 500mg 3 times a day has been shown to improve cognitive function in elderly people. Take for at least 60 days before you expect to see much improvement.

■ *Huperzine A* is an extract from Chinese moss, several studies have shown its effectiveness in improving mental accuracy and memory in elderly people. **NC**

■ Co-enzyme Q10, 100 mg a day, can improve energy production within the brain. **PN**

■ Include a vitamin B complex as B vitamins are essential for normal brain function

■ Last but not least take 1 gram of vitamin C in an ascorbate form with meals and include a multi-vitamin and mineral in this programme.

Helpful Hints

■ Exercising on a regular basis increases the amount of oxygenated blood reaching the brain. Exercise also helps lower high blood pressure which has been linked to impaired mental function.

- Keeping the brain active is another important aspect. Studies have shown that people who do not retire, but work into their late sixties or seventies have a better memory.

- Play more word games, do crosswords. During car journeys or when on a train or queuing in a supermarket add or multiply varying numbers in your head.

- Minimise aluminum exposure. This includes most deodorants, cooking pans and some cheeses (see *Alzheimer's Disease*).

- Minimise exposure to mercury.

- Never use a mobile phone for more than 20 minutes at a time and avoid using them in cars and trains which amplifies the negative affects not only for you but for those sitting around you.

- Rubbing essential oil of sage into the scalp has been shown to help prevent the breakdown of a key chemical messenger within the brain involved in storing and recalling events.

- If your memory does not improve within three months of trying these suggestions, see a nutritionist who is also a doctor (also see *Helpful Hints* under *Alzheimer's Disease*).

Sesame seeds contain far more calcium than milk.

MÉNIÈRE'S SYNDROME
(see also *Vertigo*)

This little-understood problem of the inner ear which causes recurrent attacks of vertigo, nausea, ringing in the ears and progressive deafness. People with this problem tend to feel unsteady, suffer headaches and neck pains. Causes are suggested as being linked to salt retention, food intolerances, a deficiency of nutrients from food due to poor absorption or even a spasm in the walls of small blood vessels. See also *Leaky Gut*.

Foods to Avoid
- Avoid sodium-based salt.
- Generally avoid any foods containing gluten, salt, caffeine, fried foods and alcohol.
- Reduce full-fat milk and dairy produce.

Friendly Foods
- Eat more ginger, garlic and onions which are very cleansing.
- Papaya and pineapple contain digestive enzymes which aid absorption.
- Add 2 teaspoons of cider vinegar to water and sip.
- See *Friendly Foods* under *Leaky Gut* and *Vertigo*.

Useful Remedies

■ Take a high-strength multi-vitamin and mineral.

■ The herb *Ginkgo Biloba* helps to increase circulation in the ears. Take 120mg of standardised extract daily.

■ Take a digestive enzyme capsule with main meals

Helpful Hints

■ See a chiropractor or osteopath who can check for any cranial, spinal or neck misalignments. Bowen technique has also been shown to help (see *Useful Information*).

The longer you keep fruits and vegetables, the fewer nutrients they will contain. After 3 days 50% of the vitamin C content is an orange is lost. Eat really fresh foods.

MENOPAUSE

(see also *Osteoporosis*)

The problem today is that huge pharmaceutical companies would have you believe that the menopause is some kind of illness for which you need a drug. With a market worth more than six billion dollars world-wide this comes as no surprise.

For women, menopause is a natural part of the ageing process and usually occurs somewhere between the ages of 45 to 55. At this time there is a decline in ovarian function leading to much decreased levels of the hormone oestrogen and a complete cessation of progesterone production. Common symptoms include hot flushes, night sweats, loss of libido, vaginal dryness, palpitations, depression and anxiety. Approximately one fifth of British women take HRT but up to 60% give it up within a year due to adverse side effects such as liver problems, bloating, headaches and nausea.

I do not advocate taking orthodox hormone replacement therapy (HRT) because of the increased risk of high blood pressure, weight gain, gall bladder and liver problems, not to mention breast and endometrial (womb) cancers. Orthodox HRT slows the rate of bone density loss, but only while you are taking it. If you are under a lot of stress at this time, adrenal function is greatly affected. Healthy adrenal glands continue to supply postmenopausal women with a form of oestrogen. The more stressed the adrenals, the more they are kept busy pumping the stress hormone cortisol and the less oestrogen is made.

Foods to Avoid

■ Avoid caffeine, red wine, and all spicy foods.

■ In some women, even a hot drink can trigger a flush.

■ Avoid too much caffeine, alcohol, colas and tea (see *General Health Hints*).

211

■ Generally cut down on all saturated fats found in meat, full-fat dairy, chocolate etc.

■ Recently a lot has been written about dangers of eating soya-based foods, but Dr Marilyn Glenville, the UK's leading nutritional authority on the menopause, says 'Soya in the form of tofu, miso, soya sauce, soya milk and tempeh (a fermented form of soya) are rich in isoflavones which have been scientifically shown to reduce menopausal symptoms and reduce the risk of developing cancer. But it is healthier to cook the soya first. Soya in its traditional form is definitely of benefit to menopausal women if taken in small amounts of approximately 55 grams of tofu or 600ml of soya milk, which contains 35–40 mg of isoflavones which is what I would recommended as a daily intake.'

■ In the West we tend to overload our bodies with synthetic hormones and additives from many foods, which have been sprayed with herbicides and pesticides. These compounds like lindane have an oestrogen-like effect and excessive intake of artificial oestrogens, increases the risk of breast and endometrial cancers, because these deadly toxins migrate and accumulate in fatty tissue such as our breasts.

■ Millions of cattle and chickens are regularly fed with large doses of antibiotics to reduce infection. Animals also eat grasses and feed that are contaminated with pesticides, which enter the food chain, and have an oestrogen or building-like effect within the body. Dr Glenville says 'Orthodox HRT should only be used as a last resort because it places a great strain on the liver and increases the risk of breast cancer.'

Friendly Foods

■ Isoflavones are also found in chickpeas, lentils, kidney beans, sunflower, pumpkin and sesame seeds, Brazil nuts, walnuts and linseeds. All seeds and their unrefined oils are rich in essential fatty acids which also help reduce joint pain, risk of heart disease and help lubricate the vagina.

■ Eat more oily fish, eggs and small amounts of quality meats rich in vitamin B12 which has been shown to reduce irritability, bloating and headaches associated with the menopause.

■ Potassium and panothenic acid help support adrenal function – found in whole grains such as brown rice, amaranth, barley, quinoa, salmon, tomatoes, broccoli and cauliflower, avocado, dried apricots, banana, cantaloupe melon, oranges and fish.

■ Eat organic meat, chickens, vegetables, fruits and foods to avoid ingesting too many toxins from herbicides and pesticides.

■ Also eat plenty of foods that help regulate hormone levels such as sage, broccoli, cabbage, kale, cauliflower, soya products, alfalfa, celery, beetroot and fennel.

Useful Remedies

■ A good quality multi-vitamin and mineral made especially for menopausal women such as *Femforte 11* by **Bio Care** – choose a supplement that contains at least a milligram of boron which aids absorption of other minerals and helps to balance the hormones. **BC**

■ 300iu of natural vitamin E has been shown to reduce or eliminate hot flushes.

- *Omega Plex* powders are essential fats in a powdered formula that are 100% absorbed and place no strain on the liver. This is great for keeping skin young and supple. I take half a teaspoon daily in vegetable juice or water **BC**.

- If you are under a lot of stress also take a B-complex plus 100mg of pantothenic acid.

- 1 gram of potassium daily for one month.

- Dr Glenville has formulated a herbal blend that includes agnus castus, black cohosh, dong quai, yarrow, liquorice and alfalfa which helps to restore hormone balance and reduce menopausal symptoms. One teaspoonful twice daily. Tel 01892 750511 Website: www.marilynglenville.com

- Agnus castus is a traditional European herb commonly used for many menopausal symptoms, which can be taken in conjunction with dong quai. These herbs also help with excess hair on the face and body due to the menopause **BLK**.

- *Menophase* contains Mexican yam and dong quai, plus all the vitamins and minerals a menopausal woman needs **HN**.

Helpful Hints

- Dr Marilyn Glenville has written *Natural Alternatives to HRT Cookbook*, (Kyle Cathie £10-99). For a postal consultation and more information log onto www.marilynglenville.com or for an appointment with Dr Glenville in London call 01892 750511.

- Homeopathic *Sepia 30c*, one daily for a week has been found to reduce hot flushes.

- Reduce stress levels as anxiety can trigger hot flushes. Learn to breathe and begin practising t'ai chi or yoga.

- Wear cotton underwear, especially at night.

- Women who take exercise regularly generally suffer fewer hot flushes.

- Bob Jacobs, an American naturopath and homeopath, says 'The problem with conventional HRT is that they use non-natural progesterone-like substances called progestins which are artificial hormones. These have lots of side effects such as irritability, liver dysfunction, vaginal bleeding, blood clots etc., and the positive effects of oestrogens on the heart are reversed by these progestins. Conventional HRT also uses much higher levels of oestrogen than natural HRT'. Natural *Tri-Estrogen* cream contains natural (meaning the exact molecule that is found in the human body) progesterone from wild yam and oestrogen from soya beans in the correct ratio, which not only help prevent osteoporosis but also help to relieve or eliminate menopausal symptoms. If a woman has no hormonal symptoms and good bone density there is no need for extra hormones. Women who have low-level hot flushes, insomnia, vaginal dryness or mood swings may only need natural progesterone.' The cream is available on prescription in the UK , but you can order for your own use from Pharmwest. If after using the natural progesterone for 2–3 months, there is not sufficient improvement then switch to the Tri-Oestrogen cream. For an information sheet on these creams Tel: 00 800 8923 8923. Website: www.pharmwest.com

- If you require further information on natural progesterone and a list of doctors who use it, send a first class stamp to *The Natural Progesterone Information Service*, PO Box 24, Buxton, SK17 9FB.

■ Many women become depressed during the middle years, as children leave home and some women feel their useful years are over. I became a journalist at 43 and I believe this is a time when we come into our greatest and most fulfilling years without the burden of looking after a young family. View the menopause as a positive time. If you find yourself becoming depressed, see the supplements under *Depression*, which will really help.

Eating coriander helps to detoxify heavy metals from the body.

MERCURY FILLINGS

There is now a huge body of evidence to show that mercury fillings are detrimental to health. Mercury vapour is proven to pass through the blood-brain barrier; it deposits in the brain affecting structure and function. Mercury is one of the most toxic substances known to man and is an accumulative poison. Originally it was thought that the mercury vapor could not escape as it was locked into solid metal fillings: but we now know this is not the case. The British Dental Association state that about 3% of the population are estimated to suffer from mercury sensitivity. But when the same ratio of people have flu for example, this is considered to have reached epidemic proportions. Around 1.8 million people in Britain are sensitive to mercury. Amalgam fillings are still widely used in the UK and America. Between 15–20 million amalgam fillings a year are carried out on the NHS in the UK alone.

Dr Jack Levenson, a dental surgeon based in London, has spent almost 20 years investigating the effects of the potential dangers of dental amalgam. He says 'There is a strong body of research linking mercury to heart disease, Alzheimer's, Parkinson's, multiple sclerosis, motor neurone disease, migraines, chronic fatigue, digestive disorders, infertility in men and women, antibiotic resistance, joint and muscle pain, impaired immune function, hair loss and excessive hair growth, visual disturbances, numbness, tingling and tremors.'

Are you nervous? When Jack tested my teeth, two of my amalgam fillings were 10 times over the supposed safe limit of mercury emissions. I had them removed on the spot. It would seem that the Government continues to refuse NHS patients safer, composite white fillings in order to save millions of pounds. If they admit that amalgam has poisoned millions of people the litigation bill would be huge and health insurance companies would then be forced to pay for their removal and replacement. Money, not health, it seems is once again the bottom line here.

Friendly Foods
■ Eat organic vegetables, as mass-produced fruits, grains and vegetables are often treated with a mercury-based fungicide.

■ Coriander detoxifies mercury from the body.

Foods to Avoid

■ If you have mercury fillings, avoid larger fish like cod, haddock, tuna and swordfish which often contain high quantities of mercury. (Around 20 tons of mercury plus lead, cadmium and copper is dumped into the North Sea annually from industry.)

Useful Remedies

■ If you have mercury fillings, take a good quality multi-vitamin and mineral to help support your immune system.

■ Mercury depletes the mineral selenium, which is known to reduce the incidence of cancer and heart disease. Take between 100–200mcg daily.

■ Vitamin E increases the effectiveness of the selenium – take 400iu daily.

■ Vitamin C, take 2 grams daily with food.

■ If you are having your fillings removed you will need to take extra supplements for at least a month afterwards to help eliminate any residue of mercury in the body. Dr Levenson recommends *Humet* which contains minerals to reduce heavy metals in the body. Tel: 0118 978 9604.

■ It is important that you are re-assessed by your dentist every 2–3 months as the mercury can take up to a year or so to be eliminated.

Helpful Hints

■ Many vaccines use mercury as a preservative.

■ *Tuebinger Toothpaste* has been shown to reduce the level of mercury vapour released into the mouth when used regularly. Available from health shops worldwide or call **Best Care Products** Tel: 01342 410 303. Fax: 01342 410 909.Website: www.bestcare-uk.com

■ If you would like a free mercury information sheet plus a list of dentists in the UK who specialise in safe removal of amalgam fillings send a large SAE with 3 first-class stamps to;. **The British Society for Mercury Free Dentistry** 225, Old Brompton Rd, London SW5 OEA. Or call their Information Line on 020 7373 3655. I strongly suggest you read Dr Levenson's book *Menace in The Mouth* available for £12 inc p&p from the above address.

■ A fact sheet, *Poisons in the Mouth* is available from **The Brompton Dental Clinic**, 221–225 Old Brompton Road, London, SW5 OEA. Send an A4 first-class SAE. Tel: 020 7370 0055. Website: www.mercuryfree.co.uk Email: hempleman@mercury free.co.uk

Four pieces of fruit and four servings of vegetables every day can provide a litre of water.
Patrick Holford

MIGRAINE

20% of women and 7% of men experience migraine with an average of 3 attacks per month each requiring 6 hours of bed rest. In Britain alone, the cost to society including lost working days is almost £2,000 million annually. Migraines usually occur on one side, at the back or front of the head and an attack can be precipitated by flashing lights or partial blindness. Some people are debilitated for a few hours, others several days and in addition an attack can often be accompanied by nausea and vomiting.

Migraines are linked to food intolerances and internal toxicity. See also *Leaky Gut*, *Constipation* and *Low Blood Sugar*. They are also a sign of liver congestion, so you really need to cut down on alcohol, caffeine and fats and keep the diet clean. Weather changes can also trigger migraines.

Foods to Avoid

- The foods most commonly known to trigger an attack are cheese, red wine, peanuts, chocolate, coffee, wheat and citrus fruits.

- Avoid refined sugars found in most cakes, biscuits, pastries, snacks and fizzy drinks.

- Avoid food additives, colourings, and preservatives, alcohol and caffeine as much as possible.

- Avoid hard margarines, shortenings, and any foods containing hydrogenated fats and oils.

- Cut down on red meat, full-fat dairy produce and eggs.

- Some sufferers have problems with fish such as tuna, so keep a food diary and note which foods cause the reactions.

- In one study when 54 migraine patients followed a low-fat diet the incidences of headaches were reduced from 9 monthly attacks to 3.

- If you are constipated on a regular basis, certain bacteria in the bowel can convert tyrosine (high in peanuts) to tyramine which again is thought to be a trigger.

Friendly Foods

- Eat more linseeds, sprinkled over a low-sugar breakfast cereals to keep your bowels regular.

- Drink at least 6 glasses of water daily.

- Eat more healthy grains, brown rice, lentils, barley and try amaranth, oat and rice crackers as a change from wheat.

- Eat plenty of fruits and vegetables, preferably organic.

- Make sure you eat quality protein such as fresh chicken or tofu once a day.

- Use unrefined walnut, sesame, sunflower and olive oils over salad dressings.

- Live, low-fat yoghurt contains healthy bacteria which aids digestion and keeps the bowel healthy.

- Oily fish is rich in omega 3 fats which naturally thin the blood and reduces the severity of migraines if you eat 3 portions a week.

- Drink vervain tea to help reduce head pain and add the essential oil to your bath.
- Drink more water as dehydration can trigger a migraine especially in summer.

Useful Remedies

- *Ginkgo Biloba* improves blood supply to the brain by strengthening blood vessels. It also helps to prevent the blood vessels constricting. Take 120mg of standardised extract daily.
- As all the B vitamins are vital for preventing headaches, particularly folic acid, B2, and B6, take a high-strength B complex that contains 400mcg of folic acid, 100mg of **no flush niacin**, 300mg of B2 and 50mg of B6. **BLK**
- Include 1 gram of vitamin C daily in your supplements.
- Take calcium, 1000mg with 400iu of vitamin D, plus 500–1000mg of magnesium for 2 months – a lack of these minerals is associated with migraine and they act as muscle relaxants. Many companies make combination formulas. **S**
- As digestive problems are heavily associated with migraines, take a digestive enzyme with main meals.
- If you crave sweet foods take 200mcg of the mineral chromium for at least one month to reduce food cravings.
- Omega-3 Fatty Acids (fish oils) 1000mg per day in divided doses should help relieve migraine headaches
- *Migraine Relief Formula* contains, feverfew, vitamin B6, magnesium citrate, willow bark (a natural painkiller) plus ginger, a herbal anti-inflammatory with natural calming effects. 2 tablets can be taken daily. **NC**

Helpful Hints

- Migraine is often triggered by food allergies, so keep a food diary to see if you can identify foods that trigger an attack. If this is unsuccessful, a consultation with a qualified kinesiologist is well worthwhile. See *Allergies* and *Useful Information*.
- Regular aerobic exercise has been shown to reduce migraine attacks and yoga helps reduce stress levels.
- Taken regularly, rosemary or fresh ginger tea can help bring relief from some of the symptoms.
- Grinding the teeth over many years often causes the jaw to slip out of alignment. This causes blood flow to the head to be restricted, triggering regular headaches and/ or migraines. Problems with vertebrae in the neck can also disrupt blood flow to the brain. See a chiropractor or a cranial osteopath who can re-align the neck and head (see *Useful Information*).
- Many people have found that, by wearing magnetic jewellery, pain is relieved. For details call **Magna Jewellery** on Tel/Fax: 020 8421 8848.
- Further information can be obtained from the **Migraine Action Association** Tel: 01536 41333, 9.00am-5.00pm, or write to them at 178a High Road, Byfleet, West Byfleet, Surrey, KT14 7ED Website: www.migraine.org.uk Email: info@migraine.org.uk

- Call **The Migraine Trust** Helpline. Tel: 020 7831 4818.
- There is a new device called the *Scenar* which has helped many people. (see *Electrical Pollution and Healing*).

*If you eat a non-organic diet you will consume approximately
150mcg of pesticides daily.*

MOUTH PROBLEMS

(see also *Bad Breath*)

MOUTH PROBLEMS – Burning mouth syndrome

This is most common in women especially after the menopause and may be triggered by decreased hormone production, nerve damage, stress or a sensitivity to to certain foods. In rare cases it can be due to a lack of vitamin B12 and folic acid. Symptoms can include a swollen tongue, metallic taste, soreness and a dry mouth and tongue even when the tongue looks normal. If you have a cold or flu symptoms are usually worse for a few days. This condition also denotes that your liver is under stress. If you talk a lot this dries the mouth and can exacerbate the problem.

Foods to Avoid

- It is usually made worse by highly spiced or acidic foods such as vinegar, oranges or pineapple.
- Avoid too much alcohol, black tea and coffee.

Friendly Foods

- Keep your diet clean (see *General Health Hints*) and drink plenty of water.
- Eat more nuts, seeds and fish which are high in zinc.
- Cereals, oats, alfalfa, eggs, liver, brown rice, skimmed milk and fish are all rich in B vitamins.

Useful Remedies

- A swollen tongue can be a sign of iron deficiency – have a blood test.
- A dry mouth is a specific sign of potassium phosphate deficiency – take 75 mg daily. **BLK**
- Take vitamin C, 1 gram per day, to prevent deficiency.
- Take vitamin B6, 30mg per day
- Vitamin B12, 800mcg sublingual tablet daily, to prevent deficiency.
- Take folic acid, 300mcg per day.
- As all the B vitamins work together, also take a B-complex.

- Take zinc, 22 mg per day – as lack of zinc is linked to this problem. As zinc depletes copper make sure your zinc supplement contains about 1–2mg of copper.

- GLA (evening primrose oil) – take 250mg per day to prevent deficiency which may create burning mouth syndrome. **BC**

Helpful Hints

- Mouth problems often reflect problems in the gut and digestive system. See a nutritionist who can re-balance your diet and suggest supplements to boost your immune system (see *General Health Hints*).

- Suck ice cubes if the pain is severe.

- This problem is exacerbated by stress, so learn to meditate and practice some form of relaxation.

- As nitrates and other chemicals found in drinking water are known to make symptoms worse install a good water filter. Contact *The Pure H2O Company* on 01784 221188 email: info@purewater.co.uk website: www.purewater.co.uk

MOUTH PROBLEMS – Cracked lips

Lips that are sore and cracked especially at the corners of the mouth are usually a sign of a deficiency of B-vitamins, especially vitamin B2 which is found in milk, eggs, green vegetables, liver and most fresh vegetables. They are also linked to lack of vitamin E and essential fats found in wheat germ, avocados, oily fish, seeds and their unrefined oils. Dehydration is a major cause.

Rarely, cracked lips can be a sign of vitamin A toxicity. You would need to have taken hundreds of thousands of units for quite some time for this to happen, but nevertheless if you have been taking extremely high doses of vitamin A, have a blood test.

Useful Remedies

- Take a high-strength vitamin B-complex. **BLK**

- Take a multi-vitamin and mineral that contains at least 30mg of zinc, 1–2mg of copper, 200iu of vitamin E and 500mg of vitamin C.

- Rub pure vitamin E cream onto the lips at night.

Helpful Hints

- Use a lip balm made from vitamin E and aloe vera. Body Shop make a great range.

- Take Homeopathic *Nat Mur 6 x* twice daily for 3-4 days.

MOUTH PROBLEMS – Mouth Ulcers

Mouth ulcers are quite common and usually occur on the inside of the cheek. They denote that the body is run down or under stress, but can also be caused by accidentally biting the side of mouth, excessive tooth brushing, eating food which is too hot, acidic and spicy food or from cigarette smoke. Many people suffer mouth ulcers after eating oranges and tomatoes, while others find ill-fitting dentures are the problem. I have a bridge which drives me mad and my dentist has said it is as good as I'm going to get, but when I am tired it rubs on my gums and triggers mouth ulcers. So, any chronic dental problem can trigger an outbreak. If the ulcers do not clear within 3 weeks, see your doctor.

Sodium lauryl sulphate, a foaming agent used in quite a few cosmetics, particularly toothpaste, can also trigger this problem. You might also be deficient in B vitamins and iron; so a blood test would be useful to confirm this.

Foods to avoid

■ Sugar, vinegars, pickles, tomato sauces, peanuts, strawberries, tomatoes, pineapple, plums, rhubarb, kiwi fruit, oranges and grapefruits are a problem for those who suffer mouth ulcers.

■ Avoid really hot and spicy foods. Stop smoking.

■ Reduce your intake of sugary treat foods and white-flour-based breads, cakes and biscuits which all lower immune function.

■ Avoid really salty foods like crisps, peanuts and salted meats and fish.

Friendly foods

■ Liquorice tablets or sticks can be chewed to speed up the healing of the ulcers.

■ Try a formula called *Echinacea ACE* which helps to boost your immune system. It contains the herb echinacea, vitamins A, C and E, zinc and selenium. Take once a day until the ulcers have gone **BLK**.

■ Drink more camomile tea.

Useful Remedies

■ Vitamin B complex which helps prevent and heal mouth ulcers.

■ *Lactobacillus/Acidophilus* contains healthy bacteria which help to improve the health of the digestive tract. Take 3 capsules daily.

Helpful Hints

■ Rinse your mouth out with a warm salt solution several times a day. Add 1 teaspoon salt to 1 glass boiled cooled water. Add a few drops of *Goldenseal* tincture to aid healing.

■ Crush a garlic clove and dab the tiniest amount on the ulcer and try and hold this for 30 seconds – it will sting a little – and then spit it out.

■ If stress is the culprit, exercise and relaxation may be the long-term answer.

■ Tea tree oil is a natural antiseptic and makes a marvellous mouthwash when a few drops are mixed with warm water. Some people have found they are allergic to the material that false teeth are made from. Ask your dentist to test you for an allergy – porcelain is used as an alternative material.

- Pierce a vitamin E capsule and apply the oil to the ulcers. I find that if I use toothpaste containing fluoride, I get mouth ulcers. Try to avoid all fluoride.

- Mouth problems often reflect problems in the gut and digestive system. See a nutritionist who can re-balance your diet and suggest supplements to boost your immune system (see *General Health Hints*).

> *Learn the rules so that you know how to break them properly.*
> The Dalai Lama

MULTIPLE SCLEROSIS (MS)

Multiple sclerosis is a progressive disease that affects nerve fibres in the central nervous system. It generally develops over many years and the first signs may be tingling, numbness, or weakness affecting a hand, foot, or one side of the body, double vision, or a loss of sensation in various parts of the body. These periods are often interspersed with periods of seeming recovery. After a day or two symptoms can disappear, and for some people they never return. For others, attacks are repeated which eventually leave a certain amount of disability.

The onset of MS has been attributed to viruses, and having a weak nervous system that is then aggravated by trauma, shock, infection, or toxic metals, especially mercury.

Dr Patrick Kingsley, one of Britain's leading alternative nutritional physicians specialising in cancer and MS says 'Many of my patients have high levels of mercury in their spinal fluid, and the first thing I recommend is that they have the emissions measured from any mercury fillings. Also MS symptoms can mimic those of candida, so this possibility needs to be eliminated'. (See also *Candida*) 'Many patients also have multiple sensitivities to certain foods, the most common being cow's milk and products, and I believe cow's milk to be a major trigger, but individual patients may react to almost any food, which needs to be identified on a personal basis. Many patients benefit when they follow a proper anti-candida and gluten-free diet.' (see also *Allergies*).

Foods to Avoid

- As a general rule cut down on all saturated fats especially those from animal origin, meats, and all full-fat dairy produce.

- Especially avoid cow's milk.

- Avoid all refined carbohydrates such as white bread and rice, pies, pastries, pizza, cakes and biscuits.

- As much as you can, avoid sugar.

- Stay away from all refined foods containing hydrogenated or trans fats.

- Don't fry food.

- Caffeine can irritate the bladder.

221

Friendly foods

- Eat more fish, especially oily fish.

- Eat plenty of fresh leafy green vegetables.

- GLA (gamma linolenic acid) is found in sunflower seeds and safflower oil and helps to nourish the nerve endings.

- Pumpkin, sunflower, sesame seeds and linseeds and their unrefined oils are all rich in essential fats which are vital for people with MS.

- Use more olive oil for salad dressings.

- Eat organic food as much as possible.

- People on vegan or gluten-free diets often experience some relief from symptoms – but the diet would need to be kept up for at least two years. Vegan diets are rich in essential fats needed for nerve function and low in saturated fat.

- Eat more brown rice, quinoa, kamut, spelt, lentils, barley and whole grains.

- Eat seaweeds that are rich in kelp and iodine, available from all health shops.

- Eat plenty of GM-free, organic lecithin granules which are important for the structure of the myelin sheath that surrounds and protects the nerves.

Useful remedies

- Once you have had mercury fillings removed, see under *Mercury Fillings* for the detox process.

- Take vitamin A, 10,000iu per day. Newborn infants fed a diet low in this vitamin have an increased risk of developing MS. Only take 5000iu if you are pregnant.

- Take 100mg of vitamin B-1 (Thiamine) daily which is an essential component of myelin as is vitamin B12 – Take 1000mcg per day plus 50mg of vitamin B6.

- If you prefer not to take 3 pills, and as all the B vitamins work together. Instead buy a high-potency B-complex and take one daily.

- You can take up to 3 grams of vitamin C daily, take with meals in an ascorbate formula.

- As magnesium, selenium and copper are all important – take a multi-mineral daily.

- Fish Oils, 1000 mg per day help to support nerve endings.

- As essential fats are vital try *Omega Plex* powders containing a perfect blend of omega 3 & 6 fats in an easily digestible form. Dr Kingsley says the balance of 2 parts omega 3 to 1 part omega 6 is an ideal ratio for people with MS. **BC**

- Take 2 digestive enzymes with main meals to help increase absorption of nutrients from the diet.

- Take a good quality multi-vitamin and mineral made especially for men or women. **S**

Helpful Hints

- Check the possibility of excess mercury in your diet or environment.

- Dr Kingsley has found that vitamin B12 injections help some patients. If you need to reach Dr Kingsley in the UK call his practice. Tel: 01530 223 622.

■ Make sure your body knows what rest and exercise both feel like: take three 10–20 minute rest periods every day, spaced throughout the day, and do some form of fairly vigorous exercise every day such as walking, press-ups or weight lifting. Start slowly and build up gradually.

■ Among practitioners of alternative medicine, there is a degree of consensus – not generally shared by conventional doctors – that multiple sclerosis can be controlled. This type of approach involves nutritional, environmental, and lifestyle changes. It is important that treatment be followed under the guidance of a qualified practitioner. Because multiple sclerosis affects each patient differently, treatment programmes are individualised within the same plan. Dietary and nutritional needs are often addressed, as are food allergies and environmental toxins. Recommendations may be made for detoxification therapy, as well as for the removal of mercury amalgam dental fillings. Consult a doctor who is also a nutritional physician (see *Useful Information*).

■ There is a yoga centre, which specialises in helping MS patients to recover mobility and self-confidence. For details, send a large SAE to **Yoga For Health Foundation**, Ickwell Bury, Biggleswade, Bedfordshire, SG18 9EF. Tel: 01767 627271 Website: www.yogaforhealthfoundation.uk

■ Help and advice on MS can be obtained from **The Solent Multiple Sclerosis Therapy Centre** Tel: 023 92699116 or send an SAE to 56 Hewitt Road, North End, Portsmouth, Hants, PO2 0QP. Email: solent@mstherapies.fsnet.co.uk Website: www.smstherapycentre.org.uk.

A continuously dry mouth can be a sign of potassium phosphate deficiency –
take 75 mg daily.

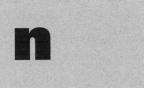

NAIL PROBLEMS

NAIL PROBLEMS – Brittle nails

This problem affects many of us as we age. It is associated with low iron levels, but always have a blood test to check if you are low in iron before taking any supplements. Anyone who has their hands in water for long periods usually has weaker nails. Lack of zinc and B group vitamins will cause nail problems. Nail-biting is another, obvious cause for poor nails.

Foods to Avoid.

■ Junk foods, fizzy drinks, white bread, biscuits and pastries: all these foods deplete the body of nutrients, especially B vitamins.

■ Reduce your intake of caffeine and alcohol.

■ Keep sugar to a minimum.

Friendly Foods

■ Make sure you eat good quality protein at least once a day, as keratin, the main substance of hair and nails is a protein.

■ Eat oily fish twice a week.

■ Eat more nuts and seeds – especially hazelnuts, Brazil nuts, walnuts plus sunflower and pumpkin seeds, and linseeds and their unrefined oils which can nourish your nails.

■ Iron-rich foods include lean meat, liver, black strap molasses, poultry and cereals.

■ See *General Health Hints*.

Useful Remedies

■ Take a good quality liquid multi-mineral that is easily absorbed. Try *ConcenTrace* in water every day. **HN**

■ Take a B-complex plus 2.5mg of biotin, a lack of which is linked to brittle nails. Take a multi-vitamin that contains 7500iu of vitamin A, a lack of which is linked to brittle nails. Only take 5000iu if you are pregnant.

■ The mineral silica is very important for healthy nails, take 75 mg daily. **BLK**

Helpful Hints.

■ The tissue salts *Combination K* helps reduce brittle nails.

■ Massage your nails regularly with jojoba or almond oil.

■ Nail-polish remover is notorious for drying nails which makes them more brittle.

NAIL PROBLEMS – Fungal infections

Fungal infections turn the nails white or at the very least they cause a discolouration and deformity in the nails. Nails tend to thicken and this usually occurs when the immune system is at a low ebb.

Foods to Avoid

■ See *Candida*.

Friendly Foods

■ Usually if there is a fungal infection in the nails, then there is a fungal infection in the digestive tract. Follow an anti-candida diet.

Useful Remedies.

■ In addition to following the anti-candida diet, take 3 x 500mg capsules of the herb *Pau D'Arco* twice daily. This has anti-fungal properties.

■ *Cat's Claw 3*, 500mg capsules taken twice daily, will reduce fungus in the body.

Helpful Hints

■ Soak nails twice a day in calendula solution or apply calendula ointment.

■ Soak the nails in white distilled vinegar for at least 10 minutes twice a day, to help eliminate any fungal infection.

■ You can also use tea tree oil or neem oil on the nails. Tea tree oil must be diluted 50% with water.

■ Tissue salts *Combination L* will help reduce this problem.

NAIL PROBLEMS – Ridges, splitting and white spots

Ridges, especially longtitudinal ridges usually denote a lack of stomach acid or digestive problems. This is helped by taking *Betaine* or a digestive enzyme with main meals. Iron deficiency is linked to nail problems and white spots denote you are lacking in the mineral zinc. Horizontal ridges denote a lack of calcium and/or magnesium.

Foods to Avoid.

■ Avoid sugar, caffeine and alcohol.

■ See *General Health Hints*

Friendly Foods

■ Zinc-rich foods are nuts, seeds and seafood.

■ Iron-rich foods are poultry, cockles, parsley, raisins, almonds, lean red meat, liver and cereals.

■ Eat pineapple and papaya which aid digestion.

■ Include more unrefined olive, walnut and sunflower oils in your diet.

■ Eat one avocado a week and sprinkle organic wheat germ over cereals and desserts as they are rich in vitamin E.

Useful Remedies.

■ A high-strength multi vitamin and mineral.

■ Calcium, magnesium and zinc – take 2 daily for two months. **S**

■ A digestive enzyme tablet with all main meals.

Helpful Hints

■ Massage olive oil or evening primrose oil regularly into the nails and cuticles, which speeds the growth of nail tissue.

■ Preventive measures include keeping nails short, wearing gloves for gardening and rubber gloves if hands are repeatedly immersed in water.

Amaranth grain was once the staple diet of the Incas. It is gluten free, high in protein and fibre and a rich source of calcium, iron, lysine and methionine. It is available from all good health stores.

NUMB/TINGLING SENSATIONS, FINGERS AND TOES

These types of symptoms are usually a sign of poor circulation (see *Circulation*), but can be caused by pressure on a nerve. These sensations are common if you sleep or sit in an awkward position, but may also be a symptom of cervical spondylosis (pressure on nerves in neck, causing numbness in hands, stiff neck or headaches) or carpal tunnel syndrome (numbness in thumb side of hand, sharp pain at night). If you suffer continually with really cold fingers and toes during the winter you may well be suffering from Raynaud's syndrome. Any conditions which reduce circulation to the nerves in the skin will produce these types of symptoms. If symptoms continue have a check up, as numbness is also linked to MS and ME.

Foods to avoid

■ See under *Circulation*.

■ Generally avoid caffeine, animal fats and smoking.

Friendly Foods

■ See also *Circulation*.

■ You are likely to be lacking in essential fats found in oily fish, linseeds, sunflower and pumpkin seeds and their unrefined oils.

■ Eat more blueberries, blackberries, sweet potatoes, cherries, apricots, spinach and leafy green vegetables. These are all rich in flavonoids which strengthen capillaries.

■ Wheat germ and avocados are rich in vitamin E which thin the blood naturally.

■ Garlic is great for circulation, while ginger will warm you.

■ Lecithin granules aid repair of the nerve endings – sprinkle on breakfast cereal or in yoghurts.

Useful Remedies

- Take a high-strength vitamin B-complex daily. A deficiency of B vitamins can cause tingling in the nerve endings. **BLK**

- Older people may also benefit from a B12 injection or a 1mg B12 tablet, a lack of this vitamin is linked to tingling in the extremities.

- Take 1–2 grams of Vitamin C with bioflavonoids daily to help repair nerve endings.

- Most people in the West are lacking in omega 3 and 6 essential fats, therefore either use a dessertspoon of *Udo's Choice Oil* over cooked foods or take *Omega Plex* powder in water daily. For details see *Fats You Need To Eat*.

- As this problem can denote a deficiency of calcium, take 600mg daily plus a multi-mineral.

Helpful Hints

- If after taking these supplements for six weeks, you still have numb and tingling fingers or toes, see your GP.

- Walking for half an hour each day, skipping, rebounding and swinging your arms full circle regularly will help to get your circulation moving.

- It is also helpful to massage your hands and feet. Obviously it is easy to massage one's own hands, however if you find it difficult to massage your feet, ask your partner, relative or friend to do it for you. Use essential oils of geranium, ginger, black pepper and lavender in a base oil. If you have no-one to massage your feet, pop a few drops of the oils in the bath and soak your feet for 10 minutes.

- If the tingling and numbness is in the feet wear some magnetic insoles to increase circulation. Call **Homedics**. Tel: 0161 798 5876 Website: www.homedics.co.uk

- Reflexology and acupuncture often helps reduce or eliminate this type of problem (see *Useful Information*).

- You may have a trapped nerve, in which case consult a chiropractor or osteopath.

OSTEOARTHRITIS

(see *Arthritis*)

Horizontal ridges in your nails denotes a lack of calcium and/or magnesium.

OSTEOPOROSIS

(see also *Low Stomach Acid* and *Menopause*)

Osteoporosis is a condition in which the bones become thin and weak, and prone to fracture, particularly in the hips and spine. The condition is more common in women, but currently 1 in 12 men suffer osteoporosis in later life.

It usually occurs after the menopause, when levels of hormones which help keep bones strong, are reduced. Women who are thin and those who smoke are most at risk, as are women who suffered anorexia when they were younger and also those who missed periods. Women who exercise to the point where their periods stop – may also be at increased risk because of low hormone levels caused by the excess exercise. A sensible balance is needed. Osteoporosis is also associated with a lack of exercise, excess animal protein in the diet, stress, low weight, low calcium consumption, too many fizzy drinks and steroids. Long-term stress causes the body to over-produce adrenalin which can dissolve bone – hence why stress levels need to be carefully managed.

Even when men and women eat a healthy balanced diet, if they are not absorbing all the nutrients needed for healthy bones, they remain at risk.

Traditionally, osteoporosis is prevented and treated by hormone replacement therapy (HRT). A study in the *New England Journal of Medicine* stated 'Women who have taken HRT for ten years or more may have a greater bone density than those who have not taken it, but lose increased density rapidly when the HRT is stopped and end up with only 3.2% higher bone density than women who took nothing. HRT can only prevent osteoporosis if taken for the rest of a woman's life'. When women exercise regularly, eat a healthy diet and take the right vitamins and minerals bone density can be increased quite dramatically, without having to endure the potential side effects of conventional HRT, which include increased risk of breast and endometrial (womb) cancers, thrombosis and strokes.

Bob Jacobs, an American naturopath and homeopath says 'The problem with conventional HRT is that they use non-natural progesterone-like substances called progestins, which are artificial hormones. These have lots of side effects such as irritability, liver dysfunction, vaginal bleeding and blood clots, and the positive effects of oestrogens on the heart are reversed by these progestins. Conventional HRT also uses much higher levels of oestrogen than natural HRT. Natural *Tri-Estrogen* cream contains natural (meaning the exact molecule that is found in the human body) progesterone from wild yam and oestrogen from soya beans, which helps to prevent osteoporosis and can with proper nutrition help increase bone density. To find out if you need this cream, have a bone density scan via your doctor and also ask for a urine DPD test to show if you are losing bone. If the bone scan is OK and the urine test shows no bone loss then you don't need extra hormones. But if your density is low and the urine test shows excessive bone breakdown, then the use of natural hormones, along with the right diet, supplements and exercise can be very useful'. For a free information sheet on *Tri-Estrogen* cream call 00 800 8923 8923. Website: www.pharmwest.com

Foods to Avoid

- Our Western diet tends to be high in acid-forming foods which cause more calcium to be excreted from the body. One of the main culprits is fizzy drinks which are high in phosphorus, an essential mineral but when taken in excess can cause bone loss.

- Acid-forming foods are meat, refined carbohydrates such as white breads, pastries, cakes and any type of sugar as well as tea and coffee – which all force the body to compensate by withdrawing calcium from the bones to re-alkalise the system.

- Many people believe that if they drink lots of milk they are helping their bones, but milk is a protein and therefore, ironically, can increase bone loss if you have an intolerance to it.

- If you drink more than 3 cups of coffee daily, you increase your risk of developing osteoporosis by as much as 82%.

- Most people, on average, eat 50% too much protein, especially animal protein, which can lead to calcium loss.

Friendly Foods

- Vegetarians generally suffer less incidence of osteoporosis.

- Dr Marilyn Glenville, the UK's leading nutritional authority on osteoporosis, says 'We all need a certain amount of protein, and studies show that women who eat less than 68 grams of animal protein daily have a lesser risk of forearm fractures.'

- Other great sources of protein are pulses, beans and lentils, seeds and nuts – but not peanuts.

- Fresh organic vegetables, fruit, broccoli, kale and seaweed all alkalise the body.

- Calcium is found in green leafy vegetables, fish and sesame seeds which contain more calcium than milk.

- Use non-dairy rice, oat or soya milk.

- Silica found in lettuce, celery, millet, oats and parsnips helps with bone regeneration.

- Kelp and alfalfa help prevent bone loss.

- Cauliflower, berries, potatoes, sweet potatoes and green leafy vegetables are all rich in vitamin C, which helps to produce the collagen that makes up 90% of the bone matrix.

- Green leafy vegetables are also a good source of magnesium and vitamin K, levels of which are often low in women with this condition.

- Boron, found in apples, pears, grapes, dates, raisins, peaches plus soya beans, almonds, peanuts, hazelnuts and honey, assists the body's uptake of calcium.

- Onions, parsley, arugula, cucumber, dill, garlic, lettuce and tomato all help to limit bone loss.

Useful Remedies

- A good multi-vitamin and mineral that contains at least 1mg of the trace element boron, which is essential for healthy bones and reduces the amount of calcium lost from the body. Try **Bio Care's** *Femforte 11*, **Lamberts** *Gynovite* or **Solgar's** *Earth Source*. **NC**

- Take 2 grams of vitamin C daily preferably in an ascorbate form with meals.

- If you are at a higher risk or have been shown to have lowered bone density – take calcium citrate 500mg, magnesium 100mg and zinc 15mg.

- Take a digestive enzyme with main meals to increase absorption of nutrients.

- Ask at your health shop for any organic green food supplement which re-alkalises your system, and sprinkle a tablespoon over breakfast cereals, desserts etc.

Helpful Hints

- Smoking can induce an early menopause and reduce bone mass. Give up for your health's sake.

- Weight-bearing exercise is absolutely crucial. Swimming and cycling are great for your heart but will not build bone. Try rebounding, skipping, walking, dancing, tennis, gentle jogging and anything that creates an impact.

- Don't over exercise as excessive exercise can deplete more calcium through sweating.

- Sunshine is essential for synthesising vitamin D in the body, which is essential for absorption and utilisation of calcium. Certain film stars and people who take absolutely no sun are putting themselves at more risk. Moderate exposure to sunshine is healthy, avoiding the hottest part of the day from 11am to 3pm.

- Dr Glenville says about HRT, 'I recommend that all women have a bone-density scan initially because if the bone density is good and the menopausal symptoms such as hot flushes can be controlled naturally – why put yourself at risk with orthodox HRT? If the bone density is at a good level then the aim is always to prevent osteoporosis. Once you have had an initial scan bone turnover can be monitored by a simple urine test where the sample can be given at home. For a postal consultation and more information log onto www.marilynglenville.com For a consultation or an appointment in the UK call 01892 750511.

- Avoid aluminium in any form, as this makes it difficult for the body to metabolise calcium. See under *Alzheimer's Disease* for a list.

- Take one tablespoon of organic cider vinegar and honey in warm water daily, to help assimilate more calcium.

- For some great bone recipes try *The Natural Alternatives to HRT Cookbook*, Dr Marilyn Glenville (Kyle Cathie) or *Body & Beauty Foods* by myself and Kathryn Marsden, (Reader's Digest Books).

Long-term stress causes the body to over-produce adrenalin which can dissolve bone.

PALPITATIONS

(see also *Tachycardia*)

This is a fairly common problem that just about everyone experiences at one time or another. If under stress, after a shock or if you are anxious, your heart begins beating faster. Once the anxiety has passed it should calm down, if it doesn't then you have a problem. Palpitations occur when the heart beats irregularly; it can skip a beat or feel like a fluttering in the chest.

If you find that you regularly suffer any of these symptoms that do not recede when you are calm, or you are regularly short of breath, then you definitely need to see your doctor. Palpitations can also indicate that there is some problem with the electrical circuitry in the heart.

Foods to Avoid

- Avoid heavy alcohol intake which can damage the heart muscle.
- Avoid stimulants such as tea, coffee, chocolates, fizzy drinks and anything containing caffeine which in itself can make you palpitate, as it stimulates the release of adrenalin into the bloodstream.
- Food additives can trigger an attack in sensitive individuals.
- Generally don't eat large, heavy meals which place an added strain on the body.
- Avoid hard fats, fried foods and eating too much meat and full-fat dairy produce.
- Avoid any energy drinks containing the plant extract guarana, which is basically neat caffeine.
- Any foods to which you have an intolerance may also cause palpitations, the most common being wheat, eggs, dairy from cows and citrus fruits.

Friendly Foods.

- See under Angina and General Health Hints.

Useful Remedies

- Irregular heartbeat is linked to a calcium, magnesium and potassium imbalance or deficiency. Take 99mg of potassium for one month. **S**
- Also take a calcium/magnesium formula that contains 100-400mg of magnesium and 200mg of calcium.
- Folic acid, 600 mcg, daily helps to stabilise the heart beat.
- Niacin, 50 mg daily, helps stabilise the heart beat. Make sure you buy the **No-Flush variety**, as niacin can cause flushing of the skin which can be rather scary if you are not aware of this effect.

- Also take a B-complex as all the B group vitamins work together to calm the nerves.
- Take a good quality multi-vitamin and mineral containing 400IU of natural source vitamin E. This helps the heart muscle to receive more oxygen.
- Co-enzyme Q 10, 60mg daily helps to regulate heartbeat. **PN**

Helpful Hints

- Learn to meditate which reduces stress, as worrying about this condition can precipitate an attack. See *Meditation* and *Stress*.
- To combat worrying, which only exacerbates the condition, learn how to breathe properly by taking yoga lessons.
- If you feel an attack beginning, splash your face with cold water, lie down, close your eyes, breathe deeply and slowly for a few minutes until the attack passes.
- Essential oil of lavender and ylang ylang have a calming effect, try a few drops in your bath. You can also inhale the ylang ylang directly from the bottle to help slow your breathing. Try regular aromatherapy massage, which is very relaxing.
- Go for leisurely walks breathing deeply.
- Avoid eating large meals if you are anxious.

*Red, green, brown and puy lentils are a rich source of low-fat,
high-fibre protein, rich in calcium, zinc, iron magnesium and folic acid – a great food
for pregnant women.*

PANIC ATTACKS

(see also *phobias*)

Panic attacks occur during periods of acute anxiety and in Britain there are approximately 10 million sufferers. Feelings of intense panic lead to the person hyperventilating which can produce feelings of light-headedness and tingling in the fingers and toes caused by too much oxygen. Panic attacks have a huge variety of causes, most of them based on fears or phobias. Obviously if a loved one dies suddenly such as a in car accident and you are with them, a panic attack would be triggered by acute shock. Some people have panic attacks if they see spiders or, if a person has had one heart attack or stroke, at the least pain because they believe another is imminent. When I had my near-death experience in 1998, for almost 2 months I suffered panic attacks, and believe me if someone tells you to pull yourself together, they are wasting their time! Reassurance and patience are what are needed. Panic attacks are also linked to low blood sugar.

Foods to Avoid

- Avoid stimulants such as caffeine, sugar and alcohol, which can cause severe mood swings and disrupt blood-sugar levels. Sugar substitutes such as aspartame are just as bad, so read labels carefully.

- Cut down your intake of animal fats, burgers, pies and processed foods.

- Tinned and pre-packaged foods are high in salt. Combine this with a panic attack and up goes your blood pressure.

Friendly Foods

- Eat calming foods that will also help to balance your blood sugar, such as brown rice, couscous, noodles, jacket potatoes, quinoa, wholemeal bread and pasta, lentil, rice and corn pastas.

- Eat small meals regularly.

- Snack on bananas, pears, apples and low-fat yoghurts.

- Eat at least one portion of quality protein such as fish, chicken or tofu once a day.

- Don't skip meals.

- There are plenty of low-sugar and low-fat seed bars available from good health stores.

- Cut down on sodium-based salts, use a magnesium/potassium-based salt.

- Generally include more fruits and vegetables in your diet.

- Eat more oily fish rich in omega 3 fats and seeds such as sunflower, sesame and pumpkin as well as walnuts, almonds and Brazil nuts which are all rich in omega 6 essential fats.

- Low levels of serotonin are linked to feelings of depression. Serotonin is made from a constituent of protein called tryptophan. Fish, turkey, chicken, cottage cheese, beans, avocados and bananas are all rich in tryptophan, which helps to keep you calm.

- Sprinkle wheat germ over a low-sugar breakfast cereal, my favourite is **Nature's Path** who make great cereals from amaranth, quinoa and kamut, that are sweetened with a little apple juice. Available worldwide. Cereals are rich in B vitamins which help to keep you calm.

- Porridge is a very calming food.

- Eat more lettuce, mushrooms, peppers and root vegetables which are also calming foods.

- For further help read *Mind and Mood Foods* by myself and Kathryn Marsden (Reader's Digest Books).

Useful Remedies

- Take a good quality B-complex daily to help support your nerves. Take *Niacinamide* (**no-flush** niacin) 500mg, which acts like a natural tranquilliser. Make sure this is a no-flush variety as this amount would cause an extreme flushing effect.

- Formulas such as *NT188* contain B vitamins and passiflora to help keep you calm. **BC**

- Take up to 2 grams of vitamin C daily with meals, as mild to moderate deficiency is associated with nervousness.

- Take 400iu of vitamin E, 1000mg of calcium and 400mg of magnesium daily. Many people who suffer panic attacks are lacking in these minerals.

- Take potassium 99 mg per day, low levels can increase susceptibility to anxiety. **S**

■ Try *L-5-Hydroxy Tryptophan* 50–200mg per day. This is the precursor to serotonin which is called the 'happy brain neurotransmitter.' Panic attacks can be reduced by increasing serotonin levels in the brain. **HN**

Helpful Hints

■ **Bach Flower remedies** are helpful for reducing panic attacks. Try *Star of Bethlehem*, *Rescue Remedy* or *Jan de Vries Emergency Essence*, and if you feel an attack coming on, treat the flower remedy as your medicine. Say to yourself as you place it under your tongue, 'This will calm me down in under 3 minutes'. Keep repeating this and it will help.

■ Regular exercise reduces stress and builds confidence. A regular aromatherapy massage with lavender oil helps you to stay calm and balances the emotions. A warm relaxing bath and sound, restful sleep does wonders to ease stress.

■ Learn how to control the attacks; fighting them will only make them worse. Tell yourself that this is just the body's way of getting you to take care of yourself. Speak to yourself gently, as you would to comfort a child.

■ Hypnotherapy and self hypnosis called *Neuro-Linguistic Programming* have proven very successful for reducing panic attacks and phobias See *Useful Information* for details.

■ If you know you are hyperventilating have a large paper bag at the ready and breathe slowly and calmly into the bag to help calm you down and stop you fainting.

■ Homeopathic *Aconite 200c* taken upon onset of an attack is a great remedy if you have intense fear.

■ **First Steps to Freedom**, a self-help group, have a helpline for people with phobias. Factsheets, self-help booklets, audio/video tapes, books and online support groups are available. For further information write to **First Steps to Freedom**, 7 Avon Court, School Lane, Kenilworth, Warwickshire, PV8 29X Tel: 01926 851608. The helpline is open 10.00am–10.00pm every day. Website: www.firststeps.demon.co.uk

Red, white and green cabbage all help to heal stomach ulcers and a leaky gut.
If cooked, drink the cooled cooking water.

PARKINSON'S DISEASE

Approximately 120,000 people in Britain have Parkinson's. It is a progressive disorder which causes deterioration of the nerve centres in the brain responsible for controlling movement. As the condition progresses muscular movement is affected. Eventually, co-ordination can become a nightmare and it is common for patients to experience tremors, rigidity, and muscular spasms in different limbs and to varying degrees. No single cause has been established, but Parkinson's is linked to nutrient deficiencies especially B vitamins, copper and iron, metal toxicity linked to aluminium, mercury and manganese, a genetic predisposition, viruses, carbon-monoxide poisoning, certain pesticides plus some drugs, particularly those used in the treatment of schizophrenia. But if drug-related, the Parkinson's usually disappears when the drug is stopped. Lack of the brain chemical dopamine makes the condition much worse and most patients take a synthetic form of the amino acid L-dopa to help restore brain function. Many of the drugs associated with Parkinson's can cause lethargy and extreme mental confusion. As every case is unique I strongly recommend that anyone with Parkinson's consult a nutritional physician as this condition needs highly specialised care (see also *Useful Information*).

Foods To Avoid

■ Cut down on all animal fats which impair the metabolism of essential fats (see *Fats You Need to Eat*).

■ Avoid sugar in any form, highly refined and processed foods and especially avoid additives and preservatives such as monosodium glutamate, and the sweetener aspartame.

■ Reduce stimulants such as coffee, tea and alcohol.

■ Under professional guidance, you may also need to eliminate gluten-containing grains such as wheat, rye, oats and barley – as the gluten can prevent absorption of nutrients and medication.

■ Cut down on peanuts, bananas and potatoes, yeasty foods, liver and meat which contain vitamin B6 which can interfere with the L–dopa. But if you are not taking L–dopa, vitamin B6 is important for Parkinson's.

■ Don't fry food.

■ Avoid all hydrogenated and trans fats.

Friendly Foods

■ As much as possible, eat only organic foods which are free from pesticides and herbicides.

■ Dr Melvyn Werbach, a respected nutritional physician based in the US suggests that restricting protein intake is helpful and that 90% of the daily intake should be eaten with the evening meal.

■ Proteins can also be found in brown rice, millet, quinoa, beans, peas and lentils.

■ Small amounts of soya, eggs, oily and white fish are fine.

■ Eat more corn-based foods and corn pasta.

■ Include apples, pears, mangos, kiwi fruit and vegetables such as cabbage, cauliflower, carrots and broccoli.

■ Broad beans are rich in L-Dopa, eat when in season as they help to replenish L-Dopa deficiency more quickly than the synthetic medication.

p

■ Use unrefined, organic sunflower, sesame and olive oil for salad dressings and drizzle over cold foods. These oils are rich in essential fats which are vital for healthy brain function.

■ Enjoy fresh vegetable juices made with carrot, beetroot, celery and fennel which are high in vitamins and minerals that help to cleanse the liver.

■ If you have mercury fillings, eat lots of coriander which detoxifies metals from the body.

■ Dried or ready-to-eat fruits such as prunes, figs and apricots help to ease any constipation.

■ Drink at least 8 glasses of water daily.

■ My thanks go to nutritionist Dr June Butlin and *Positive Health Magazine* for their help with this highly complex condition. June can be contacted via nutexcel@zoom.co.uk

Useful Remedies

■ As it is vital to take various nutrients in specific amounts for each individual case and the supplements you take also depend on the time of day and which medication you are taking, I strongly recommend that you see a qualified nutritionist or nutritional physician who can devise a programme specifically for you. Meanwhile here are some general guidelines.

■ As lack of the B group vitamins is linked to Parkinson's take a B-complex, but if you are taking L-dopa, then take the B vitamins separately excluding vitamin B6.

■ B6 is vital but should be taken under advice.

■ Studies from the *Birkmayer Institute for Parkinson's* in Vienna has shown that NADH a co-enzyme form of vitamin B3 can help increase energy levels, reduce depression and stimulate the body to produce more L-dopa. 5 mg can be taken on an empty stomach at least 40 minutes before food. Professor Birkmayer's highly absorbable NADH is called *Springfield Enada* and is available worldwide or to find your nearest stockist call **Nature's Store** on 01782 794300. **NC, FSC**

■ A multi-mineral without or with very low levels of manganese (1–2mg) as excessive manganese is linked to this condition, but minerals such as iron and copper are vital.

■ Antioxidants such as vitamin C, up to 2 grams daily with food and 600iu of vitamin E may help to slow the progression.

■ *L-Methionine*, 1000 mg per day- An essential sulphur amino acid which readily crosses the blood-brain barrier where it can be converted into **S**-adenosyl methionine (SAM-e). L-dopa supplementation reduces brain SAM-e levels. **NC**

■ *5HTP* (5-hydroxytryptophan) increases brain levels of the hormone serotonin, which helps raise mood and promotes sound sleep. 100mg twice daily. **NC**

■ Phosphatidyl serine (PS) is another vital brain nutrient. The body can manufacture PS but only if you tend to eat lots of organ meats. 100mg can be taken 2–3 times a day.

■ For those who have heard that the herb St John's wort can ease depression – it can, but should not be taken by people with Parkinson's as it can interfere with medication.

Helpful Hints

■ Mercury fillings are linked to Parkinson's (see under *Mercury Fillings*).

■ Log onto www.brainrecovery.com which gives the latest research on how intravenous anti-oxidant therapy using glutiathione is helping Parkinson's or call 0700 0781744.

■ Aluminium and mercury have been linked to Parkinson's, therefore avoid all aluminium cookware or aluminium foil. Read labels carefully as cake mixes, antacids, buffered aspirin, self-raising flour, pickles, processed cheeses, most deodorants and toothpastes contain aluminium.

■ Monosodium glutamate (MSG), the food additive, and aspartame the artificial sweetener have been linked to Parkinson's; therefore avoid all additives and preservatives whenever possible. Over 3000 foods and drinks contain artificial sweeteners.

■ Use a good quality reverse osmosis water filter system. Try *The Pure H2O Company* on 01784 221188 email: info@purewater.co.uk website: www.purewater.co.uk. As organophosphates (OPs) are now found in drinking water, many sufferers find some relief when they switch to pure water.

■ A book well worth reading is *Parkinson's Disease–The Way Forward!* by Dr Geoffrey Leader and Lucille Leader (Denor Press ISBN: 0952605686). To order call 0208 343 7368.

■ For further help contact **The Parkinson's Disease Society**, 215 Vauxhall Bridge Road, London, SW1V 1EJ. Tel: 020 7931 8080, Helpline: 0808 800 0303. Website: www.parkinsons.org.uk

Sipping organic apple cider vinegar in warm water aids digestion and absorption of nutrients.

PHLEBITIS

(see also *Circulation*)

Phlebitis is caused by inflammation of the walls of the veins, usually near the surface of the skin. It is often combined with the formation of small blood clots on the area of the inflammation. It may be caused by a sensitivity to external irritants such as washing powders or by food allergies. The condition can occur after injections or intravenous infusions and is common in intravenous drug abusers. It is more common in people who have varicose veins and also in blood vessel disorders such as Buerger's disease. Symptoms include swelling and redness along and around the affected segment of vein, which can become very tender when touched. The best way to prevent this condition is to keep your circulation in good condition by eating the right foods.

Foods to Avoid

■ Identify and avoid foods to which you have a sensitivity, the most common being wheat and dairy from cows.

- Cut down on all saturated fats found in animal produce, sausages, meat pies, full-fat cheese, milk, chocolate and hard margarines.
- Don't fry food and never use mass-produced, refined, hydrogenated oils.
- Reduce your intake of cakes, burgers, biscuits, white breads and pastas.
- Many of these foods are packed with fats, salt and sugar. Sugar turns to a hard fat in the body if not used up during exercise (see *Fats You Need to Eat* and *General Health Hints*).

Friendly Foods

- Increase your intake of oily fish which is rich in the omega 3 essential fats that help to thin blood naturally.
- Sprinkle wheat germ and lecithin granules over cereals and desserts. They help to emulsify the bad fats which aids circulation.
- Buy a packet each of organic, unsalted walnuts, Brazil nuts, almonds, sunflower and pumpkin seeds, sesame seeds and linseeds which are high in omega 6 essential fats. Whizz them all in a blender and keep in an air-tight jar in the fridge. Sprinkle over any foods you like. These add healthy fats, fibre and minerals such as zinc to your diet which are vital for skin and wound healing.
- Eat more wholemeal bread, pasta and noodles. Try lentil, corn and rice pastas that are freely available in supermarkets and health shops.
- Use skimmed milk or try organic rice or soya light milk which are both low in fat.
- Include garlic in your diet which thins blood naturally.
- Olive oil and avocados are rich in monounsaturated fats which are healthy and aid healing.
- Eat more fresh fruits and vegetables, especially pineapple and papaya which are rich in digestive enzymes that aid healing.

Useful Remedies

- Take 400iu of natural source vitamin E 400 daily to help thin the blood naturally
- Take a high-strength multi-vitamin and mineral made specially for men and/or women over 50. **S, BC**
- Some people find relief by placing raw papaya on the affected area for an hour a day.
- Bromelian extracted from pineapple has good anti-inflammatory effects. Take 2000–3000 mcu daily. **FSC**

Helpful Hints

- Basically, you need to get moving. Begin by walking for 15 minutes daily and gradually increase over a one month period to one hour a day.
- When applicable, use stairs instead of lifts.
- Swimming, yoga or Qigong (t'ai chi), an extremely gentle and easy exercise regime, would

also be helpful, as would reflexology and acupuncture (see *Useful Information*). T;ai chi can be practised by people of any age well into the eighties and nineties.

White spots on your nails can indicate a lack of zinc. Take 30mg daily.

PHOBIAS

A phobia is an extreme or irrational fear attached to a specific object or situation which is basically not life-threatening, but for the person with the phobia the fear is often overwhelming and their lives can become a nightmare. Most common phobias are fear of confined spaces, or various animals and insects such as birds or spiders. Certain social situations provoke anxiety in some people who fear that they will become trapped or embarrassed. Low blood sugar can contribute to this problem (see also *Low Blood Sugar*).

Foods to Avoid
■ As much as possible, avoid stimulants such as coffee, tea, alcohol, sugar and cut down on foods or drinks containing caffeine or sugar.
■ See *General Health Hints*.

Friendly Foods
■ Low levels of serotonin are linked to feelings of depression. Serotonin is made from a constituent of protein called tryptophan, so include more foods such as fish, turkey, chicken, cottage cheese, beans, avocados, bananas and wheat germ in your diet to raise your mood and help keep you calm.
■ Calming foods also include brown rice and pastas, noodles, couscous, potato, lettuce, mushrooms, peppers and root vegetables.
■ Sprinkle wheat germ over breakfast cereals, there are plenty available made from amaranth, quinoa and kamut, sweetened with a little apple juice. Cereals, including porridge, are rich in B vitamins that help to keep you calm.

Useful Remedies.
■ Niacinamide, vitamin B3 – 500–800 mg daily, acts as a natural anti-anxiety agent, but you must ask for the **No-flush variety**, otherwise you will find your skin looks like a cooked lobster.
■ 1000mg of calcium, 500mg of magnesium and 30mg of zinc will help keep you calmer. **S**

- *5 Hydroxytryptophan* (5HTP) is a supplement that helps to raise serotonin levels in the brain naturally, which helps to improve mood and calm you down. Start with 25 mg and increase over 10–14 days to 75mg 3 times daily.

- The **Australian Bush Essences** *Grey Spider Flower* and *Green Spider Orchid* help reduce fear and phobias. **NC**

Helpful Hints

- Learn to meditate (see under *Meditation*). People who practice regularly have lower blood pressure, are less anxious and more able to cope during stressful situations.

- **First Steps to Freedom**, a self-help group for people with phobias. Fact sheets, self-help booklets, audio/video tapes, books and online support groups are available. For further information write to **First Steps to Freedom**, 7 Avon Court, School Lane, Kenilworth, Warwickshire, PV8 29X or call their helpline, Tel: 01926 851608 which is open 10.00am–10.00pm every day. Website: www.firststeps.demon.co.uk

- Hypnotherapy is an excellent way to find the root cause of your problem and learn how to let it go so you can lead a normal life (see *Useful Information*).

- Paul McKenna the world-renowned hypnotherapist has made some great self hypnosis CDs and tapes that help to remove phobias. Tel: 01455 852233. Website: www.mckenna-breen.com

- Homeopathic *Aconite 200c* is a good remedy when you are experiencing intense fear or terror.

- *Neuro-Linguistic Programming*, has proven really quick and successful for removing phobias and is well worth trying. For your nearest practitioner write to **ANLP**, PO Box 10, Porthmadog, LL48 6ZB. Free information booklet is available. Public information line 0870 870 4970.

Avoid Korean ginseng if you suffer from high blood pressure.

PILES (HAEMORRHOIDS)

(see also *Constipation*)

Piles are formed when veins just inside the anus become enlarged. If you suffer chronic long-term constipation, then the veins can burst through the anus and protrude externally. If you feel this happening and the vein is still soft and pliable you can carefully ease the swollen vein back inside the anus. But if the pile becomes hardened and forms a clot and remains outside the anus, this calls for immediate medical attention. When you go to the loo you can often see blood in the stools and experience extreme discomfort and itching in that area. Also, if your liver is congested – which is common in this problem, it can place more pressure on your back, which in turn adds pressure to your venous system and makes piles worse.

Piles can also be caused by persistent coughing, pregnancy and childbirth, standing and sitting for long periods, overuse of laxatives and travelling long distances sitting on heated car seats, all of which raise pressure in rectal veins. If you bleed from the anus at any time, you should seek medical attention immediately.

Foods to Avoid

■ Generally you need to avoid eating too many foods based on flour – cakes, white breads, refined biscuits, pies and desserts – as flour gunks up the bowel. If you mix flour and water together you get a very sticky paste and this does not change consistency in the bowel!

■ Melted cheese and full-fat cheeses can also cause constipation.

■ Red meat takes a long time to digest. If you must eat meat only have very small portions.

■ Coffee, tea, canned fizzy drinks and alcohol all dehydrate the bowel.

■ Avoid mass-produced foods like burgers and high-fat takeaways.

■ Reduce your intake of full-fat dairy products from cows.

■ Avoid sodium-based salt.

■ For some people, eating citrus fruit and tomatoes makes the situation worse.

Friendly Foods

■ Drink at least 6 glasses of water daily even if you are not thirsty.

■ Eat far more fresh lightly cooked vegetables and salads – especially green leafy vegetables like celery, spinach, spring greens and cabbage.

■ Figs, prunes, apples, pineapples, apricots, bananas, mangos, papaya, avocados, grapes and melons will all help reduce the constipation. Strawberries, raspberries, peaches, sultanas, raisins and dates should be eaten regularly.

■ Good quality protein such as chicken without the skin, fish, tofu, beans, peas and pulses.

■ Eat more wholemeal bread, pastas and noodles.

■ Enjoy low-sugar, high-fibre cereals for breakfast. Try cereals made from kamut, spelt and quinoa which are less likely to irritate the gut than wheat bran.

■ Use oat and rice bran.

■ Try black strap molasses, honey and unsweetened jams instead of sugar.

■ Replace cow's milk with soya light and organic rice milk which are both low in fat and non dairy.

■ Almonds, sunflower, pumpkin, sesame seeds and linseeds are all rich sources of fibre.

■ Coffees made from rye and chicory, herb teas like rose hip and unsweetened fruit juices.

■ Use more unrefined organic olive, sunflower and walnut oils for salad dressings.

■ Eat live, low-fat yoghurt which is rich in friendly bacteria that encourage healthy bowels.

Useful Supplements

■ *Grapeseed Extract* acts like a natural antibiotic which helps to protect tissue and keep bowels regular. Take 100–300mg daily.

- The herb *Butcher's Broom* helps to improve circulation in the lower body and helps tone the veins. Take 500mg twice daily.

- *Horse Chestnut* capsules help to strengthen the capillaries –take 50–75 mg of standardised aescin (the active ingredient) twice daily.

- Take 2 grams of vitamin C, 1 gram of bioflavonoids and 400iu of vitamin E daily with food which help to strengthen the blood-vessel walls.

- Vitamin A, 20,000iu per day will help to repair tissue damage. Only take this dose for one month and take no more than 5,000iu if you are pregnant.

- Vitamin B-complex aids digestion which in turn aids bowel function.

- Zinc is vital for soft tissue healing, take 30mg daily with 1–2mg of copper.

- After 3 months on this regimen, switch to a good quality multi-vitamin and mineral.

Helpful Hints

- Calendula and vitamin E cream applied topically will reduce soreness.

- Apply combinations of zinc oxide, vitamin E, and aloe vera gel or olive oil to the affected area.

- Apply cold witch hazel lotion frequently to haemorrhoids to shrink the swollen blood vessel.

- In an emergency situation, or if you cannot see your doctor immediately, try dissolving one tablespoon of *Epsom Salts* into six tablespoons of luke warm water and apply with cotton wool to the affected area. This helps to reduce the swelling until you can see your GP.

- **Weleda** make *Antimony* ointment, a homeopathic preparation to help ease the discomfort of cracks and fissures. Available from health shops.

- Homeopathic remedies such as *Staphysagria* or *Aesculus Hippocastamum* (horse chestnut) can also help.

- See a qualified homeopath for individual remedies.

- Bathing the anus in cold water every morning can help prevent recurrence of piles. Bowel function can be affected by drugs such as antacids, anti-depressants, excessive iron tablets and laxative abuse. If you think these may be a factor, see your doctor.

Eating more unsalted seeds and nuts will help your hair to become shinier.

PILL, THE CONTRACEPTIVE

The progestogen (synthetic progesterone) only or mini pill, provides contraception by thickening the mucous in the cervix and making it impenetrable by the sperm. The combined pill which contains both oestrogen and progestogen prevents pregnancy by thickening the mucous and suppressing ovulation. Potential side-effects from taking the pill are an increased risk of cancers of the breast and cervix, blood clotting in the legs, high blood pressure, increased risk of heart disease and stroke, weight gain, fluid retention and migraines. Women who took the pill for 10 years or more back in the sixties have a much higher risk for developing breast cancer. The Pill depletes the body of vital nutrients such as vitamins B and C, magnesium, calcium and zinc. I took the pill for more than 10 years from the late 1960s and early 1970s which I believe was the root cause of continual heavy bleeding which at 31 caused me to undergo a hysterectomy. If you must take the Pill, then have regular breaks of several months at a time.

Foods to Avoid
■ Greatly reduce your intake of refined sugars, too much animal protein, dairy products from cows, saturated fats found in dairy and hard margarine, cakes, pastries, burgers, sausages and so on.
■ Reduce your intake of sodium-based salt, caffeine, and tobacco.
■ Reduce alcohol intake.
■ See *General Health Hints.*

Friendly foods
■ Include organic raw wheat germ in your diet as it is rich in vitamins B and E.
■ Eat far more wholegrains, brown rice, quinoa, couscous, wholemeal breads and pastas, fruits and vegetables.
■ Cereals and oats are also rich in B vitamins.
■ Cherries, kiwi fruit, cantaloupe melons, apricots and most fruit and vegetables are a rich source of vitamin C.
■ Eat more fish plus sunflower, pumpkin and sesame seeds which are high in zinc, as the pill raises copper levels which lowers zinc levels.
■ Eat more live, low-fat yoghurt containing healthy bacteria which are depleted by the pill.
■ See also *General Health Hints.*

Useful Supplements
■ Take a high-strength multi-vitamin and mineral such as *Optivite* by **Lamberts**, *Femforte 1* by **Bio Care** or **Solgar's** *Omium*. **NC**
■ Make sure any supplement you take contains at least 30mg of zinc.
■ Take a B complex as the pill depletes all the B vitamins.
■ Take vitamin C in a magnesium or calcium ascorbate form. Taking 250mg–500mg with food daily helps to prevent any deficiency caused by the Pill.
■ Support your liver with 500mg of milk thistle twice daily **BLK**

p

Helpful Hints

Studies since the 1960s have consistently shown that women are at 9.6 times greater risk of a pulmonary embolism when taking the Pill – even the lower oestrogen-containing pills.

If you are on the Pill you should not smoke, as this considerably increases the risk of some hazards, such as blood clots and heart disease.

Call the Women's Nutritional Advisory Service, Tel: 01273 487366, Monday–Friday 9am–5.30pm.

Organic wheat germ is rich in iron, folic acid and vitamin E. It also helps re-alkalise the body. Sprinkle over cereals, soups, stews and yoghurts.

PRE-MENSTRUAL TENSION and PRE-MENSTRUAL SYNDROME (PMT/PMS)

PMS causes a variety of physical and emotional symptoms in the days prior to menstruation. They vary from mood swings, food cravings and depression to breast tenderness and enlargement, fluid retention and bloating. For 1 in 10 women premenstrual mood changes are extreme. PMS is associated with low levels of progesterone and excess oestrogen (See *Menopause* for further details of natural progesterone cream.) Low blood sugar is common prior to a period and once blood sugar is balanced symptoms often disappear. (see also *Low Blood Sugar*). Many women with PMS also have candida (see also *Candida*).

Foods to Avoid
- Generally you need to cut down on animal fats, burgers, sausages, heavy rich meat-based meals that usually contain high levels of saturated fat and salt.
- All high-salt foods like crisps and salted peanuts and highly processed meat such as salami should be avoided as salt will add to the water retention problem.
- Stimulants like alcohol, tea, coffee, caffeine in any form, chocolate, snacks, cakes, biscuits and fast foods such as croissants and Danish pastries will all play havoc with your blood sugar.

Friendly foods
- Drink more water and try calming herbal teas such as camomile.
- Eat more quality protein such as fresh fish, eggs, chicken and turkey without the skin, cottage cheese and tofu.
- Foods like soya tofu, sweet potatoes, broccoli, cauliflower, Brussels sprouts all help to balance your hormones naturally.
- Lentils, barley, brown rice, oats, peas, sunflower, pumpkin and sesame seeds plus all dried beans and pulses are rich in fibre, protein and essential fats.

- Eat plenty of small snacks containing at least 55grams of protein, include plenty of fruits and vegetables.
- Add organic sunflower and walnut oil to salad dressings.
- Snack on apples, pears and bananas and try rice and oat cakes, amaranth crackers and wholemeal bread spread with a low-fat houmous or tahini.

Useful Remedies
- To be taken all the time, not only during during a period:
- A high strength B-complex containing at least 50mg of B6 per day which is needed in the liver to process oestrogens.
- Vitamin F taken 300–600iu daily, helps to reduce the symptoms of PMT.
- Take calcium at 1000mg and magnesium at 500mg per day, to reduce the symptoms of PMT as these minerals help keep you calm. Most companies now make a two-in-one formula. **FSC, S**
- Gamma linolenic acid (GLA) is the main ingredient of evening primrose oil which helps to reduce breast pain. Take 100–500mg of GLA daily. **BC**
- Also take a multi-vitamin and mineral for women that contains a further 50mg of B6 to make your total daily intake 100mg per day. **BC**.
- If your sugar/carbohydrate cravings are really bad, take 200mcg of chromium daily, which kicks in after a few days and really helps to reduce sugar cravings.

Helpful Hints
- Dr Marilyn Glenville, a leading nutritional physician and expert in women's health problems, has formulated drops containing blue cohosh, agnus castus, lady's mantle and cramp bark that help relieve breast pain, water retention, mood swings and headaches. Call 01892 750511 to order. For a postal consultation and more information, log onto the website: www.marilynglenville.com
- When you are stressed, you produce too much adrenalin, which eventually exhausts your endocrine (hormone) system and depletes calcium from your bones.
- Start taking more regular exercise to reduce stress or learn to meditate. Find some time each day to call your own, even if it's only a relaxing bath for 30 minutes.
- Treat yourself to an aromatherapy massage each month or add essential oils of rose, ylang ylang, neroli, jasmine or geranium to your bath. Clary sage is great for reducing cramping period pains.
- If you smoke, try to give it up.

Taking 200mcg of the mineral chromium daily reduces by 50% your chance of contracting late-onset diabetes. It also helps reduce cravings for sugar.

p

POST-NATAL DEPRESSION

Although the birth of a child is for most women a time of great joy, some women feel extremely low immediately after giving birth. This can be due to hormonal changes, or extreme fatigue can be due to fluctuating blood sugar levels. Also anxiety about coping with a new baby, financial problems, and of course, the realisation that life has changed for good can all add to this condition. For a few women, the feeling of depression lasts for much longer than a few weeks which can seriously undermine their ability to cope. Most doctors offer anti-depressants and tell the mother the depression will soon pass. In fact this condition can be greatly alleviated by taking the right supplements for a few weeks. Symptoms vary from increased or decreased appetite, a feeling that one is a failure and sometimes aggressive feelings towards the baby (see also *Low Blood Sugar* and *Depression*).

Foods to Avoid

■ Your enemies at this time are sugar, caffeine, alcohol and too much saturated fat.

■ See *Foods to Avoid* under *Low Blood Sugar*.

Friendly Foods

■ See *Friendly Foods* under *Depression* and *Low Blood Sugar*

Useful Remedies

■ The herb St John's wort is very useful for this problem, but not until you have finished breast feeding.

■ You can take the herb agnus castus to help re-balance your hormones even if you are breast feeding, 5mls of the tincture daily.

■ As low levels of B vitamins are associated with this condition, take a high-strength B-complex daily for at least two months.

■ Calcium 500mg, magnesium 300mg and zinc 30mg can be taken as a formula once daily. S Taking these minerals will greatly ease symptoms after a few days.

■ A multi-vitamin and mineral that contains at least 500mg of vitamin C and 150mcg of selenium.

■ **Bach Rescue Remedy**, *Star of Bethlehem* and *Gentian* help to lift the depression.

Helpful Hints

■ Taking all the above nutrients during your pregnancy (not the St John's wort) can help prevent depression especially if you suffered after an earlier pregnancy.

■ Post-natal depression is often caused by the sudden fall in progesterone levels just before birth in women whose bodies are slow to begin making progesterone again. You can use a natural progesterone cream, which is easily absorbed and will bring your progesterone levels up again until your body takes over. If you require further information on natural progesterone and a list of doctors who use it, send a first-class stamp to **The Natural Progesterone Information Service**, PO Box 24, Buxton, SK17 9FB.

■ In Britain, natural progesterone cream is available on prescription – but overseas and in Ireland it is freely available over the counter and it can be ordered for your own use. For an information sheet call 00 800 8923 8923 or log onto www.pharmwest.com **PW**

■ Homepathic *Ignatia 30c* taken twice daily for up to a week is particularly good for mothers who thought that having a baby was going to be all roses.

■ And for those who feel enveloped by a black cloud, try *Cimicifuga 30c* twice daily for up to a week.

■ Mild post-natal depression can be helped by getting more sleep, and by getting out of the house away from the baby. Don't bottle up your feelings; talk things over with a friend. By letting your feelings out it really helps to put things in perspective and to realize how many women are in a similar situation.

■ For more help and advice call the **Women's Nutritional Advisory Service** on 01273 487366. Mon-Friday 9am–5.30pm.

Judge your success by what you had to give up to get it.
The Dalai Lama

PRICKLY HEAT

This irritating condition usually affects fair-skinned people such as myself in tropical or sub-tropical climates. It initially appears as an itchy red, raised rash of hundreds of tiny bumps anywhere on the body. It has been linked to food allergies (see *Allergies*), but can just as easily be triggered by sun lotions, shower gels and soaps to which the individual becomes more sensitive in the heat and sun. I find I suffer prickly heat on my shins if I stand for too long in tropical temperatures which causes blood to 'pool' in my legs. Alcohol, antibiotics and aspirin can also trigger prickly heat.

Foods to Avoid
■ Try cutting out cow's milk and products, wheat, peanuts, tea and coffee, although the culprits could be something quite unusual like radishes or orange juice.

■ Avoid really hot drinks and highly spiced foods.

Friendly Foods
■ All foods that feed the skin such as apples, carrots, spinach, broccoli, pumpkin, apricots, mango, papaya and figs.

- Artichokes, beetroot and asparagus cleanse the liver which in turn aids healing the skin.
- Onion and garlic are rich sources of quercetin which is a natural anti-histamine.
- Avocados and oily fish are fabulous for the skin.
- Include more nuts and seeds that are rich in essential fats.
- Use more organic, unrefined virgin olive, walnut or sunflower oils over salad dressings.
- Drink lots of water.
- Muesli and most cereals are high in B vitamins, which help prevent dry skin.
- Nettle tea will help reduce the inflammation.

Useful Remedies

- Take 2–3 grams of vitamin C in an ascorbate form with meals as vitamin C acts as a natural antihistamine.
- Take natural-source carotene complex for 7 days before travel and during your holiday. BC
- Take a high-strength B-complex. **S, FSC, BC, HN**
- Take a multi-vitamin and mineral.
- Drink nettle tea.

Helpful Hints

- In most cases, prickly heat will clear up on its own in a few days if the affected area is kept cool and dry. Take regular cool showers and allow the skin to dry naturally.
- Avoid using any insect repellent on the affected areas.
- Once your skin is dry again, apply aloe vera gel.
- Don't use any type of oil-based product, which might block your sweat glands.
- If the prickly heat does not clear within 4–5 days and infection sets in, you must see a doctor.
- To prevent prickly heat, avoid situations that can lead to excessive sweating, such as hot, humid environments and strenuous physical activity.
- Wear loose-fitting cotton clothes.
- Buy products in their most natural and unadulterated state. For anyone who suffers dermatitis or skin allergies, **The Green People Company** make organic skin, hair and body lotions, sun screens, toothpaste and also have an advice line. Tel: 01444 401444. E-mail: organic@greenpeople.co.uk Website: www.greenpeople.co.uk
- Many strong antibiotics and drugs make the skin very sun-sensitive. If you are taking antibiotics, stay out of the sun.
- Stay out of the midday sun and never allow your skin to go red.
- The homeopathic remedy *Sol 30* has helped many people to prevent and heal prickly heat – but it is not a substitute for sun block.
- Avoid hot baths and showers.

A zinc deficiency causes the thymus gland – the master gland of the immune system – to shrink. Zinc is also vital for healing the skin, healthy sperm and helping reduce the incidence of colds. Take at least 10mg daily.

PROSTATE PROBLEMS

Approximately half of men over 55 suffer from enlarged prostate and 20,000 new cases of prostate cancer are diagnosed in Britain annually. The prostate is a walnut-sized gland that sits below the male bladder. The tube that takes urine from the bladder to the outside (the urethra) passes through the prostate. As men get older it is common for the prostate gland to enlarge, which places pressure on the urethra, triggering the need to urinate more often. Many men are forced to get up 3 or 4 times during the course of the night. Other symptoms include difficulty in beginning urination and dribbling at the end of urination. An enlarged prostate can also trigger urinary infections.

The majority of prostate problems are due to a condition called benign prostatic hypertrophy (BPH), but occasionally the prostate can be affected by cancer. If you have blood in your urine, difficulty in passing urine, any swelling in your testicle area, please, please go and see your doctor. Although there is now a growing and greater awareness of this problem, many men are literally dying from embarrassment when there is no need.

Foods To Avoid
- As pesticide and herbicide residues are now linked to prostate cancer, make sure you avoid non-organic foods as much as possible.
- Reduce your intake of animal fats such as meat, full-fat milk and cheeses, chocolate, hard margarines and fatty takeaways.
- Don't eat processed meat pies and pastries.
- Avoid fried foods.

Friendly Foods
- Eat organic foods as much as you can. Locally grown fruits and vegetables in season contain more nutrients than those flown thousands of miles.
- As lack of zinc is associated with prostate problems sprinkle plenty of pumpkin, sunflower and linseeds over cereals, yoghurts and soups. Heat them in a warm oven and sprinkle over salads.
- Eat more oily fish which are rich in essential fats and use organic walnut, sesame, sunflower and olive oils for salad dressings.
- Include plenty of fibre in your diet from fruits, vegetables especially broccoli, cauliflower and Brussels sprouts which balance hormones naturally.
- Include more grains such as brown rice, quinoa, millet, oats, cereals and oat and rice bran.
- Eat more pulses such as barley, kidney beans, soya beans, lentils and corn, rice and lentil pastas.

- Have one serving of cooked, organic GM-free soya tofu each week.

- The carotene lycopene is the most abundant nutrient in the prostate and studies have shown that men who eat 10 or more cooked tomatoes (in a little olive oil) weekly are 45% less likely to develop prostate cancer. The lycopene in tomatoes is released when they are heated in a small amount of oil. A great way to do this is cut the tomatoes in half, brush them with a little olive oil and add chopped garlic and basil. Grill for a few minutes and serve.

Useful Remedies

- As zinc deficiency is linked to prostate problems, take 30mg zinc daily. As zinc depletes copper levels – take a proportionate amount of copper – approximately 1mg of copper for every 15mg of zinc.

- Two of the most popular herbs used for an enlarged prostate are Saw Palmetto (take 320mg of standardised extract daily) and 50–100mg of Pygeum. Make sure you buy a standardised extract which guarantees that your tablet or capsule contains a good percentage of the active herb.

- One of the oldest remedies for enlarged prostates is nettle taken either as a tincture or as tablets. Modern research has confirmed its effectiveness. Take 5ml of tincture, or tablets 1–3 times daily.

- Omega 3 fatty acids found in oily fish or linseed oil, 1000 mg per day, help prevent prostate enlargement. Many companies now make prostate formulas that include all the above nutrients. **FSC, S, BC, NC**

- Include a natural carotene source supplement that is rich in lycopene 20-40mg daily.

- *Prostabrit* has been used successfully for over 30 years in Europe and Asia. It is a combination of extracts from the pollen of eight different plants: rye, maize, timothy grass, hazel, pine, oxeye daisy, sallow and aspen. Discovered in Sweden almost half a century ago, this non-allergenic mixture has proven effective in the treatment of BPH. Take two capsules daily. **NC**

Helpful Hints

- If you are over 50, every time you see your doctor about any health matter, just ask him to examine your prostate and testicular area. Early detection greatly increases your chances of a complete cure.

- If you are married, ask your partner to see if they can feel any abnormalities. Make this a fun thing, but try doing it once a month. The man in turn can check the woman's breasts!

- Make sure you get plenty of exercise and reduce stress levels.

- To help improve circulation to the area and reduce inflammation, lie on your back, bend your knees, bring the soles of the feet together and bring the feet as close to your buttocks as possible. Relax your legs, letting the knees fall outwards towards the ground. Hold this position for five minutes. Only attempt this exercise if you are fit and have no joint problems in your hips and legs.

- Massage a few drops of essential oils of cypress, tea tree and juniper berry mixed with a grapeseed base carrier oil into your lower back and groin areas to strengthen the prostate.

- Consult an osteopath or chiropractor to check that the pelvis and spine are not misaligned. In certain cases a major nerve connection from the lower part of the spine to the prostate becomes trapped and once this is released water can be passed normally (see *Useful Information*).

- If you have prostate cancer see *Useful Remedies* under *Cancer*.

- For further help and advice, send a large SAE to **The Prostate Help Association**, Laneworth, Lincoln, LN3 5DF. Website: www.pha.u-net.com. They also have self-help, informative books and CD-ROMS for sale. Shop website: www.prostatecharityshop.co.uk Other literature can be obtained by sending an A4 SAE with two first-class stamps to the **Prostate Research Campaign UK**, 36 The Drive, Northwood, Middlesex, HA6 1HP. Website: www.prostate_research.org.uk

Black cohosh, a member of the buttercup family has been used for centuries for reducing hot flushes, night sweats, depression, anxiety, insomnia and PMT. Available as a tincture, tablets or powder.

PSORIASIS
(see also *Candida*)

This is a chronic skin condition characterised by patches of red, raised, and scaly skin. Once it begins scaling the skin can take on a silvery, fish-like look. It does seem to have some hereditary links, but symptoms often don't appear until adulthood. It usually does not itch, but can cause discomfort and embarrassment. Areas most commonly affected are arms, elbows, behind the ears, scalp, back, legs, and knees. It may be triggered by prolonged stress, a traumatic event, food allergies, essential fatty acid deficiencies, low stomach acid levels, constipation, liver congestion and vitamin B-complex deficiencies. It is also linked to candida. Many people with psoriasis may have poor liver function, as skin problems can denote that the liver is under stress in which case you need to see a qualified nutritionist who can modify your diet to help detoxify the liver.

Foods to Avoid
- Eliminate wheat and any food containing wheat for one month and see if this helps.

- Citrus fruits and tomatoes aggravate the problem in some sufferers.

- Cut down on saturated and hydrogenated fats, especially red meat, mass produced vegetable oils, take-aways, mass-produced burgers, red meat, cakes, pastries, pies and full-fat dairy produce.

- It is likely that you are eating too many of the above foods which are all acid-forming in the body.

- Keep a food diary and note when symptoms become worse. Recall what you ate the day before and this may be your answer.

251

- As much as possible, eliminate alcohol.
- Cut down on sugary foods and drinks.

Friendly foods

- Eat as great a variety of fresh foods as possible.
- Consume fish high in omega-3 fatty acids: salmon, sardines, mackerel, herring and tuna, at least twice a week.
- Eat more brown rice, millet and buckwheat.
- Eat more pectin-rich foods such as apples and carrots. Greatly increase your intake of whole fruits and vegetables.
- Figs, prunes, kiwi and papaya are all great for the skin.
- Add unrefined, organic walnut, sunflower, sesame and olive oils to salad dressings and drizzle over cooked foods.
- Use organic rice and light soya milks instead of cow's milk.
- Pumpkin seeds, linseeds and sunflower seeds are all high in zinc and essential fats.
- Begin making fresh vegetable juices with beetroot, artichoke, carrots and apples or any vegetables you have to hand – add to this a teaspoon of green food powder which helps to re-alkalise the body , 20 drops of dandelion and milk thistle tincture and half a cup of organic aloe vera juice to help cleanse the liver – and drink immediately upon juicing.

Useful Remedies.

- Evening primrose oil, 5–6 grams or linseed oil capsules 3–5 grams per day, will help to reduce the inflammation of psoriasis.
- Take a high-strength B-complex that contains 400mcg of folic acid and 100mg of B6 which are often low in people with this condition.
- B12 injections have proved helpful to many people.
- Vitamin C with bioflavonoids, 2 grams daily to help reduce the inflammation.
- Take a multi-vitamin/mineral that contains at least 30–40mg of zinc.
- Betaine hydrochloride (stomach acid) is often useful. 1 capsule with main meals aids digestion and absorption of nutrients. If you have active stomach ulcers take a digestive enzyme instead.
- For one month take 25,000iu of vitamin A and then reduce to 5000iu daily (this amount should be in your multi). If you are pregnant do not take more than 5,000 iu of vitamin A daily.
- There has been extensive research into the healing properties of the plant *Mahonia aquifolium* in psoriasis. It is available as cream, ointment, shampoo, conditioner, scalp oil and body lotion. For details ask at your health shop or call **Taylor, Jackson Health Products** on 01923 853111 Website: www.yourskin.com

Helpful Hints

■ Sea bathing is beneficial for psoriasis. Many sufferers find relief after bathing in Dead Sea salt because of its high-mineral contents. Add 1kg to your bath and soak for ten minutes.

■ Homeopathic *Ars-iod 6x* taken twice daily for a few weeks is particularly good for dry scaly, itching skin.

■ Moderate sun exposure also helps psoriasis, but remember to wear a hypo-allergenic sunscreen.

■ Smokers run a greater risk of psoriasis.

Cat's Claw is a woody vine from Peru which increases our white cells' ability to destroy invading bacteria. It is also great for easing joint inflammation. Available as a tea, tincture or capsules.

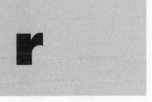

RAYNAUD'S DISEASE

(see also *Circulation*)

Raynaud's is a constriction that triggers intermittent spasms of the smaller blood vessels usually in the fingers and toes and occasionally in the nose and tongue.

Initially, symptoms occur when the extremities are exposed to cold temperatures especially if the person is stressed. The fingers become white, bluish or red and tingling or numbness are common symptoms. This condition is linked to poor circulation, a diet low in essential fats and other nutrients including iron. But never take iron supplements unless you have had a blood test showing that levels are low as iron is stored in the body and high iron levels are linked to an increased risk of heart disease. Another trigger is smoking which greatly affects micro-circulation. In rare cases the skin can ulcerate if it is starved of blood for too long (see *Circulation* and *Fats You Need To Eat*).

Foods to Avoid

■ Cut down on saturated fats found in hard margarines, fatty meats, full-fat milk and dairy produce.

■ Avoid coffee and caffeine which constricts blood vessels

■ See *Foods to Avoid* under *Circulation*.

Friendly Foods

■ You need to eat foods high in vitamin E such as raw wheat germ, avocados, nuts and seeds.

■ Rutin-rich foods help to strengthen the small blood vessels, these include buckwheat, the peel of citrus fruits, rose hips, apple peel and cabbage.

■ Make stews, soups and casseroles that are full of root vegetables, sweet potatoes, carrots, pumpkin etc – as these types of foods warm you through and are rich in minerals.

■ Iron-rich foods: lean red meat, liver, poultry, fish, broccoli and leafy green vegetables like spinach.

■ Magnesium is a nutritional vasodilator, so include more low-sugar cereals, oats, honey, wholemeal bread and pastas, almonds, Brazil nuts, walnuts, mustard and curry powder.

■ Cook with garlic and onions which help to thin the blood naturally plus fresh root ginger which warms the body.

■ Eat plenty of fruit high in vitamin C such as cherries, kiwi, and blueberries. If you hate cold food in winter make berry and fruit compotes or lightly glaze fresh fruit with a little honey and grill on kebab sticks. Serve with low-fat, live yoghurt and sprinkle with chopped coconut.

Useful Remedies

■ If you are not on blood thinning-drugs take up to 800iu of natural source vitamin E daily.

■ Vitamin C with bioflavonoids 1–3 grams a day with food. These play a key role in the synthesis of collagen, which is the key component in the walls of blood vessels. Vitamin C is essential to ensure that the small arteries that supply the fingers do not become damaged during attacks.

■ Niacin (vitamin B3), begin with 30mg and gradually increase to 100 mg per day. Beware – this really revs up the circulation and for about 15 minutes after swallowing, it can cause a pronounced red flushing effect.

■ Take a high-strength multi-mineral that contains 250mg of magnesium, 500mg of calcium and 20mg of potassium plus a trace of manganese.

■ GLA is an essential fatty acid, found in evening primrose, borage, or blackcurrant oils important for relaxing muscles. A recent study found that 12 capsules a day of evening primrose oil dramatically decreased the number of Raynaud's attacks. But as most people don't want to swallow 12 pills and the ingredient they need is the GLA, I suggest two *Mega GLA* capsules daily. **BC**

■ Take a B-complex daily and if symptoms are severe ask your doctor for a B12 injection.

■ Flax and fish oils 4,000–8,000mg per day – contain essential polyunsaturated fatty acids, known as omega 3 and omega 6 fatty acids, that have been shown to lower the bad fats and thin the blood. Fish oils also improve one's tolerance to cold – hence why Inuits rarely feel the cold!

■ The herb *Ginkgo biloba* really helps increase circulation. Take 120 mg of standardised extract daily.

Helpful Hints

■ Take regular exercise to improve circulation. Swimming, skipping and rebounding on a mini-trampoline are all wonderful ways to improve circulation. I used to suffer from this condition as a result of varicose vein surgery. I was told that I had plenty of veins left, but it reduced my circulation drastically. If you are thinking of having veins removed, you might like to keep this in mind. Wear warm socks for most of the year in bed. Never wear tight fitting shoes, which restrict circulation.

■ Magnets really help to increase circulation, which brings more oxygenated blood to the problem area. **Homedics** make shoe inserts and magnetic mitts that worn regularly should really help. For details call 0161 798 5876. Website: www.homedics.co.uk

■ Make tea infusions with fresh root ginger, cinnamon twigs or angelica root.

■ Try massaging hands and toes regularly with diluted essential oils of black pepper, rosemary, lavender or geranium or add a few drops of each oil to your bath.

■ Reflexology and acupuncture have helped many sufferers (see *Useful Information*).

■ For further Information contact **Raynaud's and Scleroderma Association**, 112 Crewe Road, Alsager, Cheshire, ST7 2JA or call their freephone no. 0800 917 2494 (24 hours with answerphone). Website: www.raynauds.demon.co.uk Email:webmaster@raynauds.demon.co.uk

Fresh radishes are great liver cleansers which also help to clear mucous from the sinuses, and purify the blood.

REPETITIVE STRAIN INJURY (RSI)

Anyone who has a job or plays a sport regularly that involves repetitive movements is at risk of contracting RSI which is basically inflammation of the tendons – tendonitis.

Tendonitis usually heals within a few weeks, but if it becomes chronic, calcium salts can deposit along the tendon fibres. The tendons most commonly affected are the Achilles, the biceps, elbow, thumb, knee, the inside of foot or the shoulder joint.

Foods to Avoid

■ Caffeine reduces the body's ability to cope with pain.

Friendly Foods

■ Eat more oily fish rich in vitamin A which aids tissue healing.

■ Eat plenty of foods high in natural carotenes which have anti-inflammatory properties. Asparagus, French beans, broccoli, carrots, raw parsley, red peppers, spring greens, sweet potatoes, watercress, spinach, apricots, pummpin, tomatoes and cantaloupe melon.

■ Nuts (unsalted) and seeds plus fish are all high in zinc.

■ Include more turmeric in food which is highly anti-inflammatory.

■Pineapple, cherries and ginger all have anti-inflammatory properties.

Useful Supplements

■ Take 2 grams of vitamin C as magnesium ascorbate daily as vitamin C plays a major role in the prevention and repair of injuries. **BC**.

■ Vitamin A 10,000iu per day is necessary for collagen synthesis and wound healing. If you are pregnant only take 5000 iu daily.

■ Zinc 30mg per day. Zinc functions alongside vitamin A. An increased copper-to-zinc ratio is often found in individuals with chronic inflammatory conditions.

■ Bioflavonoids are extremely effective in reducing inflammation. Therefore take a 1 gram bioflavonoid complex daily.

■ Include a multi-vitamin and mineral in your regimen that includes 400iu of vitamin E, 200mcg of selenium and 100–200mg of vitamin B6.

■ **Bio Care** with the help of an osteopath have formulated *Colleginase* and *Ligazyme Plus* which give maximum support to injured tendons and ligaments **BC**.

■ *Glucosamine and MSM* – 500mg daily (an organic form of sulphur) has proved useful for this problem. If you have a severe allergy to shellfish avoid *Glucosamine*. **HN**

Helpful Hints

■ Proper stretching and warming-up before exercise are important preventive measures.

■ Rest the injured part as soon as it hurts to avoid further injury.

■ Wrap some ice or a bag of frozen peas in a towel and apply to the painful area for ten minutes every hour whilst symptoms are acute. Do not wrap so tightly that circulation is impaired.

■ Compress the area with an elastic bandage to limit swelling.

■ Elevate the injured body part above the level of the heart to increase drainage of fluids out of the injured area.

■ You can also massage with essential oil of lavender in a carrier base or buy lavender cream.

■ If you sit for long hours at a desk, take regular breaks and really stretch out.

■ **Higher Nature** make an organic sulphur (MSM) and boswelia muscle balm that really helps to ease pain. **HN**

■ The Alexander Technique helps individuals learn about healthy posture and therefore, how to reduce or even eliminate RSI problems. Acute problems may benefit from treatment with osteopathy, chiropractic or acupuncture (see *Useful Information*).

■ Magnets increase circulation and bring oxygenated blood to the injury site which helps reduce pain, swelling and tenderness. For details call **Homedics** on 0161 798 5876. Fax 0161 798 5896. Website: www.homedics.co.uk

■ If, after trying all these ideas for 6 weeks you are no better then consult a specialist in sports injuries or at least have an X-ray or scan.

Every year in the UK alone we consume 76 billion cigarettes. If you are not worried about your own health, think of others and the air around the planet.

RESTLESS LEGS

This is a very distressing condition which causes tickling, burning, or pricking sensations, or involuntary twitching in the muscles of the lower legs. Also known as Ekbom's syndrome, it is more common in pregnant and middle-aged women, smokers, diabetics, people with low blood sugar (see under *Low Blood Sugar*) and in those who drink too much coffee. It could also be partly hereditary. Common causes are lack of iron, vitamin E and the mineral magnesium (see also *Circulation*).

Foods to Avoid
■ Cut down on your alcohol intake.

■ The biggest trigger is caffeine in any form, so avoid coffee, tea, fizzy drinks, chocolate and any foods containing caffeine should be eliminated.

■ Avoid too many foods containing sugar which can cause your blood sugar to fluctuate and make symptoms worse.

■ Reduce refined pastries, cakes, mass-produced pies and biscuits.

■ See *General Health Hints*.

Friendly Foods.
■ You need to eat quality protein from chicken, fish, eggs, low fat cheeses, pulses, beans peas, tofu etc. at least once a day.

■ Eat more brown rice, quinoa, couscous. For snacks eat rye crisp breads, amaranth or rice crackers which are delicious spread with a little low-fat homous or tahini.

■ Eat more leafy green vegetables, fruits and honey which are rich in magnesium.

■ Iron-rich foods are liver, lean red meat, cereals, black strap molasses and game meats such as hare, venison and pigeon.

- As essential fats are vital, include oily fish in your diet at least twice weekly and sprinkle organic unsalted sunflower and pumpkin seeds over cereals and salads.

- Eat raw wheat germ and avocados which are rich in vitamin E and healthier monounsaturated fats.

- Eat more blueberries and bilberries when in season.

- Drink herbal teas such as camomile, lemon balm or vervain.

Useful Supplements

- If you are deficient in iron take a liquid formula such as *Spatone* that is easily absorbed and does not cause constipation. Available from health stores worldwide.

- A high-strength B-complex to calm the nerve endings.

- Vitamin E 400 iu twice a day can be extremely effective in alleviating this condition. (If you are on blood-thinning drugs, vitamin E thins the blood naturally, so tell your doctor and have regular blood tests so that you can reduce your drugs.)

- The mineral magnesium is very important for relaxing muscles, so take a good quality multivitamin and mineral that contains 500mg of magnesium.

Helpful Hints

- A simple blood test will tell you if you are anaemic and actually need to take extra iron (see *Anaemia)*.

- Get plenty of exercise.

- Massage your legs and feet with essential oil of rosemary in a carrier of almond or olive oil – using kneading movements from the ankle upwards towards the knee. The legs can be bathed in alternate hot and cold water to improve circulation. Use cramp bark cream before going to bed. **NC**

- Try reflexology, acupuncture or regular aromatherapy massage to rev up the circulation.

- Take all the suggested supplements for at least three months.

- Wearing magnets in your shoes or in bed socks greatly aids circulation which can reduce the symptoms considerably at night. For details call **Homedics** on 0161 798 5876. Helpline 0161 798 5885. Web site: www.homedicsuk.

RHEUMATOID ARTHRITIS

(see *Arthritis*)

Eating a poached pear after a meal helps to improve your digestion. Pears are rich in phosphorous, iron, potassium, magnesium and calcium.

ROSACEA

A chronic acne-like eruption or flushing of the face which usually affects the area around the nose and chin, rosacea can be inherited but it is more commonly associated with drinking too much alcohol, stress, coffee, tea, spicy foods, the menopause, lack of stomach acid and B vitamins. It is a common skin disorder in adults between the ages of 30 and 50, and women are three times more likely to be affected than men. It can be triggered by a food intolerance and the most common triggers are wheat, cow's milk and oranges. Many people who suffer rosacea also suffer from migraines (see under *Migraine*). You also need to take care of your liver. Some nutritional physicians are also seeing links between rosacea and the *Helibactor pylori* bacterium which can also cause stomach ulcers.

Foods to Avoid
- Generally cut down on coffee, tea, alcohol, hot drinks and hot spicy foods.
- Keep a food diary and note as the flush appears what you were eating, drinking or feeling before the flush began.
- Don't eat heavy rich meals which place a strain on the digestion and liver.
- Don't eat too much food made from flour – these tend to be pies, cakes, etc which are often high in salt, sugar and saturated fats.

Friendly Foods
- Bitter foods such as radiccio, fennel, chicory, celeriac and young green celery stimulate stomach acid.
- Take a teaspoon of apple cider vinegar or lemon juice in warm water before a meal.
- Drink plenty of water even if you are not thirsty.
- Eat more pineapple and papaya to improve your digestion.
- Eat plenty of leafy greens especially spinach, cauliflower, broccoli, cabbage and celery.
- Eat more beetroot and artichokes to help cleanse your liver.
- Include plenty of live, low-fat yoghurt to help replenish healthy bacteria in the gut.

Useful Remedies
- If you are not suffering active stomach ulcers take one *Betaine Hydrochloride* (stomach acid) capsule with main meals. If this causes a slight burning sensation then switch to a digestive enzyme capsule from your health shop.
- Rosacea sufferers often have a decreased secretion of the pancreatic enzyme lipase. Take 1 *Lipozyme* with main meals. **BC**
- As B-group vitamins are often depleted, also take a B-complex.

- Include a good quality multi-vitamin and mineral in this regimen.
- Try using organic rice, soya or oat milk instead of cow's milk
- Amaranth, rye, rice or oat cakes make a good alternative to wheat-based breads.

Helpful Hints

- Sipping diluted lemon juice with main meals can help to treat low stomach acid, which is a factor in this condition.
- Homeopathic *Puls 6x* twice daily for a couple of weeks to reduce symptoms.
- There is a skin regime called *Sher*, which has helped many sufferers. For full details, contact *The Sher System*, 30 New Bond Street, London, W1S 2RN. Tel: 020 7499 4022. Website: www.sher.co.uk/skincare/ Email: skincare@sher.co.uk

If you take 1 tablespoon of organic cider vinegar and honey in warm water daily it helps to absorb more calcium from your diet.

SAD – SEASONAL AFFECTIVE DISORDER

SAD syndrome is a condition in which sufferers report feeling depressed and experience low moods during the winter months. Symptoms usually begin in late autumn or early winter and tend to disappear in late spring and early summer. During the winter months, the brain produces more melatonin, a hormone secreted by the pineal gland which regulates glandular function and makes us feel more sleepy. In countries where sunshine is rare during the winter months, suicide rates increase. Not everyone experiences the same symptoms, but common symptoms of SAD syndrome include cravings for sweet or starchy foods, weight gain, low energy levels, lethargy, a tendency to oversleep, mood swings, irritability and an increased feeling of being 'no use' to anyone.

Foods to Avoid

■ During the winter months, reduce your intake of stimulants such as tea, coffee, chocolate, caffeine and sugary based foods and drinks.

■ Alcohol lowers brain levels of the neuro-transmitter serotonin which helps keep us positive.

Friendly Foods

■ Eat foods that help the body to produce more serotonin – fish, turkey, chicken, cottage cheese, beans, avocados, bananas and wheat germ.

■ 60% of the brain is fat so eat plenty of oily fish which is rich in omega 3 fats. Add linseeds to your breakfast cereal as they are also rich in essential fats.

■ Include more organic tofu and beans in your diet. Kidney, cannellini and black-eyed beans are a rich source of fibre and protein to help raise your mood.

■ During the winter make rich stews with plenty of green and root vegetables, add brown rice and pasta.

■ Low-sugar oat-based muesli and cereals are rich in B vitamins which are great mood foods.

■ Reduce your intake of refined, sugary foods, and if you crave sugar use a little honey or brown rice syrup as a sweetener, both of which are rich in magnesium.

Useful Remedies

■ Firstly take a good quality multi-vitamin and mineral supplement that contains at least 200 mg of magnesium plus 30mg of zinc.

■ Add to this a B-complex, as lack of vitamins B3, 6, 12 and folic acid are all linked to depression. **BLK**

■ *5-Hydroxy Tryptophan* (5-HTP) is derived from an African plant griffonia which helps boost serotonin levels. This supplement has been shown to be as effective as orthodox anti-depressants, without the negative side effects. 100mg can be taken twice daily. **HN**

■ St John's wort has proven very effective and you will need 500-1000mg a day. Not to be taken with blood-thinning drugs. If you are on any drugs check for contraindications with your GP.

■ Cod liver oil is rich in vitamin D, a lack of which is associated with SAD syndrome – 2 capsules or a teaspoon of the oil daily.

Helpful Hints

■ Tanning beds should not be used to treat SAD. The light sources in tanning beds are high in ultraviolet (UV) rays, which harm both your eyes and your skin. Light boxes emit full spectrum light. Use Biolight's full spectrum lightbulbs. **HN**

■ Exercise as much as possible during daylight to increase production of serotomin – the feelgood hormone.

■ Take a winter holiday in the sunshine.

■ *The SAD Association (SADA)* have a support network, and by sending a large SAE to PO Box 989, Steyning, BN44 3HG you will receive a SADA information pack, which contains full details of SAD treatments, where to obtain light therapy equipment, how to adapt your lifestyle, clinics, meetings and books. Tel: 01903 814942.

Avoid shampoos, bubble baths, shower gels and cleansers containing sodium laurel (and laureth) sulphate SLS which has been shown to damage eye tissue.

SCALP PROBLEMS

SCALP PROBLEMS – Dry, flaking, itching scalp (Dandruff)

This condition occurs when the tiny cells in the outer layer of skin are shed at a faster rate than normal. Dandruff usually results from a malfunction of the sebaceous glands, affecting the amount of sebum or oils they produce. If too little sebum is secreted, the hair becomes brittle and dandruff appears. Dry skin on the scalp is also linked to eczema and psoriasis. An itchy scalp can also be linked to candida. Dandruff is also associated with food intolerances.

Foods to Avoid

■ I'm afraid it's the usual culprits of highly refined foods, high in animal fats and sugar. See also *General Health Hints*.

Friendly Foods

■ You need to increase your intake of healthier fats found in oily fish, sunflower, pumpkin and sesame seeds.

■ Use organic walnut and olive oils, not only for salad dressings, but also drizzled over cooked dishes. *Udo's Choice Oil* is a perfect blend of omega 3 and 6 fats that will help to feed the skin from the inside out. See *Fats You Need to Eat*.

■ Eat more whole foods, brown rice and bread, barley, quinoa, millet, brown bread and pasta.

■ Greatly increase your intake of fresh fruits and vegetables.

■ Eat pineapple and papaya with main meals to aid digestion.

■ Include more low-fat, live yoghurt in your diet to also aid digestion.

■ Eat more wheat germ and avocados rich in vitamin E.

■ Dry skin denotes dehydration, so drink at least six glasses of water daily.

Useful Remedies

■ Take a good quality multi-vitamin and mineral that contains 30mg of zinc (vital for healing skin).

■ Take a high-strength B complex.

- Vitamin E aids healthy skin, take 300iu daily.

- *Omega Plex* is a powered formula containing a perfect blend of omega 3 and 6 fats. Mix half a teaspoon daily in a small glass of water. **BC**

- Your multi will contain some vitamin A – but make this up to 10,000 iu per day. If pregnant take no more than 5000iu altogether.

Helpful Hints

- Use natural-based shampoos that contain no chemicals and colourings. *Blackmores*, *Aveda* and the *Body Shop* make excellent ranges.

- For organic shampoos and hair products try **The Green People Company** products. To find your nearest stockist call 01444 401444. Website:www.greenpeople.co.uk

- Massage the scalp with pure rosemary oil mixed with jojoba or olive oil and leave on overnight.

- Homepathic *Ars-alb 6x* can be taken once or twice daily for a week.

SCALP PROBLEMS – Greasy scalp

Greasy hair and scalps are usually caused by overactive sebaceous glands, which produce a waxy natural oil known as sebum to keeps hair supple. This problem is more common during the teenage years but as we age for most people the scalp becomes drier. It is far more common in men and teenagers and is linked to acne and hormonal changes. See also *Acne*. It can be aggravated by frequent washing with strong shampoos, which will destroy the acid balance of the scalp. Always use a pH balanced shampoo or add a little vinegar or lemon juice to your final rinse.

Foods to Avoid

- Cutting down on refined carbohydrates especially sweets, chocolates and soft drinks often helps. Reduce intake of red meats which take a long time to digest and can putrefy in the gut.

- Cut down on alcohol, caffeine and saturated fats which place an extra strain on the liver.

Friendly Foods

- Eat more organic tofu, broccoli, cauliflower, Brussels sprouts, lentils and beans which will help to regulate hormone levels.

- Drink at least 6 glasses of water every day.

- Eat more fish and oily fish, avocados, sunflower, pumpkin and sesame seeds and linseeds. Also use their unrefined oils for your salad dressings.

- See also *General Health Hints*.

Useful remedies

■ Vitamin A, 5000iu a day helps balance oil production

■ Take an essential fatty acid formula such as *Omega Plex*. **BC**

■ Take a multi-vitamin and mineral plus 2–3mg biotin, the B vitamin that is often deficient with this problem.

Helpful Hints

■ Wash hair regularly with mild or very dilute shampoo (try a herbal shampoo such as seaweed or rosemary).

■ Take plenty of exercise which will help to reduce overproduction of sebum.

■ Massage your scalp regularly. Many companies now make mild astringents that can be used for massage.

■ Homeopathic *Nat Mur 6x* can be taken once daily for 7–10 days.

■ Dandruff which sticks to the hair and scalp can be loosened by rinsing the scalp with sour milk or a mild solution of lemon juice (2 tablespoons lemon juice to 0.5 litre cooled boiled water).

■ Apply *Calendula* ointment to itchy areas.

■ Consult a qualified nutritionist who can help you to rebalance your diet (see *Useful Information*).

Avoid toiletries containing propylene glycol which is linked to dermatitis, kidney and liver problems.

SCALP PROBLEMS – Head lice

This is a common problem especially in school age children. The most obvious symptom is a constantly itching scalp and upon examination grey coloured insects can be seen. These are the adults. The lice eggs (nits) are white and stick to the hair. As the eggs have a 7–14 day incubation period, patience and regular daily treatments are necessary. Many orthodox treatments contain organophosphates (pesticides) which are now linked to cancers.

Foods to Avoid

■ See *General Health Hints*.

Friendly Foods

■ See *General Health Hints*.

Useful Remedies

- The spray *Nice N Clear* contains tea tree, lavender, citronella, nettle, thyme, orange and neem oil which help to kill the lice. For details call 020 8875 9915.

- *Chinese Whispers* is a herbal formula that has been shown in medical trials to kill the lice. For details of your nearest stockists call **Nature's Store** on 01782 794300.

Helpful Hints

- Comb the hair daily with a fine-toothed comb to remove the lice.

- Check the head daily as simply leaning close to someone who is infested can spread the lice.

- Wash all clothing in a really hot wash and then leave in the freezer for 2–3 days to kill any remaining lice.

- Combine one part lavender oil and one part tea tree oil to 3 parts of olive oil. Massage into the head and then rinse with vinegar.

During the winter months, get out in the sunshine and natural daylight as much as possible to avoid the winter blues.

SCIATICA

Sciatica is usually a symptom of a structural problem in the lower back, where the sciatic nerve becomes trapped or pinched. The pain tends to affect the buttocks and back of the thighs, can travel down the back of the leg and in some cases as far as the feet. It may also cause numbness, pins and needles and/or weakness in those areas. The most common cause is a trapped nerve but it can also be caused by a slipped or bulging disc in the lower back which causes pressure on the sciatic nerve. Other causes include an abscess, an inflammation of the sciatic nerve, or the after-effect of minor injury to the back, for instance lifting too heavy a weight in the gym, or sitting in an awkward position.

Foods to avoid

- Avoid excessive consumption of foods that drain the body of thiamine and magnesium, such as coffee, tea, colas and fizzy drinks, chocolate and refined sugars which reduce the body's ability to cope with pain.

- Lack of magnesium and thiamine can also contribute muscular pain and spasms.

Friendly foods

- Cereals, wheat germ, meats, *Bovril*, fresh peanuts, brewer's yeast and Brazil nuts are all rich in thiamine.

- Magnesium-rich foods are cereals, honey, wheat germ, soya flour products, almonds, Brazil nuts, mustard and curry powder.
- Eat plenty of green leafy vegetables, yellow peppers and fresh fruits, which are all nutrient rich, to support your nerves.
- Add more turmeric and cayenne to foods.
- Ginger helps to reduce pain, so add to cooking or make fresh ginger tea.

Useful Remedies

- Take NT188 containing B vitamins and passiflora to help calm the nerves. **BC**
- Magnesium malate 500mg twice daily to help relax the nerve endings.
- Calcium has anti-spasmodic properties; take 400–600mg daily.
- 100mg daily of Thiamine (vitamin B1) to nourish the nervous system.
- Vitamin B12 injections may be helpful in some cases.
- As all B vitamins work together, include a B-complex.
- Take 200iu of vitamin E which helps to reduce any inflammation.
- Organic sulphur (MSM) plus the amino sugar glucosamine have shown great results in reducing this type of pain. Take 500mg twice daily until symptoms ease (if you are highly allergic to shellfish avoid glucosamine). **HN**
- DLPA, an amino acid, encourages the production of the body's own pain-killing chemicals. 400mg can be taken 3 times daily until symptoms ease. Also helps to lift your mood. **FSC**
- Take 1–3 grams of vitamin C with bioflavonoids to aid tissue healing.

Helpful Hints

- To reduce pain and discomfort, prepare an ice pack plus a hot-water-bottle wrapped in towels. Place each alternately on the site of the pain for ten minutes; try this twice daily.
- To relieve sciatica, lie down on your back with your knees bent, feet flat on the floor. Place your hands underneath your buttocks (palms down) beside the base of your spine. Close your eyes, and taking long, deep breaths, rock your knees from side to side for two minutes. Reposition your hands every few minutes to enable different parts of the buttocks muscles to be pressed. Gently move your legs from side to side with your knees pulled into your abdomen and your feet off the floor and support your legs by holding them with your palms just behind your upper legs.
- Many alternative practitioners have found that regular deep-tissue massage gives enormous relief to sciatica sufferers, as muscular spasms in this area can be mistaken for sciatica.
- Essential oils of Roman chamomile and lavender are very useful for reducing pain.
- Homeopathic *Lach* is good for right-sided sciatica. Take 30c 3–4 times daily for up to 4 days.
- See a qualified osteopath, chiropractor or Bowen Technique therapist as soon as possible and then try acupuncture for further relief of pain. See *Useful Information*.

- Join a local yoga class to keep your spine and joints in great shape.

- When sleeping or resting, lie on your side with a pillow between your knees to minimise pelvic strain. If you sleep on your back put a soft pillow under your knees.

If you can't eat it, don't breathe it into your body.

Alfred Zam

SHINGLES (HERPES ZOSTER)

Shingles is caused by the same virus that causes chickenpox. The basic rule is that you cannot contract shingles if you have not had chickenpox, as the virus lies dormant for many years in a nerve root in the spine. There is anecdotal evidence that a person suffering from shingles can pass the virus, especially to a young child, and give them chickenpox. Also, if a child who has chickenpox is in contact with an elderly relative who has also suffered from the disease the contact may reactivate the virus in the form of shingles.

Shingles is common after the age of 60 but younger people are beginning to suffer shingles. It can be activated by shock, stress or lowered immune function. As the virus multiplies and attacks the nerve, it can cause searing pains along the nerve pathways. After a few days, the skin erupts in itchy blisters. These generally heal within a week, but nerve pains may last for several weeks. If the facial nerves are affected, there may be temporary paralysis. If the optic nerve is affected, the cornea may be damaged. It usually affects one side of the body or face.

Foods to Avoid

- Foods which are rich in arginine, an amino acid found commonly in chocolate, carob, lentils, beans and nuts.

- Avoid sugar, refined foods made with white flour and high-saturated-fat foods which again have a negative effect on the immune system.

- Some people suffer an attack when they eat too much dairy produce from cows.

Friendly Foods

- Eat good-quality protein such as lean meats including turkey, duck, lean pork plus fish, corn and soya, all of which are rich in lysine, an amino acid which has been shown to interfere with replication of the virus.

- Most people feel very poorly indeed with shingles, therefore home-made vegetable soups that are easy to eat and rich in nutrients would be very beneficial.

- Live, low-fat yoghurts aid digestion and replenish the healthy bacteria in the bowel.

- See *General Health Hints*.

Useful Remedies

■ At the onset of symptoms begin taking 500–1000mg of *Lysine* daily. If you are already suffering take up to 4 grams daily.

■ Take up to 5 grams of vitamin C daily in an ascorbate form whilst the situation is acute. This may trigger loose bowels, in which case reduce the dose until this stops.

■ Also apply pure vitamin C cream topically as soon as the sores begin to form but not if the skin is broken. **BC**

■ Pierce a 600iu vitamin E capsule and apply directly to the sores. Leave it on for about 15 minutes and generally within 8 hours the pain is greatly reduced.

■ Zinc in the form of a cream applied regularly can help fight the virus. Also take 30mg daily internally in the form of a multi-vitamin and mineral.

■ Liquorice applied topically and internally can also help to kill the virus.

■ During an attack take 30,000iu of vitamin A daily for one month (only 5000iu if you are pregnant). This aids skin healing and boosts immune function.

■ Sold as *Larreastat*, a new extract of the larrea bush has had a 97% success rate in treating all types of herpes. It is available in capsules or a lotion. Take one capsule up to 3 times daily and apply the lotion topically. **NC**

Helpful Hints

■ Take as much bed rest as possible when the attack starts.

■ The herb St.. John's wort is very useful for relieving the depression associated with shingles. If you are not on blood-thinning drugs, take 500mg 3 times daily.

■ Make sure you change your toothbrush and face towels regularly as these can harbour the virus.

■ *Calendula* tincture can be dabbed directly on to the sores.

■ Homeopathic *Rhus Tox 6x* taken 3–4 times daily for 3 days will help reduce the pain.

■ Apply plain yoghurt mixed with a little zinc oxide cream along the path of the affected nerve 2–3 times daily can clear herpes zoster in 24–48 hours, if you start the regimem at the first sign of an outbreak.

■ Hot and cold compresses help relieve nerve pain.

Men who eat organic foods have a higher sperm count.

SINUS PROBLEMS

(see also *Allergies, Allergic Rhinitis* and *Catarrh*)

Sinusitis is an inflammation of the mucous membranes in the sinuses. It usually occurs after a viral or bacterial infection, such as a cold or flu, which has affected another part of the respiratory system. It can also be caused by injury to the nose, dental treatment or swimming. Common symptoms are a blocked nose, nasal-sounding speech, often accompanied by facial pain and headaches, which can be made worse by bending forward. If you suffer chronic sinus problems they may be linked to food intolerances and stress.

Foods To Avoid

- At the onset of an acute sinusitis attack, try eating really lightly. This clears the body of toxins and gives the digestive system and liver a rest, which boosts immune function.
- Avoid sugar in any form for at least 6 days, as sugar greatly impairs your immune functioning and encourages bacterial growth.
- At all costs avoid mucous-producing foods such as full-fat milk, cheese, chocolate, white bread, croissants, pastries, cakes and anything else containing white flour and milk. Try the detox diet from Stephanie Lashford (see also *Allergies*).

Friendly Foods

- For 3 or 4 days live on really thick soups that are full of fresh vegetables and a little chicken, lentils, brown rice or barley.
- Eat more garlic and onions.
- Hot curries also help clear the sinuses.
- Drink plenty of freshly blended vegetable juices.
- Snack on fenugreek seeds and add fresh root ginger to meals.
- Drink lots of water and elderflower tea to help to reduce congestion.

Useful Remedies

- The B-group vitamins are often lacking in this condition and while symptoms are acute take 250mg of pantothenic acid (B5) twice daily, B6 – 50mg daily, and 1000mcg of B12.
- Vitamin C – take up to 3grams daily to boost immune function and reduce allergic responses to foods and external allergens.
- Take a multi-mineral that contains magnesium and zinc to boost immune function.
- The bioflavonoid quercetin, 400mg one to three times daily acts as a natural anti-histamine.
- Echinacea and golden rod help reduce mucous– available in tincture 5mls a day.

Helpful Hints

- Inhaling steam is another useful treatment. Add a few drops of mint or eucalyptus oil to boiling water, place a towel over your head and inhale for 5 minutes.
- Avoid dry atmospheres and humidify rooms. Blow your nose very gently as some people can suffer nosebleeds when this area becomes infected.

S

If you are having an argument – deal only with the current problem.
Don't drag up the past.

SLEEPING PILLS, ADDICTION

(see also *Insomnia*)

Sleeping pills have their place for short-term relief of chronic insomnia, which is commonly caused by chronic stress, exhaustion, anxiety, an inability to shut the mind down at night and so on. Once we begin taking sleeping pills, they alter brain chemistry and over time this situation gets worse until your brain can literally keep you awake most of the night if it does not receive its hit. If you find that you cannot go to sleep without first taking a pill and if you believe that you are only able to sleep if you take a drug, then you are addicted. There are some newer sleeping pills available on prescription that are not as addictive as the older ones like temazepam, valium and rohypnol. Nevertheless if you take any sleeping pills in the long term, they can affect your memory and cause mood swings. Natural remedies may not work for the first couple of weeks due to the toxic residues left in your brain and liver from the drugs you have taken. It takes a month for the brain to register that it is no longer going to get its hit, you can then establish a healthier sleep pattern. Whatever – be patient with yourself. A good time to try and get off the pills would be when you are on holiday, when you are not so worried about sleeping.

Foods to Avoid

■ Avoid eating late at night and eat at the same time every evening to establish a routine.

■ Don't eat heavy, rich meals late at night, they are difficult to digest and can keep you awake.

■ Greatly reduce your alcohol intake – drinking can make you drowsy initially but can cause you to wake in the early hours feeling very dehydrated.

■ Avoid all caffeine, cola, coffee, tea and cocoa. If you are really sensitive then even a few cups of coffee in the morning can interfere with the quality and quantity of sleep at night.

■ Generally avoid sugar, but if you find you cannot still your mind, then a small amount of sugar satisfies the hypothalamus area in the brain which can help you to get off to sleep.

Friendly Foods

■ Eat more pasta, wholemeal bread, bananas, wheat germ, avocados and cottage cheese at night. They are rich in a substance called tryptophan which encourages natural sleep.

■ Organic porridge made with rice milk makes a great breakfast cereal but it is also a calming food later in the day, packed with the B vitamins that nourish your nerves. Make some before bed and add half a chopped banana and a little honey to sweeten; which really helps you relax.

■ As a bedtime drink, try herbal teas such as camomile, valerian, passionflower or skullcap.

■ To ease the load on your liver eat more beetroot, artichokes, celeriac and celery.

Useful Remedies

■ Niacinamide (vitamin B3) 500 mg before bed, acts as a natural sleeping pill, but be certain to buy the **no-flush** variety, as niacin can cause a nasty flushing affect which would keep you awake ! This is particularly helpful for those who fall asleep readily but can't return to sleep after waking up during the night.

■ Vitamin B-12; take 1000 mcg daily to aid natural sleep.

■ As all B vitamins work together, also take a B-complex with breakfast.

■ Take magnesium, nature's tranquillizer; 500 mg before bed.

■ *5-Hydroxy Tryptophan* helps to raise serotonin levels and re-establish normal sleep patterns. Take 50–200 mg before bed. **HN**

■ *Alpha Lipoic Acid* is a great antioxidant. 100mg taken per day helps detoxify the liver from sleeping pills.

■ 1200mg of *N-Acetyl Cysteine* per day is a great liver cleanser.

Helpful Hints

■ There are many alternative remedies which you can find at your local health store.

■ Stop working an hour before bedtime and read something light; take more exercise, preferably earlier in the day.

■ Turn your bedside clock to the wall, stop worrying about the time.

■ For over 20 years I have had a problem sleeping, but find when I am on holiday I sleep like a log. Most of us today lead very stressful lives and have a lot on our minds, and at night our brains seem to wake up. If this is your problem, I strongly suggest you learn to meditate and include more regular exercise, which reduces stress (see under Meditation).

■ **Potter's** *Nodoff Mixture* is a traditional herbal remedy to promote natural sleep. It tastes ghastly but helps a lot of people. Available from all good health stores For your nearest stockist contact **Potter's (Herbal Supplies) Ltd** Tel: 01942 405100 Website: www.pottersherbal.co.uk

■ **Bioforce** also make an excellent tincture called *Dormesan* containing hops, lemon balm and valerian, all of which have sedative properties. This is useful for people who tend to wake during the early hours. There are literally dozens of natural sleep remedies – ask for advice at your local health store.

Dandelion leaves are rich in potassium and act as a safe, natural diuretic
to relieve water retention.

S

SMOKING

If you smoke, the best favour you can do for yourself and those around you is to give it up. Every cigarette you smoke takes eight minutes off your life. A pack a day equates to losing a month of life each year. One cigarette can increase your heart rate by twenty beats a minute and can also increase blood pressure. Smoking one packet of cigarettes a day depletes 500mg of vitamin C from your body – the average daily intake is 60–100mg.

Cigarettes increase carbon monoxide levels in the blood and it takes the circulatory system six hours to return to normal after you have smoked a cigarette. Perhaps now you understand why heart disease, cancer, strokes as well as high blood pressure and numerous other chronic diseases are linked to smoking. It's also worth noting that smoking ages your skin and tests have shown that the skin of a 40 year old smoker is comparable to that of a 65-year-old non-smoker. A recent study showed that pregnant women who smoked more than 20 cigarettes a day, more than doubled their son's risk of arrest for violent crime in later life.

The more you can control your blood sugar, the easier it will be to give up smoking for good and avoid mood swings associated with withdrawal.

Foods To Avoid

■ Cut down on the foods that you have just prior to enjoying a cigarette, such as wine or beer.

■ Cut down on saturated animal fats which will harden your arteries over time.

■ Cut down on caffeine, colas, sugar, tea and other stimulants.

■ See also *Heart Disease*.

Friendly Foods

■ Eat plenty of foods that re-alkalise your body, such as fruits, vegetables, millet, buckwheat and wheat germ.

■ Begin using unrefined walnut, sunflower and olive oils for salad dressings and use sunflower and pumpkin seeds and linseeds over breakfast cereals and salads.

■ Eating more leafy greens such as cabbage, spring greens, spinach or kale reduces your risk of lung cancer.

■ Cantaloupe melons, apricots, carrots, French beans, mangos, raw parsley and watercress. These are all high in natural source carotenes that help protect the delicate tissue in the lungs. Eat more oily fish rich in vitamin A.

■ Generally eat small meals regularly to control blood sugar (see *Friendly Foods* under *Low Blood Sugar*).

Useful Supplements

■ Take a B-complex daily.

■ Take at least 2 grams of vitamin C daily with meals.

■ Take vitamin A 10,000iu to protect lung tissue. If you are pregnant you should not be smoking, and the dose would need to be no more than 5000iu.

■ Take a high-strength antioxidant formula containing vitamins A, C, E plus zinc and selenium plus natural source beta carotenes. **NL**

■ Magnesium taken daily – 500mg – helps ease breathing.

■ Take *N-Acetyl Cysteine*, 1200mg per day. This amino acid helps bronchial conditions as it loosens mucous and strengthens tissue.

■ The amino acid tyrosine – 500mg per day – helps reduce the craving for nicotine.

■ 200 mcg per day of the mineral chromium helps to keep your blood sugar on an even keel, thus reducing the cravings. Take between meals.

Helpful Hints

■ A herbal extract made from crushed lobelia leaves, which Mexican Indians used to chew as a tobacco substitute, is available from health stores, or by mail-order from **Fresh and Wild** in London. Tel: 020 7229 1063. Website: www.freshandwild.com

■ The medical herbalist Andrew Chevallier suggests this remedy: Mix one heaped teaspoon of coltsfoot and half a teaspoon of thyme into a teapot of boiling water, cool and sip. Coltsfoot strengthens the lungs and thyme is antiseptic and healing.

Sugar interferes with the ability of white blood cells to kill invading bacteria.

SORE THROATS

(see also *Colds and Flu* and *Immune Function*)

If you tend to suffer a persistent sore throat it usually denotes that your immune system is struggling to cope. When I become overtired and my throat becomes sore, I know that if I were to eat some foods high in sugar, this can send my immune system off the deep end and I will end up with a cold or infection. I now know my limits and listen to my body. Regular bouts of tonsillitis mean that your lymphatic system is under stress and your body is telling you to detoxify. Regular sore throats are also associated with the yeast fungal overgrowth candida (see *Candida*).

Inflammation and pain in the throat can trigger symptoms such as pain upon swallowing or speaking, a dry tickling feeling, build up of mucous in the nose and sinuses and occasionally a husky voice or loss of your voice. These types of infections are caused by bacteria or viruses.

A sore throat caused by a streptococcal infection (often called strep throat) needs to be identified and treated, or it could trigger rheumatic fever. So if symptoms are severe, please see your doctor.

Foods to Avoid

- Eliminate sugar in any form for 7 days to give your immune system a chance to fight infection.
- Greatly cut down or avoid all white-flour-based products, snacks and burger-type meals.
- Tea, coffee, sugary drinks and alcohol dehydrate the body and act as stimulants – if your adrenal glands are exhausted they will add to the problem.
- Cut down on all full-fat dairy produce.

Friendly Foods

- Increase fluid intake, include lots of filtered water, herbal teas, diluted fruit juices, and broths.
- Sip warm water mixed with powdered vitamin C plus lemon, ginger and/or garlic with a little honey.
- See *Friendly Foods* under *Colds and Flu*.

Useful Remedies

- While symptoms are acute take 10,000iu of vitamin A daily to boost your immune system (if pregnant only 5000iu).
- Take at least 2–3 grams of vitamin C daily with meals.
- Take a B-complex to support your adrenal glands.
- Take vitamin E – 400iu. A deficiency is associated with increased infections.
- Low levels of selenium are linked to viral infections. Take a multi-vitamin and mineral that includes 200mcg of selenium and 30mg of zinc.
- *Chloride compound*, 200mg daily, helps to clear lymphatic congestion and relieve sore throats. **BLK**
- A natural source beta-carotene complex boosts immune function and fights infection. **BC FSC HN S**
- Zinc Gluconate Lozenges really help reduce a sore throat – take 3–4 daily.
- If you end up taking antibiotics, make sure you replenish healthy bacteria by taking acidophilus/bifidus capsules twice daily for 6 weeks.

Helpful Hints

- Crush fresh sage, make into a tea, allow to cool, gargle and swallow. Sage is antiseptic and eases the soreness. If the throat is really sore, soak a cloth in the sage mix and apply to the throat area.
- You can also crush an onion and wrap in a cloth and place on the throat.

- *Propolis* tincture can be diluted in water and used as a gargle.

- Change your toothbrush regularly.

- At the onset of a sore throat use homeopathic *Aconite* or *Belladonna 30c* – every few hours for 2 days. For children's sore throats, a hacking cough and swollen tonsils try Chamomila 30c – 3 times daily for 2 days.

- The herb thyme is a natural antiseptic. It can be made into a solution and used as a gargle for sore throats or sipped as a tea mixture to help relieve sore throats and coughs.

- *Bee Propolis* throat spray and lozenges also help relieve a sore throat.

- Tea tree oil is a natural antiseptic, use diluted with a little sea salt as a gargle, but do not swallow. Gargle with a mixture of hot water and a quarter teaspoonful of turmeric powder and a pinch of salt.

Keep an open mind.

SPIRITUAL EMERGENCY

Spiritual emergency is a well-known phenomena in the East and as our spiritual awakening gains pace it is becoming more common in the West. I have yet to meet an orthodox doctor (apart from my own GP) who has heard of this condition, but believe me it does exist.

I experienced a huge spiritual emergency during 1998. I began affecting electrical equipment, I could clearly see people's energy or auric fields, I became super psychic, telepathic, and could clearly hear people from the spirit world. I received huge amounts of information which placed an enormous strain on my brain and nervous system. The full story is told in my book *Divine Intervention* (Cima Books), and is available from all major book shops.

People experience various phenomena such as seeing auras and hearing other realms during spiritual development courses. We all have psychic abilities and are capable of miracles, but most of us don't truly comprehend this ultimate truth. The problem being that when you undergo this type of experience you need to turn to someone who can determine whether you are psychotic or having a genuine spiritual breakthrough. At this moment in our evolution the average human uses between 3–5% of their brain's potential capabilities. Certain highly evolved spiritual people use up to 50% and are capable of incredible feats which need to be seen to be believed.

If during your spiritual growth, you begin to feel ultra-special and your ego comes into play – you need to ground yourself. Find your nearest spiritualist church who will undoubtedly know of someone who can help you. Hands-on healing would definitely be of benefit during a spiritual emergency – see under *Healing*.

It's your choice whether to turn to an orthodox doctor, but you may end up on huge amounts of medication and be admitted to a psychiatric hospital. If I had not had tremendous support from my family and friends this could have easily happened to me.

Foods to Avoid

- Sometimes, during this type of situation you don't want food, but it is imperative you eat to help ground yourself.

- The last thing you need is stimulants, so avoid caffeine, sugar and alcohol.

Friendly Foods

- If your brain is in absolute overdrive and feels as though it's on fire, eat some sugary food quickly. The brain uses pure glucose as a fuel, and as you may be processing huge amounts of information, your brain will need an energy supply. It is always preferable if you can eat small healthy meals regularly, but if the situation is acute then eat sugar or a banana.

- Generally eat what I term 'earthy' grounding foods such as porridge made with organic rice milk, stews and thick vegetable or grain-based soups.

- You may not want it, but you need protein which helps balance your blood sugar levels for longer periods. Fish and animal products might repulse you, in which case eat some beans, pulses and brown rice with plenty of fruits and vegetables.

- Drink plenty of water and as many calming herbal teas as you like.

- Your digestion may be upset, so include fresh ginger in soups and make ginger teas.

- If you simply cannot eat at least make yourself some fresh vegetable juices with added aloe vera juice and a green food powder, which will keep you going for 2–3 days.

Useful Remedies

- Begin taking **Bach Rescue Remedy**, *Star of Bethlehem* immediately every 2 or 3 hours.

- Also begin taking homeopathic *Arnica 30c* every few hours.

- *Aurum Metallicum* can help to balance your aura.

- **Australian Bush Essence** *Mint Bush* is made specifically for a time of spiritual turmoil. Available from all health shops. **NC**

- Take a high strength B-complex to support your nerves. Try an extra 1000mg of pantothenic acid (vitamin B5) daily to support your adrenal glands which are most probably working over time.

- Take a multi-vitamin and mineral formula daily.

Helpful Hints

■ **Runnings Park** in Malvern is one of the few places in the UK that specialises in helping people who are 'hearing voices'. They have psychiatrists on hand who can determine whether a person is having a spiritual experience or a psychotic one. Tel: 01684 573868. E-mail: info@runningspark.co.uk

■ If you want to know more about how to channel spirit guides in a safe and controlled way call **The School of Channelling**, Tel: 01684 573868. E-mail: schoolofchannelling@fsmail.net

■ In London call **The College of Psychic Studies** which takes students from all over the world. Tel 0207 589 3292. Website: www.psychic-studies.org.uk

■ At this time, you need all the support and patience friends and family can provide, as you may say and do many things – like levitate or produce ash – which can initially be quite frightening. You may also experience periods of complete and utter bliss and might find it hard to remain physical at this time. If you feel yourself moving into another dimension, eat something sugary as fast as you can and ask a friend to come and stay with you.

■ Avoid negative thoughts at all costs. For every negative thought replace it with a positive one.

■ Try not to panic – the experience will pass – it just takes time. See also *Panic Attacks*.

■ Read *Spiritual Emergency* by Stanislav and Christina Grof MD. ISBN 0-87477-538-8 To order in the UK call 0207 323 2382. This book really helps when personal transformation becomes a crisis.

Men who eat at least three portions of oily fish a week are helping to protect their prostate against cancer.

STITCH

This is a sudden, sharp pain in the side or abdomen, triggered by exercise that wears off after a few minutes when we rest. The pain is almost certainly caused by a spasm in the gut wall. Stitch is the body's way of telling you it needs more oxygen, so stand still and breathe deeply. It can also be triggered by too much exercise after a heavy meal.

People who tend to be sedentary, eat insufficient fresh fruit and vegetables but too much sugar, caffeine and animal protein are often lacking in calcium and magnesium, which causes a build up of lactic acid, resulting in regular attacks of muscle cramps or stitch.

Foods to Avoid

■ Avoid sugar and highly refined foods such as croissants, biscuits, cakes, pizza and white-flour-based foods in general.

Friendly Foods
■ Magnesium-rich foods such as green leafy vegetables, fruits plus brown rice, barley, lentils and whole grains rich in fibre will give you more protection in the long term.
■ Include good quality protein in the diet such as fresh fish, tofu, lean meats at least once a day.

Useful Remedies
■ Take a vitamin B-complex.
■ Calcium 1000mg and 500mg of magnesium to help reduce spasm and relax the muscles.

Helpful Hints
■ A stitch is more likely to occur if you exercise while food is still digesting in the gut. Avoid strenuous exercise for an hour or two after a substantial amount of food.
■ Generally take regular exercise to avoid lactic acid accumulation in the body.
■ Do not sit for long periods without going for a walk or a good stretch. Breathe deeply more often.
■ Bend down and touch your toes to relieve a stitch.

*Duodenal ulcers are more common in men, stomach ulcers
are more common in women*

S

STOMACH AND DUODENAL ULCERS
(see also *Acid Stomach*)

Stomach ulcers are small raw areas on the walls of the stomach where the protective mucous coating has been worn away. This can be due to excessive stomach acid production, insufficient mucous lining and regurgitation of bile from the duodenum, which are linked to heavy smoking, alcohol, erratic eating habits and a diet high in acid forming foods. They are painful immediately upon eating.

Duodenal ulcers are small raw spots in the lining of the duodenum eroded by stomach acid. They usually trigger pain 3 hours or so after eating a meal.

A bacterium called *Helicobacter pylori* has been found in over 90% of duodenal ulcers and 80% of gastric ulcers. This bacteria is also linked to stomach cancers, low energy levels, skin conditions such as rosacea and urticaria. Inflammatory conditions such as migraines and Raynaud's are also linked with *Helicobacter pylori*. Treatment with high dose antibiotics usually kills the bacteria.

Stress is a major factor in any type of ulcers as when you are stressed the body produces more stomach acid. Food intolerances to foods such as wheat, cow's milk and prescription drugs, plus long-term use of aspirin, steroids, and non-steroidal anti-inflammatory drugs such as ibuprofen are also linked to ulcers.

Foods to Avoid

- There is a proven link between over consumption of caffeine and ulcers, so avoid all coffee, black tea and colas. De-caffeinated coffee is also a problem.
- Eliminate all dairy produce from cows for at least one month.
- Alcohol stimulates stomach acid production.
- Don't eat too much sugar and rich fatty foods which again tend to increase acid production.
- Avoid spicy foods which can aggravate the gut lining.
- Avoid eating late at night which places a great strain on your digestive system.
- Avoid citrus fruits, raw tomatos, rhubarb, plums, and pineapple.
- Avoid all refined white-flour-based foods.

Friendly Foods

- Eat lots more fresh cabbage which is rich in L-glutamine, an amino acid that helps to heal the gut. Eat raw, added to fresh vegetable juices. If you cook the cabbage then use the cooking water for gravy or drink it once it has cooled.
- Replace cow's milk with soya light or organic rice milk
- Eat plenty of vegetables and fruits such as bananas, figs, lychees or pears.
- Include barley, brown rice and wholemeal bread, pastas and noodles plus lentils, millet, amaranth and couscous in your diet.
- Eat more jacket potatoes, peas, corn and apples which are high in fibre.
- Add seaweed such as kombu to your bean dishes as it contains healing properties.
- Fish, nuts and seeds are high in zinc which aids tissue healing.
- Eat more live, low-fat yoghurt, manuka honey and liquorice which all help to heal the gut.
- Add cinnamon to fruit dishes and eat more garlic.

Useful Remedies

- Chew 1 to 2 tablets of deglycyrrhized liquorice twenty minutes before food. This encourages healing of the stomach lining and helps to eradicate the *Helicobacter* if this is present. **FSC**
- Vitamin A is vital for the stomach lining to be able to heal. If you are not pregnant take 20,000iu daily for the first month and then reduce to 10,000iu.
- B vitamins aid digestion and reduce risk of ulcers. Take a B-complex daily.
- Take vitamin C as magnesium or potassium ascorbate 500 mg before meals and at bedtime, as most ulcer patients are lacking this vital vitamin. **BC**
- *Mastica* is an extract of the mastic gum tree found in the Greek Aegean sea. 500-1000mg per day for two weeks has been shown to rapidly heal gastric ulcers. **NC**
- Take L- glutamine 500 mg x 4 daily, 1 hour before meals to speed the healing process.

279

Helpful Hints

- Chew food thoroughly. Never rush a meal as digestion is made difficult when you are stressed or in a hurry.

- Don't drink too much with meals as this dilutes digestive juices.

- Ulcers can be encouraged to heal by eating only small quantities of food at a time.

- Avoid stress and rushing as much as possible as stress over a prolonged period can cause great harm to our digestive system.

- Smoking greatly increases the risk of ulcers.

- *Slippery Elm Food*, taken every 2 hours, helps soothe the gut.

- Drinking 75ml of concentrated aloe vera juice twenty minutes before meals also helps to soothe the digestive tract.

- Homeopathic *Nit-Ac 6x* can be taken twice daily for a week.

Continually puffy eyes may denote a food intolerance or an underactive thyroid

STRESS

Stress can be good or bad for you depending upon your reaction to it. Stress in the short term helps keep you sharp and alert but in the long term it can destroy your health. In the short term if we are faced with a crisis, our adrenal glands begin pumping the powerful hormones adrenaline and cortisol. This increases blood pressure, tenses the muscles and thickens the blood. In days gone by, this would have given us the energy to run faster, and if we suffered an injury, our blood would clot more quickly.

But in today's environment, most people when stressed don't go for a run, and if levels of these hormones remain high, they eventually become toxic to the body which can damage every major organ. When you are under constant stress the body's ability to cope with pain is greatly reduced. I believe that 85% of most chronic disease is triggered by stress.

Symptoms of excessive stress include a chronic sore throat, urgency to urinate – which denotes the adrenal glands and kidneys are in trouble. Palpitations, shallow breathing, losing your temper for no good reason, constantly tapping fingers and feet and nervous twitching of the eyelids. Perhaps you are also unable to sleep at night but can easily nod off during the day. And if you tend to wake between 3–5 am in the morning this denotes your adrenal glands and/or your liver are struggling.

In his book *Mental Health, the Nutrition Connection* (ION Press), nutritionist Patrick Holford writes about people who are addicted to stress saying, 'As a consequence of prolonged stress your energy level drops, you lose concentration, get confused, suffer from bouts of brain fog, fall asleep after meals, get irritable, freak out, can't sleep, can't wake up, sweat too much, get headaches'.

If any or all of these symptoms sound familiar, you need to stop and rest, because the next stage could be total burn out, a heart attack or stroke. Have a break and take a really good look at your life. You can choose. Low Blood sugar can result from stress (see also *Low Blood Sugar*).

Foods to Avoid

■ Avoid any foods and drinks containing alcohol, caffeine and sugar which are all stimulants that cause the adrenal glands to overwork and interfere with normal brain chemistry.

■ Especially avoid artificial sweeteners.

■ Cut down on heavy meals especially red meat which is hard to digest.

■ The more refined and processed food you eat, the more stress you place on your liver, digestive system and ultimately your adrenal glands.

Friendly Foods

■ Eat more oats, especially porridge made with rice milk, as oats are a rich source of B vitamins that help you to stay calm.

■ Make sure you eat breakfast – a low-sugar muesli, eggs or wholemeal toast would be fine.

■ Liquorice tea helps to support adrenal function.

■ Valerian and camomile teas help to calm you down.

■ Fruit compotes are easier to digest than raw fruit if you are really stressed.

■ Wholewheat pasta, noodles and breads, couscous, amaranth or oat crackers, brown rice and barley are all calming foods.

■ Avocados, turkey, cottage cheese, bananas, potatoes, ginger, yoghurt, leafy green vegetables, lettuce and low-fat milks will also help to de-stress you.

■ Eat more oily fish such as tuna, sardines and salmon and use organic, unrefined walnut and sunflower oils for dressings.

■ For more help on calming recipes try my cook book *Mind and Mood Foods* by myself and Kathryn Marsden, Readers Digest Books.

Useful Remedies

■ Firstly, support your adrenal glands by taking *Liquorice Formula Tincture* 1–3 mls daily in a freshly made vegetable juice. **FSC**

■ Begin taking a high-strength B-complex to support your nerves plus 500mg of vitamin B5 pantothenic acid four times a day which really helps adrenal function.

■ Urinary excretion of vitamin C increases with stress, so take 1–2 grams of vitamin C plus 400iu of vitamin E to thin your blood naturally – as stress also thickens the blood.

S

- You also need calming minerals, so take 750mg of calcium and 500mg of magnesium – the mineral magnesium is usually very depleted in a stressed person. Take this supplement at night.

- *5-Hydroxy Tryptophan* (5 HTP) 50-200 mg helps to increase the hormone serotonin in the brain which helps to raise mood.

- A high-strength fish oil containing EPA and DHA essential fats that thin the blood naturally and help keep blood pressure down.

- The fish extract *Garum Stabilium* helps you to feel more calm, reduces the feeling of being overwhelmed and helps you to feel more positive. Initially take four capsules on an empty stomach in the morning for 15 consecutive days. After two weeks, the dose should be reduced to two capsules every morning. **NC**

Helpful Hints

- Take stock of your life.

- Laughter releases stress – learn to lighten up.

- You will find that what you tend to resist the most, is what you need in your life.

- Make a space and time between what stresses you and your reaction to it. Think about this. Concentrate on what you can change in your life; let go of the things you have no control over.

- Nearly every one of us suffers stress but it's how we react to the stressful situation that's important. Stay calm and sleep on the problem.

- Make sure you get at least 8 hours' sleep every night.

- Stop cramming in appointments – learn to say 'no' and not feel guilty.

- Learn to meditate – see under *Meditation*.

- Get plenty of exercise: relaxed muscles mean more relaxed nerves, which reduces stress. Take yoga lessons and learn how to breathe properly which helps reduce stress. Lying down, take a deep breath into your stomach (place your hand on your tummy and actually feel the breath going into the abdomen as it rises) to a count of 6 and slowly breathe out to a count of 10.

- Have a massage using a mix of essential oils of lavender, valerian, frankincense, neroli, jasmine or ylang ylang which will all help to calm you down. As the oils are absorbed into the body, leave them on overnight to increase their effectiveness.

- *Neuro Linguistic Programming* or hypnotherapy on a weekly basis will really help to calm you down (see *Useful Information*).

*As many as eight toxic pesticides are sprayed on apples before you eat them –
eat more organic foods.*

STROKE

(see also *Angina* and *Heart Disease*)

As we age, arteries gradually narrow due to a build of up of sticky cholesterol-like substances. Approximately 80% of strokes are caused by blood clots which prevent oxygenated blood reaching vital areas of the brain. 20 % are caused when a blood vessel bursts. Depending on the part of the brain affected, there may be sudden loss of speech or movement, heaviness in the limbs, numbness, blurred vision, confusion, dizziness, loss of consciousness or coma. Symptoms can last for several hours or the rest of one's life depending on the severity of the stroke.

High risk factors for stroke are high blood pressure, eating too much salt, smoking , too much saturated fat, high oestrogen levels, stress, high LDL cholesterol levels and being overweight. People who tend to be angry or aggressive much of the time are at a higher risk – as stress and anger raise LDL (the bad) cholesterol level which thickens the blood.

High levels of homocysteine, a toxic by-product of the metabolism of proteins, can cause increased blockages in the arteries.

Foods to Avoid
- Avoid all carbonated, fizzy drinks.
- Greatly reduce your intake of saturated fats from full-fat dairy produce, cheeses and chocolates.
- Goat's cheese is extremely high in saturated fats.
- Cut down on red meats, sausages, meat pies and mass produced white-flour-based foods, such as croissants which are usually high in saturated fat and salt.
- Enjoy the odd glass of wine or coffee but be aware that caffeine can drive up blood pressure.
- Eliminate sodium-based salts from your diet, replace with a little magnesium or potassium-based salt such as *Solo Salt*.
- Avoid all highly preserved meats, salted nuts and smoked foods.
- Don't eat fried foods or hard margarines.

Friendly Foods
- Eat plenty of fresh fruits and vegetables and their freshly made juices. Especially good are whole grains such as brown rice, barley, lentils plus broccoli, sprouts, carrots, watercress, fresh and dried apricots, spinach, cabbage, spring greens, mangos, cantaloupe melon and tomato purée.
- Eat more oily fish and use unrefined olive, walnut and sunflower oil for salad dressings.
- Eat more raw, unsalted nuts and seeds which are a rich source of essential fats.
- Garlic and onions help to thin the blood naturally.
- Magnesium-rich foods include honey, kelp, raw wheat germ, winkles, almonds, Brazil nuts and curry powder.

S

- Low-sugar cereals are high in B vitamins which help reduce homocysteine levels.
- Drink at least 8 to 10 glasses of water a day.
- Sprinkle raw wheat germ over cereals and soups as it is high in vitamin E.

Useful Remedies

- Take a B-complex to help control homocysteine levels.
- Take fish oils 1–3 grams daily to thin the blood naturally.
- Take 1 gram of vitamin C, plus 400iu of vitamin E which protect against clotting.
- Co-enzyme Q 10, 30–60mg per day, helps support the heart, people high in co-Q10 are less prone to strokes.
- Bioflavonoids – 1000 mg taken daily helps to strengthen capillaries.
- The herb *Ginkgo Biloba* 120 mg of standardised extract helps to increase micro circulation.
- A good quality antioxidant formula that contains at least 200mcg of selenium. **NL**
- *Evolve* (*P25 Tocotrienol*), is an extract of rice bran which helps to reduce the stickiness in the blood. It is an excellent alternative to aspirin, particularly where patients suffer stomach irritations. Take one capsule daily. **NC**

Helpful Hints

- Many doctors have found that anyone who has suffered a stroke caused by a clot in the brain should be given intravenous magnesium as soon as possible after the stroke. Magnesium has a powerful dilatory action on the arteries and helps restore blood flow to the damaged tissue.
- Research shows that people living in soft water areas are more prone to high blood pressure, which can lead to strokes, as soft water can be low in magnesium; therefore, if you live in an area of soft water, take 250mg of magnesium daily.
- Homeopathic *Arnica 6x* – take 3 times daily for 2-3 weeks helps to reduce the shock and speeds the recovery rate.

There are currently more than 500 million mobile phones in use worldwide.
The frequencies they emit and receive now cover the globe. To reduce the risk of cancer
and ill health, reduce your calls.

SWOLLEN FEET and ANKLES

(see *Foot Problems* and *Water Retention*)

TACHYCARDIA (RAPID HEART BEAT)
(see also *Palpitations*)

Tachycardia is a sudden increase in heart rate to over 100 beats per minute in an adult. It occurs in healthy people during exercise but if tachycardia occurs when you are resting then you should consult a doctor as a matter of urgency. Symptoms may include palpitations, breathlessness and lightheadedness, sweating and dizziness (see also *Low Blood Sugar*).

Foods to Avoid
- Avoid drinking too much alcohol which can damage the heart muscle.
- Avoid caffeine which causes more adrenaline to be released into the bloodstream and can precipitate an attack.

Friendly Foods
- Eat potassium-rich foods. These include all leafy green vegetables, bananas, fresh and dried fruits, nuts, fish and sunflower seeds.
- See *Friendly Foods* under *Heart Disease*.

Useful Remedies
- Take a high-strength B-complex
- Co-enzyme Q 10, 60mg daily helps strengthen the heart muscle. **PN**
- Natural source vitamin E helps the heart muscle get oxygen and naturally thins the blood. Take 400iu daily.
- The mineral magnesium is often deficient. Take 300–600 mg daily.

Helpful Hints
- To combat worrying, which only exacerbates the condition, learn how to breathe properly by taking yoga lessons.
- Practice meditation, which teaches you how to stay calm when stressed. If you feel an attack beginning, splash your face with cold water, then lie down, close your eyes, breathe deeply and slowly for a few minutes until the attack passes.
- Essential oil of lavender or ylang ylang has a calming effect, so add a few drops to your bath – never use it neat. Try regular aromatherapy massage, which is very calming.
- Go for leisurely walks, breathing deeply.

If your gums bleed regularly you may be depleted in vitamin C

TASTE AND SMELL, LOSS OF

Loss of taste and smell occurs if we have a cold or blocked sinuses. If the nose becomes too dry and 'stuffed up' then the sense of smell can be impaired. It is generally easier to smell and taste in warm moist atmospheres rather than cold, dry ones. Hay fever, allergic rhinitis, nasal polyps, and smoking can all interfere with taste and smell. Lack of zinc is associated with this condition. Certain heart drugs can also cause a loss of taste and smell.

Foods to Avoid

- Generally you need to avoid mucous-forming foods, such as full-fat milk and dairy produce.
- Sugar will also make the situation worse.
- See *Foods to Avoid* under *Colds and Flu*.

Friendly Foods

- Keep your diet clean, with plenty of fresh fruits and vegetables.
- Eat more brown rice, barley, lentils, cereals, oats and wholemeal bread and pastas.
- Zinc-rich foods include lean steak, lamb and beef, calf's liver, raw oysters, fresh peanuts, hazelnuts, ground ginger and dry mustard.
- Sunflower, pumpkin and sesame seeds and linseeds all contain fair amounts of zinc.
- Try rice milk as a non-dairy substitute.

Useful Remedies

- Take 15–30 mg of chelated zinc or zinc picolinate which can be useful in helping to restore the sense of smell.
- If an infection triggers a loss of taste and smell take 10,000iu of vitamin A which helps support the upper respiratory tract. If you are pregnant, take no more than 5000iu.
- Include a high-strength multi-vitamin and mineral, plus 1 gram of vitamin C daily. **HN**
- If the problem is linked to an infection, take *echinacea*, 500 mg twice daily to boost your immune system.

Helpful Hints

- Tap water is often contaminated by chemicals which can exacerbate this problem. Invest in a reverse osmosis water filter system which is far more effective than over-the-counter carbon filters. For details contact *The Pure H2O Company* on 01784 221188 email: info@purewater.co.uk website: www.purewater.co.uk

■ See a qualified nutritionist who will help rebalance and detoxify your system.

■ Homeopathic *Nat Mur*, *Silica* or *Pulsatilla* are also very useful for loss of taste, *Belladonna* or *Hyos* are useful for loss of smell (see *Useful Information*).

THROAT PROBLEMS
(see *Sore Throat*)

The mineral silica helps to strengthen brittle hair and nails – take 200mg daily.

THRUSH
(see also *Candida* and *Cystitis*)

Vaginal thrush is caused by the same fungus, *Candida albicans*, which causes oral thrush. Infections develop when the acid-producing bacteria in the vagina are destroyed. This happens if we take too many antibiotics, eat too much sugar and junk-type food, become very run down, use highly perfumed soaps and deodorants etc. Symptoms can range from an itchiness or general soreness of the vagina, and sometimes the vulva swells and is accompanied by a thick, whitish discharge which smells rather yeasty. You may feel the need to urinate more regularly and there could be some slight stinging when you pass urine. If the infection takes hold, the lymph glands in the groin can swell. If this happens you must see a doctor (see also *Candida*).

Foods to Avoid
■ See *Foods to Avoid* under *Candida*.

Friendly foods
■ Eating 250 grams of plain, live yoghurt daily really helps to clear thrush.

■ See *Friendly Foods* under *Candida*.

Useful Remedies
■ Take 1000mg 3 times daily of the herb *Pau D' Arco* – which has anti-fungal properties.

■ *Grapefruit Seed Extract*, 800–1200 mg is anti-fungal. It also acts like a natural antibiotic.

■ Take a course of acidophilus/bifidus – healthy bacteria which really help to kill the yeast overgrowth. **BC**

■ Try tea tree oil or neem oil suppositories – use 1 at night before bed for at least 7 days.

■ Douche with yoghurt (1 pot natural live yoghurt to 1.75 litres boiled cooled water) Douche with apple cider vinegar diluted into water (4 tablespoons to 1 litre of boiled cooled water). This helps to re-acidify the area.

■ Include a high-strength multi vitamin and mineral in your regimen. **S**

Helpful Hints

- While an attack, lasts avoid sexual intercourse which could be extremely painful. Your partner will also need to be treated for candida as you are more than likely passing the problem back and forth.

- Douche in luke-warm water with a few drops of tea tree oil, a crushed garlic clove and a little organic cider vinegar.

- Wear cotton underwear and change it every day, and do not use vaginal deodorants, perfumed bath salts, or talcum powder.

- Only use pH balanced soaps.

- Avoid all vaginal deodorants, perfumes and bubble baths.

- Vitamin E or calendula cream may relieve itching.

- Homeopathic *Nat Mur* or *Kali Mur 6x* take 2–3 times daily for up to a week will help to reduce symptoms.

- For oral thrush use *Borox 6x* twice daily for up to a week.

Fresh root ginger is rich in zinc, copper, calcium, iron, magnesium and potassium. It helps reduce inflammation, feelings of nausea, has antibiotic properties and helps to lower LDL cholesterol levels.

THYROID, UNDERACTIVE AND OVERACTIVE

The thyroid gland lies in the neck, just below the Adam's apple. It produces the hormone thyroxine which controls the rate of metabolism in the body. Under- or over-production of this hormone can slow down or speed up all metabolic processes in the body. To produce these vital hormones, the thyroid needs the trace element iodine, which is ingested from food and water.

When the thyroid is underactive (hypothyroidism), it produces too little thyroxine which causes the body to slow down, producing symptoms such as extreme tiredness, an intolerance to cold, mental drowsiness, a slower heart rate, thinning hair, constipation, dry swollen skin, a deeper voice, low libido, weight gain even with a poor appetite, women can also suffer heavier periods.

An overactive thyroid (hyperthyroidism) means you are producing too much thyroxine which can cause symptoms such as a goitre, when the thyroid itself becomes more prominent, bulging eyes, over anxiety, an inability to relax or sleep properly, shakiness, sweating, feeling hot – even on cold days, rapid heart rate, palpitations, breathlessness and weight loss despite a healthy appetite. Stress, adrenal malfunction and a diet high in stimulants such as coffee, sugar and alcohol are all linked to an imbalance in the thyroid.

As thyroid imbalance is a highly complex situation, consult a nutritional physican who can totally change your diet and help you to control the symptoms (see *Useful Information*).

Food intolerances are linked to thyroid problems. There also appears to be a greater incidence of thyroid conditions in areas of fluoridated tap water.

Foods to Avoid

■ Tea, chocolate, coffee, and cigarettes contain caffeine, theobromine or nicotine which all stimulate the release of adrenalin and make an overactive thyroid worse.

■ Soya products, turnips, mustard, pine nuts and the cabbage family can decrease thyroid function.

Friendly Foods

■ If **underactive** eat more seaweeds such as wild sea kelp, kombu, arame, dulse, and swiss chard.

■ Minced beef, egg yolk, lecithin granules, sesame seed butter, artichokes, onions and garlic, and raw, organic seeds and nuts are all rich in iodine.

■ If you have an **overactive thyroid**, eat more turnips, cabbage, mustard, soya-based foods, pine nuts and millet which contain goitrogens – substances that interfere with thyroid function. It would be advisable to consult a qualified nutritionist. See *Useful Information*.

Useful Remedies for an underactive thyroid

■ Take a vitamin B-complex

■ Take 1–2 grams of vitamin C daily in an ascorbate form with meals.

■ Vitamin E 400iu is required for proper endocrine function.

■ 30 mg daily of Co-enzyme Q 10 helps to support energy production in the body.

■ The minerals zinc 30 mg, selenium 200mcg and copper 2mg daily are vital for a healthy thyroid.

■ The body makes thyroxine from the amino acid tyrosine, the enzyme that turns tyrosine into thyroxine needs Iodine, zinc and selenium, therefore take 500mg of *Tyroplex* twice daily containing the amino acid tyrosine **HN**

■ Take 150mcg of kelp daily.

■ *Thyro Complex* is a formulation by natureopath Martin Budd, an established authority on thyroid health. He has spent 15 years researching the nutritional support required for healthy thyroid function, and his formula containing magnesium, vitamin C, L–tyrosine, calcium, iodine, liquorice, B vitamins, zinc, manganese, dong quai, carnitine and phenylalanine which all help to balance the thyroid. Take 1–3 tablets daily 30 minutes before food. **NC**

Useful Remedies for an overactive thyroid

■ *Thyrotoxcurb (TTOX 69)* contains the herbs damiana, nettles, Irish moss, thyme, yarrow, valerian and pulsatilla which help to calm an over active thyroid. 1–3 capsules twice daily with food. **NC**

t

- If you are not pregnant you could try taking 25,000iu of vitamin A daily for one month, which helps regulate thyroid function.

- Calcium absorption is often impaired with thyroid problems, therefore to help protect your bones take 200 –500 mg of calcium.

- The herb *Lycopus* helps to calm an overactive thyroid – try 5mls of tincture daily. **NC**

Helpful Hints

- Many readers have found that taking stabilised aloe vera juice has helped their overall health when suffering thyroid problems. If you have thyroid problems, it would be wise to consult a doctor who is also a qualified nutritionist (see *Useful Information*).

- Smoking is known to make an underactive thyroid worse – so give up smoking.

- Read **Hypothyroidism, the Unsuspected Illness** by Borda O'Barnes and Lawrence Galton, (Harper and Row) Tel: 0207 323 2382.

- Others who are taking a natural progesterone supplement instead of HRT have also seen improvements (see Menopause for details of natural progesterone).

- *Siberian Ginseng* 1–3 grams, or 2-6mls daily can help balance an under- or overactive thyroid. Avoid *Korean Ginseng* if you suffer high blood pressure.

In life, try not to neglect the people who you love, and who love you the most – don't take them for granted.

TINNITUS

Tinnitus is a chronic and distressing condition when the patient suffers a ringing, buzzing or humming in one or both ears. This condition can have a variety of causes, which include exposure to loud noise or an explosion, long-term use of aspirin, use of beta blockers and antibiotics, compacted ear wax, spinal or cranial misalignment which can reduce circulation to the ears, or food intolerances. Tinnitus is more common in older people, but is appearing in younger people who are exposed to excessively loud music.

Foods to avoid

- Avoid alcohol, smoking and caffeine, all of which may aggravate the condition.

- Cut down on salt, which may increase fluid build up in the ear.

- Avoid all full-fat cow's milk and produce for two weeks as they are mucous forming which can block the ears and sinuses.

- Generally cut down on saturated fats such as red meat, cheese, chocolate, highly refined white-flour-based foods, pies, pastries, biscuits and so on.

- Yeast-based foods such as *Marmite*, *Bovril* and yeasty breads can also make this problem worse.

- Don't use hard margarines or highly refined cooking oils and eliminate fried foods.
- Read labels carefully and avoid any foods containing hydrogenated or trans fats.

Friendly Foods
- Eat plenty of garlic and onions which are very cleansing.
- Choose low-fat dairy options such as fully skimmed milk or cottage cheeses.
- Use organic rice milk for making porridge and with cereals, and try live, low fat yoghurts in desserts instead of creams.
- Generally increase fruits and fresh vegetables and include more nutritious foods such as lentils, barley and corn, rice and spelt-based pastas in your diet.
- Jacket potatoes are a wonderful food, but add yoghurt instead of lots of butter or use a non-hydrogenated spread such as *Vitaquell* or *Biona*.

Useful Remedies.
- For one month take 25,000iu of vitamin A to nourish the inner ear nerve cells. (If you are pregnant limit to 5000iu.)
- Take 30mg of zinc in a multi-vitamin and mineral, as lack of zinc is associated with tinnitus. For the first month take 30mg three times daily until symptoms ease.
- Taking vitamin B12 – 1000 mcg a day helps noise-induced tinnitus.
- As all the B vitamins work together, also take a B complex.
- Taking *Ginkgo Biloba* 120–240mg of standardised extract daily increases circulation to the ear.
- Try garlic and horseradish tablets or tincture which act as decongestants. **FSC**

Helpful Hints
- Recordings of soothing music or sounds help mask the unwanted noise, especially when you are trying to get to sleep.
- Regular exercise may provide relief by increasing blood circulation to the head.
- Practice relaxation techniques.
- Impacted wisdom teeth and tooth decay can cause this problem. When we grind our teeth over many years, the jaw can be misaligned, this is known as TMJ (Temporo-mandibular joint Syndrome). Dentists who specialise in treating TMJ problems can make a small brace to be worn at night that holds the jaw in its correct position, which often alleviates tinnitus. There is now a craniofacial pain clinic in Surrey which is dedicated to the treatment of head, neck and facial pain; call 01737 767100, The Purlew Centre, 11 Devon Crescent, Redhill, Surrey, Mr Sean O'Geary.
- Cranial osteopathy or chiropractic can release built-up tensions in the head and neck, which can trigger tinnitus. Acupuncture has proved beneficial to some sufferers (see *Useful Information*).
- You can call the **Tinnitus Helpline**, c/o **RNID**, for up-to-date research. Tel: 0345 090210, 10.00 am-3.00 pm, Monday to Friday, freephone number 0808 808 6666.

If you want something badly enough
you have to be willing to work hard to make it happen.

TONGUE PROBLEMS

The tongue is a great indicator of overall health. A tongue should be moist and clean, with little or no coating. A white coating usually denotes the digestive system is not working as it should, liver and bowels are sluggish, and you are eating too many mucous-forming foods; such as full-fat dairy food, sugar and red meat. Smokers are more likely to have a coated tongue. Candida can cause a thick white coating on the tongue (see also *Candida*).

Foods to Avoid
- Red meat, full-fat dairy produce and most foods made with white bread can add to the mucous load in the body and slow digestion.
- Reduce alcohol, caffeine, fried foods and junk-type takeaways which place strain on the liver.
- See *General Health Hints*.

Friendly Foods

- To clear the coating you would need to keep your diet really clean for 7 days. Try the *Lashford Technique* detox diet, (see also *Allergies*).
- Drink plenty of fresh vegetable juices made with garlic, ginger and any fresh vegetables you have to hand. Celery, artichoke, celeriac and beetroot are great liver cleansers.
- See Friendly Foods under *Constipation*.

Useful Remedies
- Take acidophilus/bifidus for at least 6 weeks to replenish healthy bacteria in the bowel.
- Take a digestive enzyme with main meals. **BC**
- The herb milk thistle 500mg three times daily will help to improve liver function.
- The mineral sodium phosphate, 600mg daily, helps to reduce a cream coating. **BLK**

TONGUE PROBLEMS – Geographical tongue
This is so named because the tongue often resembles a map, when discolouration forms irregular shapes on the surface. Usually it disappears of its own accord, but sensitivity to certain foods can make it worse (see *Allergies*). I have had letters from pregnant women whose geographical tongue disappeared once the baby was born, also linked to iron and/or vitamin B deficiency. The patches can be caused by infection or irritants such as vinegar.

Foods to Avoid.

■ Cut down on caffeine, highly spiced foods, vinegar, pickles, pineapple and plums.

■ Alcohol will also irritate the delicate tissues in the mouth.

Friendly Foods

■ Include more ginger and live, low-fat yoghurt in your diet which is very soothing.

■ Garlic and onions are very cleansing.

■ Drink plenty of water.

■ See the cleansing *Lashford Technique* under *Allergies*.

Useful Remedies

■ *CT 241* is a formula of herbs such as horsetail, silica, kelp, vitamin C, boron and digestive enzymes which improve absorption of nutrients from food and encourages soft tissue healing. **BC**

■ Take a B-complex.

■ Ask your doctor to check if you are low in iron, in which case take a liquid formula such as *Spatone* which will not cause constipation.

■ **New Era** *Calcium Fluoride Tissue Salts* 4 times a day.

Helpful Hints

■ Tea tree oil can be used as a mouthwash as well as 1% hydrogen peroxide in water.

■ Some sufferers report an improvement after taking a garlic capsule before breakfast every day.

Lettuce contains the sedative lactucarium which helps to calm the nerves.
No wonder the Duchess of Windsor ate lettuce every night to help her sleep.
Eating with the Season, by Paula Bartmeus

TRAVEL SICKNESS

This is extremely common especially in children and older people. Just worrying about a journey can be sufficient to trigger symptoms in a sensitive individual. Eating a large meal prior to travelling and stuffy atmospheres can also make symptoms worse. Some people can read while moving, but for others if you try and focus on something stationary while in a moving vehicle this can disturb the balance in the inner ear resulting in nausea. Symptoms include looking pale, feeling clammy and sometimes nausea and vomiting.

Food to Avoid

■ On short trips avoid eating and drinking anything.

Friendly Foods

- On the day prior to travel, eat light foods, salads, fresh fruit compotes or grilled fruits, soups and low-fat yoghurt.

- If you are on a long trip and can face food – eat really light, low-fats foods such as a rice or oat cakes. Otherwise try dry toast or a cheese biscuit.

- Sip small amounts of fresh lemon or lime juice in warm water.

- Peppermint and ginger herbal teas can also be sipped to calm the digestive tract and stomach.

Useful Remedies

- Magnesium is nature's tranquillizer. If you tend to get nervous the day before your trip begin taking 200mg of magnesium a couple of days prior to travelling.

- Ginger is really successful at reducing the feelings of nausea and you can take 4 ginger capsules two hours prior to travel – but it is often more effective when you can taste the ginger.

- Make tea with a small piece of fresh root ginger and a little honey and take in a flask to sip during your journey or take 1–2ml of the tincture in a little water.

- Take a B-complex daily to support your nerves.

- *Motion Mate* is a mixture of natural herbal oils that have been used for centuries to combat dizziness and nausea. It includes oils of chamomile, frankincense, myrrh, birch, ylang-ylang, lavender and peppermint. Apply to the skin behind the ears. **NC**

Helpful Hints

- Stay fairly still and breathe calmly. Look ahead to the horizon and not downwards to help keep the fluid in the ears balanced.

- Try to sit at the front of any vehicle.

- If possible, open a window.

- Avoid the company of people eating strong-smelling foods.

- A drop of peppermint oil on the tongue helps reduce feelings of nausea.

- Acupressure can help control motion sickness. See a reflexologist who will show you which points to treat, or wear *Sea Bands*, which work on a similar principle; available from most large chemists.

- Try homeopathic *Petrol* or *Cocculus 30c* – take one before travelling and one every few hours during the journey.

*Drinking a glass of freshly made vegetable juice every day will
rebalance the pH levels of your body which will help you to heal or avoid many chronic
conditions such as arthritis.*

TREMORS

This problem can be triggered by a huge variety of symptoms such as extreme nervousness, excessive consumption of caffeine or alcohol or an overactive thyroid gland. Recovering alcoholics and drug addicts often suffer tremors. If the tremors occur when resting or you suffer involuntary jerking, this is associated with conditions such as Parkinson's Disease and rheumatic fever. On rare occasions tremors can be inherited. As mercury and heavy metal toxicity are linked to tremors, cigarettes are high in cadmium, so stop smoking. If you have mercury amalgam fillings – see under *Mercury Fillings*. If you suffer blood-sugar problems this could make symptoms worse (see *Low Blood Sugar*).

Foods to Avoid

- Any foods or drinks containing aluminium (see *Alzheimer's Disease*).
- Greatly reduce any foods or drinks containing caffeine, this includes chocolate, fizzy canned drinks, guarana, coffee and strong tea.
- Avoid alcohol and spicy foods which are stimulants.
- Don't eat too many high sugary foods which can make you feel more hyper.
- Avoid preservatives and additives.

Friendly Foods

- Generally you need calming foods such as potatoes, pasta, wholemeal bread, brown rice, lentils, barley, cereals and oats.
- Porridge made with organic rice milk, add a chopped raw apple or banana and a little honey to sweeten makes a very calming breakfast or supper.
- Turkey, chicken, tofu, bananas, wheat germ, sunflower, pumpkin seeds and linseeds and oily fish are all calming foods – and the oily fish and seeds help to nourish your nerves.
- Almonds, soya flour, dates, Brazil nuts, mustard, curry powder and all green leafy vegetables are a good source of magnesium which calms the muscles.
- Drink more water.

Useful Remedies

- Take a high strength B-complex to nourish your nerves. **BLK**
- Include a multi-vitamin and mineral that contains 20mg of zinc.
- Calcium and magnesium help to reduce muscle spasms. Most vitamin companies supply them in one formula. Take 500mg of calcium with 300mg of magnesium.
- Either take 4 evening primrose oil capsules (250–400mg) daily or 2 mega GLA (a fatty acid found in evening primrose oil that helps to reduce tremors). **BC**

Helpful Hints

■ Some people report relief when they plunge the limb into cold water for a few minutes each day.

■ Acupuncture and reflexology have also helped many people (see *Useful Information*).

*Bee propolis is a sticky substance which bees use to sterilise their hives,
it is rich in vitamins and minerals and is anti-viral, anti-bacterial and anti-fungal, and
makes a great natural alternative to antibiotics.*

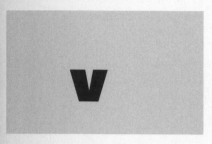

VARICOSE VEINS

(see also *Circulation, Constipation* and *Raynauds*)

Varicose veins are caused by weak valves in the veins and the most commonly affected areas are the legs. Eventually the veins can clearly be seen on the skin and over time can bulge, swell and become painful. If not treated they can also ulcerate.

This condition is closely linked to constipation, and if you strain when you go to the toilet – then blood is forced into your lower body which makes the problem worse. Vein problems are also linked to standing or sitting for long hours, being overweight, pregnancy and crossing your legs too much. You can inherit the tendency to varicose veins from your parents but by practising prevention in your teens this will greatly reduce your chances of developing veins in later life.

When I became pregnant in my late teens, I worked for 12 hours a day in a supermarket filling shelves, which was just about the worst thing that I could have done. In my twenties I worked for 9 years as an air stewardess and had to be on my feet for 15 hours at a stretch. Today I often sit at a desk for 10 hours at a time. And my mother and father both had vein problems. In my forties I had the worst veins stripped and the surgeon assured me I had plenty left and it would not affect my circulation, but it did. Today I look after my diet and take regular exercise but suffer poor circulation and cold feet. Hence, prevention will pay you huge dividends in later life. Even if you have varicose veins there are plenty of ways to reduce and protect them from getting worse.

Foods to Avoid

- Generally cut down on heavy meals, red meat and cheeses which takes a long time to pass through the bowel.
- Reduce your intake of white-flour-based foods.
- Coffee, tea, colas and alcohol all dehydrate the bowel.
- Reduce your salt and sugar intake.
- See *Foods to Avoid* under *Constipation*.

Friendly Foods

- Eat more foods containing the bioflavonoid rutin which helps to strengthen your veins, Buckwheat makes great pancakes and can be added to breads and biscuits and is high in rutin.
- Apricots, rose hips, apple peel, cabbage, blackberries, bilberries, cherries, sweet potatoes, squash and pumpkin are all rich in vitamin C and make healthy vein foods.
- Avocados and raw wheat germ are high in vitamin E which helps to thin the blood naturally.
- Garlic, onions, ginger, and cayenne pepper all aid circulation
- Eat plenty of fish especially oily fish.
- Drink more water – 6-8 glasses a day.
- Herbal rose hip tea will help toughen up your veins.
- See also *Diets* under *Circulation* and *Constipation*.

Useful Remedies

- Take 1000mg of rutin daily which helps reduce swelling and strengthen the vein walls.
- Silica is an excellent mineral for toughening up veins. Take 200mg of silica compound daily or take Vein Support. **BLK**
- 1000 mg per day of citrus bioflavonoid complex – will help strengthen your veins.
- Take a B complex daily.
- Take 1-2 grams of vitamin C daily with meals.
- Take 400iu of natural source vitamin E to help protect blood vessels.
- Horse chestnut really does strengthen the veins and capillaries. You need 50–75mg of aescin twice daily, this is the active ingredient in horse chestnut. In tincture 1-4 mls twice a day. **FSC**
- A formula called *V Nal* contains horse chestnut and the herb butcher's broom which helps to increase lower limb circulation. Take one daily. Available from all good health stores.

Helpful Hints

- If veins are sore and swollen apply witch hazel in a tincture form directly to the veins. witch hazel in capsules and tincture can also be taken internally to reduce the swelling. **NC**

- Get plenty of fresh air and walk for at least 30–60 minutes every day.

- Any pounding exercise that helps move the blood such as walking, rebounding, skipping, tennis, jogging and dancing are all wonderful for supporting veins.

- Apply a little vitamin E cream mixed with two drops of juniper oil topically where the skin is sore.

- If the veins are sore and throbbing, make a warm water compress with added cypress and geranium essential oils.

- Use cold compresses to reduce swelling.

- Reflexology and acupuncture can help to increase circulation.

- Wear support tights and for 10 minutes daily place your feet above your head level to give the veins a rest.

- The herbs butchers broom, witch hazel and horse chestnut can help reduce varicose veins and haemorrhoids

VEGETARIANISM

After the BSE and CJD crisis in the UK and Europe, more and more people are turning to a vegetarian diet, which basically means not eating any foods or products derived from the slaughter of animals.

Vegetarians generally suffer less ill health, heart disease and cancer than meat eaters, mainly because vegetarian diets tend to be higher in fibre and low in saturated fats. Many parents worry that their children will become deficient in nutrients, especially vitamin B12, iron and vitamin D – but this is only a problem for vegans who eat no dairy produce. Simply make sure you or your children eat as great a variety of foods as possible.

Foods to Avoid
- Don't go overboard on full-fat cheeses which are high in saturated fats.

- Products that are high in coconut or palm oil should be kept to a minimum as they are also very high in saturated fats.

Friendly Foods
- Green leafy vegetables, sesame seeds, low-fat yoghurts and parmesan cheese are all high in calcium.

- For protein, eat lentils, beans, soya-bean products such as soya milk and flour, tofu and textured vegetable protein or TVP, rice, cereals, corn, almonds, Brazil nuts, peanuts, sunflower seeds and sesame seeds which also contain good levels of zinc.

- Eggs and dried skimmed milk plus soya milk are rich sources of vitamin B12. Alfalfa sprouts, comfrey and spirulina contain small amounts.

- For carbohydrates, eat cereals, oats, wholemeal bread, brown rice and pasta, barley, millet, buckwheat and rye.

- Potatoes, parsnips, turnips and swedes are also good sources of carbohydrates.

- Red or yellow vegetables, carrots, tomatoes, pumpkin, sweet potatoes, dried apricots, leafy green vegetables are all rich in vitamin A

- Nuts and seeds are high in essential fats.

- Wheat germ can be sprinkled on cereals and desserts as a rich source of B vitamins.

- Mushrooms and peas also contain the B-group vitamins.

- Use unrefined walnut, sunflower and olive oils for salad dressings

- Iron is found in leafy green vegetables, wholemeal bread, molasses, eggs, dried fruits (especially apricots), beans, seeds, pulses, nuts, chocolate and cocoa.

- Eat plenty of fruits rich in vitamin C such as kiwi and cherries, as vitamin C aids absorption of iron from foods.

Useful Remedies
- Take a high strength B-complex.

- Take a multi-vitamin and mineral.

- If you have been found to be low in iron, take a formula such as *Spatone* – available worldwide from health stores.

*If your eyes are twitching because you are tired and stressed take
500mg of magnesium which relaxes the muscles.*

VERRUCAS

(see also *Immune Function*)

Verrucas are 'plantar warts' that occur on the soles of the foot. They are extremely common and highly contagious and can be very painful. Verrucas are essentially a viral infection and you are more likely to contract them if you are really run down.

Foods to Avoid
- Reduce your intake of all foods and drinks containing sugar which lower immune function.

- Reduce caffeine, alcohol and all highly processed white-flour-based foods.

Friendly Foods
- Eat lots of garlic, asparagus, parsley, avocados, sea vegetables such as kelp, whey, apples, cucumbers, millet, rice bran and sprouts.

- See *Friendly Foods* under *Immune Function* and *General Health Hints*.

Useful Remedies

■ To fight the virus take 20,000iu of vitamin A daily for one month and then reduce to 5000iu daily in a multi-vitamin and mineral. (If you are pregnant take no more than 5000iu).

■ Take a garlic capsule daily.

■ Vitamin C is vital for boosting your immune system, take 2 grams daily with food.

■ Take a high-strength antioxidant formula that contains 200mcg of selenium. .**NL**

■ Take 500mg twice daily of the anti-viral herbs – *Maitake* and *Echinacea*.

■ Take 30mg of zinc daily for its anti-viral properties.

Helpful Hints

■ Apply a tiny amount of crushed garlic or tea tree oil into the affected area twice a day.

■ If you don't like garlic, dab undiluted essential lemon oil onto the verruca twice daily for a few days.

■ There is an enzyme in banana skin, which can attack the verruca. Many people have written to say that, although somewhat bizarre, this remedy really does work! Apply the inside of the banana skin to the verruca and tape on, change every 2 days until the verruca disappears.

■ Homeopathic *Thuja 6C* can be helpful as well as *Thuja Mother* tincture applied directly onto the warts and covered with a plaster.

Some breakfast cereals contain more salt than an average bag of crisps.

VERTIGO

(see also *Ménière's Syndrome*)

Vertigo is a sensation of moving or spinning, a feeling that you are losing your balance even when you are standing or sitting still. It can be accompanied by nausea. Vertigo usually lasts for a few minutes, but can continue for hours and even days. It can be caused by impacted ear wax, blockage of the Eustacean tube, or by a viral infection of the balancing mechanism of the inner ear (see under *Catarrh* and *Sinus Problems*). Vertigo can also be triggered by high blood pressure and iron deficiency (see *Anaemia*). It is also linked to blood sugar problems (see *Low* and *High Blood Sugar*) and poor circulation. Vertigo is also a symptom of Ménière's syndrome. Beta blockers and some prescription drugs can trigger an attack, make sure you carefully note any contraindications on drugs.

Foods to Avoid

■ Generally, you need to cut down on saturated fats found in full-fat milk and dairy produce, cheeses, meat, chocolates, cakes, biscuits, pies, sausages and so on.

■ Goat's cheese is also very high in saturated fats and excessive intake of high-fat foods is linked to ear problems.

■ Avoid caffeine, especially cappuccinos and chocolates, fizzy drinks, sodium-based salt, fried foods, alcohol and aspartame.

■ Cut down your intake of sodium based salts; there are now plenty of magnesium and potassium-based salts available from health stores.

Friendly Foods

■ Vitamin A and carotene-rich foods are needed for sensory cells in the inner ear to function normally. Eat more oily fish and fish oils, sweet potatoes, pumpkin, apricots and sweet potatoes.

■ Eat more garlic, onion and ginger.

■ Calf's or lamb's liver, eggs and leafy green vegetables are a rich source of iron and vitamin A.

■ Use organic rice milk instead of cow's milk.

■ Eat more sunflower or pumpkin seeds and linseeds which are rich in essential fats and zinc and use their unrefined oils for salad dressings.

■ Eat more bananas, dried fruit, fish and sunflower seeds which are rich in potassium.

■ See *General Health Hints*.

Useful Remedies.

■ Vitamin A, 25,000iu per day. The inner ear needs a high concentration of vitamin A and sensory cells are dependent upon vitamin A. If you are pregnant only take 5000iu daily.

■ A B-complex helps nourish the nerve endings in the inner ear

■ Take a multi-mineral that contains at least 100mg of calcium and 99mg of potassium, the potassium reduces the sodium (salt) levels in the body – high levels of sodium in the blood can make symptoms worse. **S**

■ The herb *Ginkgo Biloba* helps to improve circulation to the inner ear. Take 120–150mg of standardised extract daily.

■ A vitamin C and bioflavonoid complex – up to 2000mg daily.

■ Ginger capsules can be taken 4–6 times daily during an attack to help reduce feelings of nausea.

Helpful Hints

■ If you smoke, stop.

■ Avoid rapid body movements, especially of the head.

■ Generally reduce stress and make sure you are getting sufficient sleep.

■ See a chiropractor or cranial osteopath to make sure your neck and spine are not misaligned which can trigger problems in the ear. Hypnotherapy and acupuncture have helped in some cases (see *Useful Information*).

■ High blood pressure and beta-blockers have been known to trigger vertigo in some people. If you have been taking prescription drugs for a long period of time, check with your GP.

VIRAL INFECTIONS

(see under *Immune Function*)

Vitamin B1 – 100mg daily taken for one week before travelling to the tropics helps deter mosquitoes.

VITILIGO

A condition in which white patches appear on the skin when pigment production stops. The darker the skin colour the more obvious and distressing the appearance of the skin. This condition has been linked to low stomach acid levels, stress, low levels of the B-group of vitamins, pernicious anaemia and an overactive thyroid gland. It could also be triggered by nutritional deficiencies or a fungal overgrowth.

Foods to Avoid
■ Alcohol, caffeine, processed foods and sugar all deplete the body of B vitamins.
■ See *General Health Hints*.

Friendly Foods
■ Papaya and pineapple contain enzymes which aid digestion and absorption of nutrients.
■ Foods rich in B vitamins include wheat germ, brewer's yeast, **Bovril**, calf's liver, eggs, whole grains such as brown rice, nuts, fish, chicken, turkey, dates, oats, cereals, mushrooms, green vegetables, molasses, dried skimmed milk and fruits, plus apricots.
■ As low zinc levels are linked to vitiligo eat more fish, shellfish, sunflower and pumpkin seeds.
■ Live, low-fat yoghurt also aids digestion.
■ Drink plenty of water – at least 6 glasses daily.

Useful Remedies
■ Khella, a South African herb has been shown to help restore pigmentation. Take 100mg daily. **NC**
■ As lack of stomach acid is linked to this problem, take *Betaine* (HCl) for up to 2 years with main meals. **FSC**
■ If you have active stomach ulcers take a digestive enzyme capsule instead of the betaine.
■ Take a high strength B complex plus 400mcg of folic acid and 500mcg of vitamin B12.

- Include 1–2 grams of vitamin C daily – which is vital for collagen production.

- Copper 2mg per day. Copper is needed for certain enzymes that are required for skin pigmentation.

- PABA is a B vitamin, take 100mg, 3–4 times daily to help re-pigment the skin.

- The amino acid phenylalanine 50mg per kilo of body weight taken on an empty stomach with careful sun bathing helps to re-pigment the skin. Use a high factor sunscreen and don't sit in the midday sun. Just take 15 minutes twice daily for a few days and gradually the skin should re-pigment.

Carrot juice is rich in carotenes and vitamin A which is great for the skin, but don't go overboard as too much carrot juice can thicken your blood.

VOMITING

Vomiting can have many causes, the most obvious being food poisoning or food allergies, but it could also be prescription drugs that disagree with you – certain antibiotics have this affect on me. Morning sickness, migraines, bulimia, drinking too much alcohol and eating a really high-fat, rich meal can all trigger nausea. If an infant vomits violently within a few minutes of being fed – you would need to seek medical attention. If a child drinks a poison such as bleach, or swallows an object and begins to vomit, urgent medical attention is needed.

Dehydration is the biggest concern with vomiting. If the person is small, also has diarrhoea, and cannot keep any fluids down, obviously the rate of dehydration will be much faster than in a tall, weighty person. If I get sick, I have low blood pressure and if I vomit regularly, I pass out and need a drip which brings me round very quickly. If you suffer low blood pressure and begin vomiting frequently, call a doctor. If you have severe abdominal pain or begin vomiting any blood, have a fever and the vomiting has continued for more than 24 hours seek urgent medical help . Nausea after fatty foods can be related to liver congestion, in which case you need to greatly reduce your intake of fats, coffee and alcohol.

If a baby or small child suffers frequent vomiting and diarrhoea they are at a greater risk for dehydration and need immediate medical attention.

Foods to Avoid

- If you are tempted to eat pink or uncooked chicken, don't.

- When abroad, avoid reheated rice dishes.

- Make sure eggs are fresh.

- If any food smells 'high' such as prawns, don't be polite, refuse to eat it.

- Avoid tap water that is questionable.

- Don't eat heavy, fried, fatty meals, especially if you suffer a hiatus hernia or stomach ulcers.

Friendly Foods

■ Sip clear fluids such as boiled water, fruit juices, or an electrolyte powdered drink called *Re-hydrate*, available from all chemists..

■ If you can tolerate it, sip a little ginger ale or ginger tea.

■ Don't drink more than a couple of tablespoonfuls of liquid at any one time.

■ Once vomiting has stopped gently increase your fluid intake. No coffee or black tea for 24 hours.

■ Sip apple cider vinegar while feeling nauseous or vomiting. Put one teaspoon of apple cider vinegar in a glass of water and sip. This helps settle your stomach and flush out the toxins from the digestive system.

■ Slowly begin eating again: fresh soups, a little poached fish with mashed potato, low fat yoghurts or brown rice.

Useful Remedies

■ Don't take these supplements until at least 24 hours after the vomiting has stopped.

■ A vitamin B-complex to calm down the digestive system.

■ Deglycerrhized liquorice – 15 drops twice daily helps to soothe the digestive tract.

■ Acidophilus/ bifidus, take 2 capsules daily for a couple of weeks to replenish healthy bacteria in the bowel.

Helpful Hints

■ Place some essential oils of ginger and peppermint under your nose, this helps to reduce the dreadful nauseous feeling.

■ Homeopathic *Aconite 30C* can be taken every 5 minutes up to 10 doses and *Arsenicum Album 12C* – take one dose every 30 minutes up to 10 doses daily until symptoms ease.

Dandelion Root liquid makes a great cleanser and tonic for the liver, which can help problems ranging from gallstones and constipation to acne and weight loss.

WARTS

Warts are caused by a varied assortment of viruses which invade the skin, causing cells to multiply rapidly forming raised lumps. When your immune system is at a low ebb, warts are contagious, and touching warts can transfer viruses to new sites, and new warts to develop. They are commonly found on the soles of the feet (see *Verrucas*) and on the hands or arms.

Foods to Avoid
- See *Foods to Avoid* under *Immune Function*.

Friendly Foods
- As vitamin A and carotenes are vital for healing the skin, eat more leafy greens, pumpkin, apricots, tomatoes, cantaloupe melon, oily fish and liver.
- Sulphur-containing foods such as onions, garlic, Brussels sprouts, cabbage, and broccoli.
- Eat more low-fat, live yoghurt.
- See *Friendly Foods* under *Immune Function*.

Useful Remedies
- If you are not pregnant take 20,000iu of vitamin A daily for one month to help fight the virus.
- Take 400iu of natural source vitamin E daily.
- Take 2 grams of vitamin C daily in an ascorbate form to boost your immune system.
- Take a high-strength multi-vitamin and mineral that contains 200mcg of selenium and 20mg of zinc.
- The herb *Echinacea*, *St John's wort* and *Goldenseal*, are all anti-viral. Take 1–2 grams of each for one month.

Helpful Hints
- Soak a plaster with apple cider vinegar and place over the wart. Change the plaster regularly and keep adding more vinegar. The wart should disappear within 2 weeks.
- *Dandelion Tincture* can be added to the wart through a small piece of card in which you have cut a small hole. Dab on the tincture for 3 days.
- Apply the following mixture twice daily for up to ten days: add a little freshly crushed garlic to the contents of one vitamin E and one vitamin A capsule and mix with some zinc cream. Add only to the site of the wart and cover with a dressing. If the skin surrounding the wart becomes inflamed then eliminate the garlic.

■ Homeopathic *Thuga 6x* can be taken twice daily – but you must stop this remedy as soon as you see an improvement.

Drink the juice of half a lemon in warm water before breakfast,
this is a great liver cleanser.

WATER ON THE KNEE

Inflammation of the little fluid-filled sacks that surround the knee joint. This problem is usually triggered by a knock, a fall or by a chronic condition such as arthritis.

Foods to Avoid
■ Avoid meat, salt, caffeine, black tea and all highly processed foods.
■ Avoid foods from the nightshade family, tomatoes, potatoes, eggplant and sweet peppers. See *Foods to Avoid* under *Bursitis*.

Friendly Foods
■ Eat foods high in magnesium, dark leafy greens, squash, fruits, vegetables and honey.
■ Add a teaspoon of apple cider vinegar and a touch of honey to boiled water and sip throughout the day.
■ Take 2 grams of cod liver oil daily.
■ Eat plenty of potassium-rich foods, bananas, linseeds, sunflower and pumpkin seeds and nuts.
■ Eat more avocado and raw wheat germ which are rich in vitamin E.
■ Pineapple is a rich source of bromelain which has anti-inflammatory properties.
■ Eat oily fish such as tuna, mackerel, herrings, salmon or sardines twice a week.
■ Drink plenty of water.

Useful Remedies
■ Chloride compound helps to lessen the inflammation. 200mg daily. **BLK**
■ Silica helps to strengthen the tissues in the knees. 200mg daily. **BLK**
■ Take 2 grams of vitamin C with bioflavonoids to help reduce the swelling.
■ Take 400–600iu of natural source vitamin E to help reduce the inflammation.
■ Take zinc 22mg per day – zinc helps the body fight inflammation.
■ The amino acid DL-Phenylalanine, 1000–2000mg per day, will help to reduce the pain.

Helpful Hints

■ At the onset of inflammation rest the affected area and avoid putting pressure on the joint for a few days.

■ Hot or cold compresses can help to disperse the swelling.

■ Homeopathic *Ruta 6x* taken twice daily for 3–5 days really helps reduce knee problems.

■ Perseverance with this regime is important as knee problems can take some time to heal. Acupuncture and homeopathy have proved helpful to many sufferers (see *Useful Information*).

■ Drink strong camomile tea, particularly at bedtime, to help relieve pain.

If you suffer thrush regularly, have a urine test – you may be diabetic.

WATER RETENTION (OEDEMA)

This problem is commonly seen in the hands, feet or around the eyes. The most common cause is a food intolerance, the usual culprits being wheat and dairy. It can be triggered by a sodium, potassium imbalance, pregnancy, the Pill or HRT and is very common in women, especially over 60. Another trigger can be standing for too long in hot weather.

Occasionally, fluid retention can denote more serious problems that affect the heart, kidneys or liver. Therefore if these ideas do not work after 2–3 weeks please have a thorough check up. Some people mistakenly think that if they cut back on their fluid intake their water retention will disappear, but in fact the opposite is true.

Foods to Avoid

■ Cut down on high-salt foods and don't add salt to meals.

■ Meat pies, cheese, sauces, pizza, crisps, preserved meats and pickles can all be high in sodium.

■ Some breakfast cereals contain more salt than an average bag of crisps.

■ Don't add salt to cooking unless it's a potassium and magnesium-based salt.

■ Even some chocolate drinks and breaksfat cereals can be very high in salt.

■ Alcoholic and caffeinated foods and drinks increase dehydration.

Friendly Foods

■ Eat lots of fresh fruit and vegetables as they are very rich in potassium.

■ Include more spinach, celery, kale, cabbage, bananas, bilberries, and blueberries.

■ Add the spice curcumin to your meals which helps strengthen the kidneys.

■ Drink at least 6–8 glasses of filtered water daily.

■ Eat good quality protein such as fish, chicken, turkey or tofu at least once a day.

Useful Remedies

- *Dandelion Leaf* tea or tincture. 1ml can be taken 3 times a day, this is a gentle diuretic which puts more potassium into the body than it takes out.

- Take 1–2 grams of vitamin C as potassium ascorbate which can help lymph drainage. **BC**

- Take a B complex that contains 100mg of B6 which is a natural diuretic.

- *Celery Seed Extract* – one capsule twice daily. Celery is a natural liver and kidney cleanser and helps to neutralise excess acid in the tissues. **BC**

- The herb *Gota Kola* stimulates circulation in the lower limbs and improves lymph drainage. Up to 500mg twice daily when symptoms are acute. **S**

- *Sodium Sulphate* is known as the problem-fluid remover. Take 200mg three times daily. **BLK**

Helpful Hints

- Try to elevate your feet for at least 15 minutes every day.

- Rebounding on a mini-trampoline is particularly good for enhancing lymph drainage. Have regular lymph drainage massage (see under *Useful Information*).

- Take regular exercise such as swimming, walking, skipping or jogging.

- If you are overweight, try to lose weight.

Sodium Sulphate *is known as the problem-fluid remover.*
Take 200mg three times daily. **BLK**

WEIGHT PROBLEMS

(see also *Allergies, Candida* and *Low Blood Sugar* and *Thyroid Problems*)

62% of men and 53% of women are now overweight and the problem is escalating. Being overweight is a contributing factor to high blood pressure, heart disease, arthritis, water retention and late onset diabetes.

This problem deserves a book in its own right, and let's face it, there are thousands of them. What I do know is that constantly trying various diets, going on a diet one month and off the next and so on is not a long-term solution to control your weight.

We also need a lot more honesty. During my years as a health writer I think I have heard every excuse in the book, 'It's in my genes, I have a chemical imbalance in my body, I eat so little, and I never touch bread and cakes.' When I meet such people in a coffee bar, I find them stacking up on chips and puddings – and they say 'Oh this is the first time I've had a meal like this in years'. And of course I believe them!

I am not asking everyone to live on lettuce leaves, of course you can have treats, but you cannot live on them. All that is needed is a sensible balance.

The basics of finding your perfect weight and maintaining it are controlling your blood-sugar levels, eating a varied diet that contains plenty of fibre and taking sufficient exercise.

If you feel that you have truly tried every diet and you are still finding it hard to lose weight, then you may have candida, an underactive thyroid or a chronic food intolerance that is causing water retention. Also, as we age our metabolism slows down and everyone has their own unique metabolic rate.

If you try and survive on only 1000 calories a day, your brain will begin craving more glucose which is the only form of fuel it utilises, and the more sugar you eat, the more this affects blood sugar levels and the more you will go on craving sugary foods.

Recent research from America, Japan and France has confirmed that a tendency to overeat and to store fat is largely controlled by biochemical signals emitted by a part of the brain called the hypothalamus. As well as governing many important processes such as temperature and hormone balance, the hypothalamus also controls the feeling of being satisfied. It also interprets emotional upset, stress or low blood sugar as hunger, and sends a message to the body to eat.

Snacking on sugary foods gives the brain a quick energy boost for a short time, but then triggers a further drop in blood sugar levels, which causes the hypothalamus to demand more fuel. This vicious cycle can trigger numerous symptoms ranging from chronic exhaustion, mood swings and brain 'fog' to black outs. The answer is to keep the hypothalamus happy by controlling blood sugar levels.

Nutritionists have known for years that the most effective way to control blood sugar is to eat small amounts of foods such as fruit, vegetables, wholemeal bread and pasta or brown rice regularly, which release their natural, complex sugars more slowly into the bloodstream – but the reality is that the huge majority turn to a snack bar to feed the sugar craving, and the average person eats 12kg of snacks a year. Is it any wonder so many people are struggling with their weight.

Don't cut all your favourite foods at once; this will cause you to become despondent and binge. The slower you do this, the easier it will be for your body to adjust. Sugar is addictive and it takes a good month to educate your body to a new way of eating.

Foods To Avoid

- Cut down on fried and fast foods, croissants, Danish pastries, meat pies, burgers, pizzas and melted cheese type snacks.

- Artificial sweeteners, now found in over 3,000 foods and low calorie drinks place a great strain on the liver and can actually slow weight loss. The worst offender is aspartame.

- As much as you can, reduce foods high in sugar which turns to a hard fat inside the body if it is not used up during exercise.

- Avoid salted nuts and highly preserved meats.

- Reduce sodium-based table salt.

- If you eat meat, make sure it's a lean cut and remove all skin and fat before putting it on your plate.

- Many foods labelled 'low fat' have a high sugar content – start reading labels.

- Avoid all hard margarines, full-fat milk, chocolate, full-fat cheeses and Greek yoghurts.

Friendly Foods

■ Use organic rice milk, skimmed milk or soya light instead of full-fat milk.

■ Instead of white-flour-based foods, use wholemeal bread which is more filling and experiment with various pastas made from corn, rice, lentil and potato flour.

■ Eat more brown rice, lentils, chick peas, barley and dried beans.

■ Instead of wheat-based breads, try amaranth crackers or rice cakes, spread with a little low fat houmous or cottage cheese – add a tomato and cucumber for a quick snack.

■ Eat plenty of fresh fruits and vegetables – the more fibre the better. Cabbage, broccoli, Brussels sprouts, cauliflower, onions, ginger, beans, spring greens, spinach, pak choi, fennel, celery and apples are all great foods for assisting weight loss.

■ Include kiwi fruit, cherries, papaya, blueberries and mangoes.

■ Eat at least one portion of quality protein a day, such as fish, eggs, chicken or tofu, as protein balances blood sugar levels for a longer period. Try to eat the protein at lunchtime.

■ A jacket potato is fine, but fill it with low-at yoghurt and chives instead of butter.

■ Always eat breakfast, there are dozens of organic low-sugar cereals now available and a great breakfast is organic porridge made with half water and half rice milk. Use a couple of ready-to-eat apricots or prunes to sweeten it plus a chopped raw apple.

■ Drink lots of herbal teas and at least 6–8 glasses of water a day. Water suppresses appetite, reduces fat depositing in the body, reduces water retention, and encourages toxins to be flushed through the body.

■ Essential fats are vital if you want to lose weight. Use a little unrefined, organic walnut, sunflower or olive oil for your salad dressings.

■ Sprinkle a teaspoon each of linseeds and sunflower seeds over your breakfast cereal.

■ You can also add a tablespoon of rice or oat bran for extra fibre.

■ Begin drinking dandelion tea, eat more fennel, radiccio, chicory, celeriac and young green celery which are great liver cleansers.

■ If you are desperate for sugar, use a little organic honey or brown rice syrup as a sweetener.

■ Ask at your health shop for a magnesium and potassium-based salt.

Useful remedies

■ To reduce cravings for sweet and refined foods take 200mcg of chromium twice daily in between meals. This mineral is usually depleted in people who eat too many refined foods. It takes a while to kick in, but it really does help to reduce sugar cravings.

■ Take a B-complex to support your nerves and aid digestion. **BLK**

■ Try the *Satisfy System* which is based upon keeping the hypothalamus happy by taking a glucose tablet, that contains under 10 calories. This satisfies the cravings and helps you to stop snacking on higher calorie snacks. The system also contains herbs that help to increase your metabolic rate. **PW**

■ Include a good quality multi-vitamin and mineral in your regimen. **S**

■ Research from Professor Mike Pariza of the University of Wisconsin in America has found after 20 years of research, a new essential fatty acid called Conjugated Linoleic Acid CLA which helps to burn fat while increasing muscle mass. **BC**

Helpful Hints

■ To kick-start your diet see the *Lashford Technique* under *Allergies*.

■ Regular exercise increases your metabolic rate, decreases fat deposits and reduces food cravings. Regular exercise also increases muscle mass which burns more energy just to keep the muscles functioning properly.

■ Begin by walking for 30 minutes every day. Join any local dance, aerobic, yoga, t'ai chi or any exercise classes. It helps if you work out with people who have the same goal in mind.

■ Think positive and try not to get despondent.

■ Eat the majority of your food before 7 pm if possible and try to make lunch your main meal.

■ An excess of oestrogen can cause weight gain and water retention if your body is low in progesterone. If you would like a Progesterone Factsheet, send a first-class stamp to **The Natural Progesterone Information Service**, PO Box 24, Buxton, SK17 9FB.

■ For details of natural progesterone cream, see under *Menopause*.

■ One of the best books I have seen which clearly explains how to permanently control your weight is *Body Wise* by Dr John Briffa (Cima Books).

■ Another great way to lose weight is through food combining. Read *The Complete Book of Food Combining* by Kathryn Marsden, Piatkus or log onto www.kathrynmarsden.com

■ If you suffer from eating disorders contact The Eating Disorders Association. A membership scheme is available. 1st Floor, Wensum House, 103 Prince of Wales Road, Norwich, NR1 1DW Tel: 01603 621414, Monday–Friday, 9.00am–6.30pm, Youth helpline, Tel: 01603 765050, Monday–Friday, 4.00pm–6.00pm. Website: www.edauk.com E-mail: info@edauk.com

Well, after almost 6 months of research and typing, much soul searching and a growing desire to throw my computer out of the window – this is the end of the Hints Section. I apologise if your specific condition is not mentioned, but if I tried to help every illness this book would be thousands of pages thick. What we have tried to do is to give you a good basis to enable you to become your own health detective.

Due to my work schedule I can no longer answer individual letters, but you have plenty of names and addresses to turn to for more help.

Remember, you can still enjoy plenty of treats but just balance them out with plenty of healthy foods. It's never too late – and your body is perfectly capable of healing itself, when given the right tools for the job. Above all, reduce the stress in your life, exercise regularly and as much as possible enjoy your journey.

Good luck and Good health.

Hazel Courteney and Gareth Zeal.

INDEX OF USEFUL INFORMATION AND ADDRESSES

ACUPUNCTURE

Practitioners use fine, sterile needles inserted into specific points to stimulate energy to move more easily around the body, which encourages the body to heal itself.
To find your nearest practitioner, send an SAE to
British Acupuncture Council,
63 Jeddo Road, London, W12 9HQ. Tel: 020 8735 0400 Fax: 020 8735 0404
Website: www.acupuncture.org.uk E-mail: info@acupuncture.org.uk

ALEXANDER TECHNIQUE

Teaches you how to use your body more efficiently and how to have balance and poise with minimum tension in order to avoid pain, strain and injury.
To find your nearest practitioner or list of affiliated societies worldwide, contact
Society of Teachers of the Alexander Technique,
129 Camden Mews, London, NW1 9AH Tel: 020 7284 3338 Fax: 020 7482 5435
Website: www.stat.org.uk E-mail: enquiries@stat.org.uk

AROMATHERAPY

The use of essential oils to improve health and well-being, by massage, inhalation, compresses and baths. Excellent for reducing stress and anxiety.
For a register of practitioners, contact the
International Federation of Aromatherapists (IFA),
182 Chiswick High Road, London, W4 1DD. Tel: 020 8742 2605
Website: www.int-fed-aromatherapy.co.uk E-mail: ifa@ic24.net
Or contact
The International Society of Professional Aromatherapists, ISPA House,
82 Ashby Road, Hinckley, Leicestershire, LE10 1SN. Tel: 01455 637987. Fax: 01455 890956.
Website: www.the-ispa.org Email: lisabrown@ispa.demon.co.uk

BACH FLOWER REMEDIES

A healing system used to treat emotional problems such as fear and hopelessness. The liquid remedies are made from the flowers of wild plants, bushes and trees.
For further information contact
The Bach Centre, Mount Vernon, Bakers Lane, Sotwell, Oxfordshire, OX10 0PZ.
Tel: 01491 834678, Monday to Friday, 9.30am-4.30pm, Fax: 01491 825022.
Website: www.bachcentre.com E-mail: mail@bachcentre.com

BOOKS

If you have difficulty finding any of the recommended books, or simply want to find a book on your condition, the Nutri Centre bookshop in London have an extensive library of self-help books and would be happy to order for you, or give assistance on specific subjects.
Tel: (011 44) 020 7323 2382

BOWEN TECHNIQUE

Devised by Australian Thomas Bowen, this is a gentle system of muscle manipulation where therapists roll the muscles and ligaments back into alignment. Suitable for children and adults.
To find your nearest therapist contact The Bowen Therapist European Register on Tel: 01458 252599. Or send a SAE to Ian Robins, BTER Admin Office, Homelea, Bow Street, Langport, Somerset, TA10 9PQ. Email: bowen@bter.freeserve.co.uk

CHELATION

Chelation, an intravenous treatment using the synthetic amino acid EDTA, has been proven to improve blood flow in blocked arteries in heart, diabetic and stroke patients. When combined with antioxidants and other substances the healing and anti-ageing effects are amplified. It is very useful if you have any of the above complaints, plus senile dementia, Alzheimer's, Parkinson's, ME, Chronic Fatigue, arthritis, multiple sclerosis or want to prevent cancers. It is now being called IVAT, Intravenous Antioxidant Therapy. For further details, read *Forty-Something Forever* by Harold and Arline Brecher, Healthsavers Press; to order, Tel: 0207 323 2382 or call **Dr Keith Scott-Mumby** on 0700 078 1744 or log onto www.anti-ageing-uk.com or www.brainrecovery.com or call **Dr Rodney Adenyi-Jones** on 0207 486 6354.

CHINESE HERBAL MEDICINE

The concept of restoring an uninterrupted flow of chi, the vital energy of the body. Be aware that if you are taking large doses of herbs they are extremely potent and you may want to have a liver function test at regular intervals during your treatment.
For further information contact
Register of Chinese Herbal Medicine, PO Box 400, Wembley, Middlesex, HA9 9NZ.
Tel/Fax: 07000 790332 Website: www.rchm.co.uk E-mail: herbmed@rchm.co.uk

CHIROPRACTIC

Manipulation to treat disorders of the joints and muscles and their effect on the nervous system. Chiropractors treat the entire body to bring it back into balance and restore health. I visit my chiropractor once a month who keeps my spine and neck mobile and almost free of pain after an injury several years ago.
To find a practitioner in your local area, contact
The British Chiropractic Association, Blagrave House,
17 Blagrave Street, Reading, Berkshire, RG1 1QB. Tel: 0118 950 5950. Fax: 0118 958 8946.
Website: www.chiropractic-uk.co.uk E-mail: enquiries@chiropractic-uk.co.uk
Or send a SAE to
McTimoney Chiropractic Association, 21 High Street, Eynsham, Oxford, OX8 1HE. Tel: 01865 880974. Website: www.mctimoney-chiropractic.org
E-mail: admin@mctimoney-chiropractic.org

COLONIC HYDROTHERAPY

A method of cleansing the colon to gently flush away toxic waste, gas, accumulated faeces and mucous deposits. Check with your GP before undertaking this therapy. Colonics are very useful if you are chronically constipated or have taken antibiotics or painkillers, which can cause constipation. I have a colonic whenever I have taken antibiotics or had any kind of surgery – to help remove the toxins from my system. I visit Margie Finchell who is brilliant. Tel: 020 7724 1291. To find your nearest practitioner, send an SAE to
Colonic International Association, 16 Drummond Ride, Tring, Hertfordshire, HP23 5DE.
Tel: 01422 876687 Web: www.colonic-association.com

COLOUR THERAPY

There is plenty of evidence to show that colour affects our mood and behaviour, as different colours emit different frequencies which our bodies absorb. For good health, we need to be exposed to all the colours which are in natural daylight.
To find your nearest practitioner, contact
The Colour Bonds Association,
137 Hendon Lane, Finchley, London, N3 3PR. Tel/Fax: 020 8349 3299.

COUNSELLING

If you, or a member of your family, are in need of professional counselling, send an SAE to
British Association for Counselling (BAC), 1 Regent Place, Rugby, CV21 2PJ
Tel: 0870 4435252 Website: www.counselling.co.uk E-mail: bac@bac.co.uk

CRANIAL OSTEOPATHY

A gentle method of osteopathy concentrating on nerves and bones in the head, neck and shoulders.
Many readers have reported relief from ME (Chronic Fatigue Syndrome), facial pain, jaw pain and
arthritis from this therapy.
To find your nearest practitioner, send a SAE to
International Bio-Cranial Academy,
1 High Street Manor, Comber, Co. Down, BT23 5TF.
Tel: 028 9187 0837. Fax: 028 9187 0838. E-mail: bcranial@aol.com

FLOWER ESSENCE PRACTITIONER

Traditionally flower essences have been used to heal emotions and act as a catalyst for healing. They
work on subtle energies of our bodies and help to unblock emotional or personality problems.
Specific flower essences are available to suit your particular condition from Serena Smith who is a
holistic therapist and healer. For further information write to
Serena Smith at Little Miracles, PO Box 3896, London, NW3 7DS.
Tel/fax: 020 7435 5555 Website: www.littlemiracles.co.uk E-mail: info@littlemiracles.co.uk

GENERAL ORGANISATIONS

If you want to know more about specific alternative therapies, the following organisations will be
happy to give you advice and put you in touch with the practitioners and societies that now meet
with their high standards of practice and therapy.
Institute for Complementary Medicine, PO Box 194, London, SE16 1QZ. Tel: 020 7237 5165
Fax: 020 7237 5175 Website: www.icmedicine.co.uk E-mail: icm@icmedicine.co.uk

HALE CLINIC

This clinic is the largest alternative treatment centre in Europe with over 100 practitioners, many of
whom are also qualified medical doctors. Some of the best people working in alternative medicine in
the UK are based at The Hale.
The Hale Clinic, 7 Park Crescent, London, W1N 3HE. Tel: 020 7631 0156
Fax: 020 7637 3377 Website: www.haleclinic.com

HEALING

A healer channels healing energies through their hands and into the patient's energy field which
encourages the body to heal itself. Especially good for chronic fatigue and for raising energy levels
when you are under the weather or suffering any illness.
To find your nearest practitioner, send a SAE to
National Federation of Spiritual Healers, Old Manor Farm Studio, Church Street, Sunbury-on-
Thames, Middlesex, TW16 6RG Tel: 0845 1232777 Fax: 01932 779648
(Monday to Friday, 9.00am-5.00pm).

HEALING, REIKI

The Reiki Association,

Cornbrook Bridge House, Clee Hill, Ludlow, Shropshire, SY8 3QQ.
Tel/Fax: 01584 891197. Send a large SAE for list of practitioners.
Website: www.reikiassociation.org.uk

HERBALISM

The practice of using plants to treat disease. Treatment may be given in the form of fluid extracts, tinctures, tablets or teas.
For further details a register of qualified members send a SAE to:
The National Institute of Medical Herbalists, 56 Longbrook Street, Exeter, Devon, EX4 6AH
Tel: 01392 426022 Fax: 01392 498963, office hours: Mon/Fri 10.00am–5.00pm,
Tues/Weds/Thurs 9.30am–3.30pm.
Website: www.nimh.org.uk E-mail: nimh@ukexeter.freeserve.co.uk
Potter's make one of the most comprehensive ranges of herbs available in the UK and for a list of their remedies and a stockist near you, call
Potter's (Herbal Supplies) Ltd, Tel: 01942 405100 Fax: 01942 820255
Website: www.pottersherbal.co.uk

HOMEOPATHY

Works in harmony with the body to stimulate the body's natural healing mechanisms. Fiona J. McKenzie L.LB.LCH.MHMA, is a highly qualified homeopath who has helped me with all the homeopathic remedies in this book. Tel: 020 7229 6689 or Tel: 01242 890 532.
For a register of professionally qualified homeopaths and general information about homeopathy contact The Society of Homeopaths, 4A Artizan Road, Northampton, NN4 4HU.
Tel: 01604 621400 Fax: 01604 622622, opening times: Monday to Friday, 10am-1.00pm and 2.00pm-4.00pm. Website: www.homeopathy-soh.org E-mail: info@homeopathy-soh.org
Or send a SAE to
Homeopathic Medical Association (HMA),
6 Livingstone Road, Gravesend, Kent, DA12 5DZ.
Tel: 01474 560336 Fax: 01474 327431 Website: www.the-hma.org E-mail: info@the-hma.org

British Homeopathic Association (BHA) formerly Homeopathic Trust
15 Clerkenwell Close, London, EC1R 0AA. Tel: 020 7566 7800 Fax: 020 7566 7815 Website:
(likely to change) www.trusthomeopathy.org

HYPNOTHERAPY

By allowing external distractions to fade, the therapy allows you to fully relax and understand the root cause of many of your problems, phobias and addictions.
To find your nearest practitioner, send an SAE to
The General Hypnotherapy Register, PO Box 204, Lymington, Hants SO41 6WP. Tel/Fax (24 hour answerphone): 01590 683770 Website: www.general-hypnotherapy-register.com
E-mail: admin@general-hypnotherapy-register.com
I visit Leila Hart in London – she is a brilliant therapist who helps me to really relax. Monday-Friday 9am-5pm Tel: 0207 402 4311.

INSTITUTE OF OPTIMUM NUTRITION

The Institute of Optimum Nutrition prints a wonderful quarterly booklet which is packed with up-to-date health news and the latest research in alternative medicine. The Institute also holds seminars on health and have in-house nutritionists. For details, contact:
Institute for Optimum Nutrition (ION), 13 Blades Court, Deodar Road, Putney, London, SW15 2NU Tel: 020 8877 9993 Website: www.ion.ac.uk E-mail: info@ion.ac.uk

IRIDOLOGY

A method of analysis rather than treatment, based on the theory that the whole body is reflected in the eyes. Using a magnifier, the practitioner examines the visible parts of the eyes to pinpoint physical weaknesses or potential areas that might cause you problems in the years to come.
Send an SAE for a list of qualified practitioners to the
Guild of Naturopathic Iridologists Int., 94 Grosvenor Road, London, SW1V 3LF
Tel: 020 7821 0255 Website: www.gni-international.org

KINESIOLOGY

The science of testing muscle response to discover areas of impaired energy and function in the body. Kinesiology is especially useful if you think you have an allergic reaction either to a food or an external allergen.
To find your nearest practitioner, send 4 loose first-class stamps to the
Association for Systematic Kinesiology, 19 Westfield Lane, St Leonards-on-Sea, East Sussex TN37 7NE Tel: 01424 753375 Email: info@kinesiology.co.uk Website: www.kinesiology.co.uk

MANUAL LYMPHATIC DRAINAGE

A very gentle pulsing massage, which helps to drain the lymph nodes, thereby reducing swelling and pain related to the lymph glands.
To find your nearest practitioner, send an SAE to
MLD UK (Manual Lympatic Drainage UK), PO Box 14491, Glenrothes, Fife, KY6 3YE
Tel: 01592 840799 Website: www.mlduk.org.uk E-mail: admin@mlduk.org.uk

NATUROPATHY

Practitioners use diet, herbs, natural hormones and supplement therapy to treat the root cause of any illness, thereby boosting the immune system and restoring health.
For details of qualified practitioners, contact the
General Council and Register of Naturopaths (GCRN),
Goswell House, 2 Goswell Road, Street, Somerset, BA16 0JG Tel: 08707 456984
Website: www.naturopathy.org.uk E-mail: admin@naturopathy.org.uk
In central London contact
The Society of Complementary Medicine, 3 Spanish Place, London W1U3HX
Tel: 0207 487 4334.

NEURO-LINGUISTIC PROGRAMMING

This is a profound and yet simple way to re-programme any negative thoughts or habits to more positive ones. Great for phobias, panic attacks and for attaining your goals in life. The Society of NLP in the UK is at: **Mckenna-Breen, Society of NLP, Aberdeen Studios, 22-24 Highbury Grove, London N52 EA0. Tel: 0207 704 6604. Fax: 0207 704 1676**
Email: happening@mckenna-breen.com Website: www.mckenna-breen.com

NUTRI CENTRE, THE

The Nutri Centre, located on the lower ground floor of the Hale Clinic at 7 Park Crescent, London, is unique in being able to supply almost every alternative product currently available from any country, including specialized practitioner products. The Nutri Centre offers an excellent and reliable mail order service worldwide for all its products. For supplements
Tel: 020 7436 5122 Fax 020 7436 5171; for books Tel: 020 7323 2382
Website: www.nutricentre.com E-mail: enq@nutricentre.com

NUTRITIONAL THERAPY

To find your nearest qualified nutritionist who can help you to balance your diet and suggest the correct vitamins and minerals etc. Send £2 plus a A4 SAE to

The British Association of Nutritional Therapists, 27 Old Gloucester Street, London WC1N 3XX Tel: 0870 606 1284 Website: www.bant.org.uk

Contact **The Institute for Optimum Nutrition.** For a directory of nutritionists send £5-00 to **ION, 13 Blades Court, Deodar Road, Putney, London SW15 2NU** Tel: 020 8877 9993, Fax: 020 887 9980. www.ion.ac.uk

NUTRITIONIST WHO IS ALSO A DOCTOR

You will need to be referred by your own GP who will be able to find the address of your nearest practitioner by contacting

British Society for Allergy Environmental and Nutritional Medicine (BSAENM), PO Box 7, Knighton, LD7 1WT.

Tel: 01547 550380 Fax: 01547 550339 Website: www.jnem.demon.co.uk

ORGANIC PRODUCE

The Soil Association has published an Organic Directory, which is packed with information on where to buy organic produce throughout the country. To obtain a copy, send £7.95 plus £1.00 postage and packing to the

Soil Association, Bristol House, 40-56 Victoria Street, Bristol, BS1 6BY

Tel: 0117 929 0661 Fax: 0117 925 2504 Website: www.soilassociation.org.uk

E-mail: info@soilassociation.org.uk

OSTEOPATHY

A system of healing that works on the physical structure in the body. Practitioners use manipulation, massage and stretching techniques. To find your nearest practitioner, contact the

Osteopathic Information Service, Osteopathy House, 176 Tower Bridge Road, London, SE1 3LU Tel: 020 7357 6655 Ext. 242

Website: www.osteopathy.org.uk E-mail: info@osteopathy.org.uk

PILATES

This is a great, low impact, isometric form of exercise which you can practise even if you have suffered some kind of injury. Very powerful but gentle. **Pilates Foundation, PO Box 36052, London SW6 1XQ** Tel: 07071 781859

Website: www.pilatesfoundation.com Email: admin@pilatesfoundation.com

POLARITY THERAPY

A therapist will use bodywork, awareness skills, diet and stretching exercises to help the body and mind heal itself naturally. A very relaxing rebalancing therapy useful for extreme stress and fatigue. To find your nearest practitioner, send an A5 SAE to the

United Kingdom Polarity Therapy Association, Monomark House, 27 Old Gloucester Street, London, WC1N 3XX Enquiry line: 0700 705 2748

Website: www.ukpta.org.uk

QIGONG (T'AI CHI)

An extremely gentle form of exercise, which helps people with impaired mobility like severe arthritis. Anyone can practise qigong and no special clothes are needed. For further information contact **TSE Qigong Centre, PO Box 59, Altringham, Cheshire, WA15 8FS.** Tel: 0161 929 4485 Fax: 0161 929 4489 Website: www.qimagazine.com. E-mail: tse@qimagazine.com

317

READING

Here's Health is a marvellous magazine for anyone who really cares about their health and wants to know more about alternative ways to become and stay well. It's packed with new ideas plus reader's and therapists case studies, £2.40 per month. **Tel: 020 7208 3209**, Subscriptions **Tel: 01858 438869** Website: www.ukmagazines.co.uk

Optimum Nutrition is a brilliant quarterly magazine from
The Institute of Optimum Nutrition, £3.50 Tel: **020 8877 9993**

Patrick Holford's newsletter *100% Health* is a goldmine of easy to read information and up to the minute research results. **Fax 020 8874 5003** Website: **www.patrickholford.com** I would highly recommend all of Patrick's books which will change your life.

Positive Health is one of my favourite monthly magazines. It is excellent for practitioners and public alike, and keeps you abreast of the latest research, therapies, books and nutritional developments that really work. Costs £3-50 and can be ordered from anywhere in the world. They also have a brilliant Website.

Positive Health Publications,
1 Queen Square, Bristol, BS1 4JQ Tel: 0117 983 8851 Fax: 0117 908 0097
Website: **www.positivehealth.com**

What Doctors Don't Tell You is a monthly newsletter packed with alternative health information, up to date health news and warnings about the side effects of prescription drugs. Lynne McTaggart is famous throughout the health industry as not being afraid to tell the truth. They also have an extensive range of books on subjects ranging from Cancer to the dangers of Vaccinations. For details, write to

What Doctors Don't Tell You,
Satellite House, 2 Salisbury Road, London, SW19 4EZ. Tel: 0870 444 9886.
Fax: 0870 444 9887. Website: www.wddty.co.uk E-mail: office@wddty.co.uk

REFLEXOLOGY

Works on the principle that reflex points on the hands and feet correspond to every part of the body. By working with pressure on these points, blockages in the energy pathways are released which encourages the body to heal itself. This is a great way to boost circulation and really relaxing.

To find your nearest practitioner, contact **Association of Reflexologists,**
27 Old Gloucester Street, London, WC1N 3XX. Tel: 0870 567 3320.
AOR is a member of **Reflexology in Europe Network and International Council of Reflexology.**
Website: **www.aor.org.uk E-mail: aor@reflexology.org**
The British Reflexology Association, Monks Orchard, Whitbourne, Worcester, WR6 5RB Tel:
01886 821207 Fax: 01886 822017 Website: www.britreflex.co.uk E-mail: bra@britreflex.co.uk

WHAT DOCTORS DON'T TELL YOU –

See *Reading* in this section.

YOGA

The ancient principles of yoga are beneficial for staying healthy and supple well into one's 80's and beyond. Yoga teaches relaxation and breathing techniques, together with gentle stretching exercises, which help keep the 'whole' self fit for life. Especially useful for keeping the spine strong.

To find your nearest class, send an A5 SAE to
The British Wheel of Yoga, 25 Germyn Street, Sleaford, Lincolnshire, NG34 7RU.
Tel: 01529 306851 Fax: 01529 303233
Website: **www.bwy.org.uk E-mail: office@bwy.org.uk**

ALPHABETICAL LIST OF ENTRIES

Acid Stomach (*see also* Indigestion and
    Low Stomach Acid)
Acne (*see also* Rosacea)
Ageing
Alcohol
Allergic Rhinitis (*see also* Allergies and Hayfever)
Allergies (*see also* Leaky Gut)
Alzheimer's Disease (*see also* Memory)
Anaemia
Angina (*see also* Cholesterol)
Antibiotics (*see also* Candida and Thrush)
Aphrodisiacs, Male
Arthritis, Osteo and Rheumatoid
    Arthritis – Osteo
    Arthritis – Rheumatoid
Asthma (*see also* Allergies and Leaky Gut)
Athlete's Foot
Autism
Back Pain
Bad Breath (see Halitosis)
Bereavement
Bladder (see Cystitis, Incontinence and Prostate)
Bleeding Gums (*see also* Fluoride)
Blepharitis (see Eye Problems)
Bloating (see Constipation and Flatulence)
Body Hair, Excessive   Hirsutism
Body Odour
Boils (Furuncle)
Breast Cancer (see Cancer of the Breast)
Breast Pain and Tenderness (*see also* Cancer of the
    Breast)
Brittle Nails (see Nail Problems)
Bronchitis
Bruising
Burns, Minor
Bursitis

Cancer (*see also* Cancer of the Breast)
Cancer of the Breast – Prevention of
Candida (*see also* Allergies)
Carpal Tunnel Syndrome
Cataracts
Catarrh
Cellulite
Chilblains
Cholesterol, High and Low
Chronic Fatigue (see Exhaustion and ME)
Circulation (see Chilblains and Raynaud's Disease)
Coeliac Disease
Colds and Flu
Cold Sores
Conjunctivitis
Constipation and Bloating (*see also* Flatulence)
Coughs
Cramps
Crohn's Disease
Cystitis

Depression
Dermatitis
Diabetes (Diabetes Melliitus)
Diarrhoea
Diverticular Disease or Diverticulitis
Dizzy Spells (see Low Blood Sugar, Low Blood Pressure
and Vertigo)

Ear Ache (*see also* Glue Ear, Tinnitus and Vertigo)
Eczema
Electrical Pollution and Electrical Healing
Emphysema
Endometriosis
Exhaustion (*see also* ME and Stress)
Eye Problems – (*see also* Cataracts)
    Blepharitis
    Itchy Eyes
    Macular Degeneration
    Optic Neuritis
    Puffy Eyes
    Red Rimmed Eyes

Fatigue (see Exhaustion and Stress)
Fats You Need to Eat
Fibroids
Flatulence (*see also* Constipation and Bloating)
Flu (see Colds)
Fluoride (*see also* Bleeding Gums)
Foot Problems
    Fallen Arches
    Hot Burning Feet
    Numb/Tingling Feet
    Swollen Feet and Ankles
Frozen Shoulder

Gall-bladder Problems
Gall-stones
General Health Hints
General Supplements For Better Health
Glandular Fever (Mononuecleosis)
Glue Ear.
Gout
Gums (see Bleeding Gums)

Haemorrhoids (see Piles)
Hair Loss
Halitosis (Bad Breath)
Hangovers (see Alcohol)
Hay Fever (*see also* Allergies and Allergic Rhinitis)
Healing and Healers
Heartburn (see Acid Stomach, Indigestion and Low
    Stomach Acid)
Heart Disease (*see also* Angina, Cholesterol, Circulation
    and High Blood Pressure)
Head Lice- see under Scalp problems.
Herpes
Hiatus Hernia
High Blood Pressure